Forensic Child Psychology

Forensic Child Psychology

Working in the Courts and Clinic

Matthew Fanetti
William O'Donohue
Rachel Fondren Happel
Kresta Daly

WILEY

Contents

Preface

The field of forensic psychology has grown slowly over the past century. From the early debates by Hugo Munsterberg and Sigmund Freud that psychology should play a larger role in the legal system, to the use of psychology in advocating the elimination of segregation in schools in the U.S. Supreme Court case *Brown v. Board of Education*, psychology has struggled to help legal decision makers be better informed. The past five decades have seen an exponential growth in the use of scientific research to answer important questions in forensics, from matters such as bystander inaction to the strengths and frailties of the memories of eyewitnesses. In the 1990s, psychology responded to a rash of well-publicized day-care child sexual abuse scandals, with a push for scientific understanding of children's allegations of sexual abuse. In just 25 years, the applied field of child sexual abuse assessment has come from an ad hoc and unstandardized approach to assessment, characterized by wild disagreements and untrained assessors, to a (mostly) highly controlled approach, which is informed by research with an aim to understand and reduce error. In our estimation, this is a very desirable outcome of mere decades. Psychology can work with the applied community and it can help to work toward better responses to real problems. Ultimately, this was the position of Munsterberg and Freud, though the field at the time was not ready to provide the necessary support.

College instructors today have an interesting problem: finding a text that supports the goals of their classes in forensic psychology. Unlike courses such as the typical general Introduction to Psychology experience (for which available texts are plentiful and varied), undergraduate texts in forensic psychology are rare. Even worse, those with a focus on child issues are even more rare. Compound this with the fact that most available texts are written for students with strong backgrounds in psychology (or graduate students and professors in psychology) and what does an instructor do for a forensic psychology course filled with sophomores in social work, criminology, nursing, premed, and so on? These students need to understand some basic principles, because these principles affect an everyday working environment. However, many students do not have sufficient background in psychology to use an advanced forensic psychology text. Furthermore, they have little need of many of the specific topics discussed in those texts.

The overarching goal of this text is to provide an accessible and basic examination of psychology and law pertaining to children so that students who will enter into the workforce with need of this kind of information will be better prepared. We have focused on writing style and ease of use. Rather than a text that explores every permutation of every relevant concept, we focus on a clear and well-explained iteration of basic ideas. The goal is clarity and understanding, not comprehensive depth.

The first focus of the text is a basic review of some concepts in psychology that may be important to those who actually work in forensic environments, including (1) why psychology is a science and why that is important, (2) relevant social and learning psychology, (3) relevant psychopathology, and (4) basic concepts in memory as applied to forensics.

The second focus of the text is an examination of specific topics and concepts related to child forensics, including (1) an overview of child abuse and exploitation, (2) child abuse in the modern technological world, (3) pedophilia and child molestation, (4) assessment of child sexual abuse, and (5) treatment of children who have been abused.

The third and final focus of this text is to provide a basic understanding of the legal world related to child forensics, including (1) basic concepts in law, (2) mandated reporting, (3) juvenile justice systems, and (4) the role of psychological expert witnesses in child abuse cases.

Ultimately, we hope that the text provides a sound framework for building new courses that are specifically designed for those who will be working directly with children. We are hoping to have built an accessible entry point into the field for some and an understandable set of working principles for others.

We welcome feedback about how to revise this text to help serve the needs of instructors and working professionals. We would also welcome inquiries from instructors hoping to create courses in forensic child psychology. The process may be easier than you think, and finding community resources to assist in the endeavor is often a productive way to engage a department in the public affairs of its own community. Our team has been able to enlist the support of (and directly include) powerful community agencies that can rally around a common goal: to make our professionals more effective and thus strengthen the fight against child abuse.

For correspondence:
Matthew Fanetti, PhD
Professor
Coordinator of Child Forensic Psychology Certification
Department of Psychology
Missouri State University
Springfield, MO 65897
mfanetti@missouristate.edu

Acknowledgments

The authors wish to acknowledge the Greene County (Missouri) Prosecutor's Office and the Child Advocacy Center of Springfield (Missouri), Inc., for the leadership they have provided in the cause of safeguarding our children. Specifically, Darrell Moore, Dan Patterson, Jill Patterson, and Barbara Brown-Johnson have been instrumental in bringing valuable resources together in this effort and heroically dedicated to the never-ending fight against child abuse.

Many thanks also go to the research assistants in the Forensic Child Psychology Laboratory at Missouri State University who participated in the development of this textbook. Specifically, we would like to acknowledge the hard work and the contributions of Tabitha Carwile, Shannon Nicholson, Emily Rader, Rebecca Pearson, Katie Plasmeier, Jamie Thayer, Mariah Turner, and Kathy Robitsch.

Finally, we also wish to acknowledge the Sacramento Children's Receiving Home for the care and compassion they provide in helping victims of abuse and neglect.

Basic Principles

Introduction to Forensic Psychology

GOALS OF THIS CHAPTER:

1. To understand the basic definitions, development, and role of psychology as a *science*.
2. To explore the important social events that caused the focus on forensics in psychology.
3. To understand the broad range of activities a forensic psychologist might engage.

Within the past few decades the label *forensic psychology* has become more common than it might have been prior to the 1980s. Within the past decade, more researchers and practicing professionals may be using the more specific label *forensic child psychology*. A quick review of articles listed in *PsycInfo* revealed that articles containing the keywords "forensic psychology" increased from 156 during the 1960s to 8,117 during the 2000s. A similar review using the keywords "Child" (and) "Forensic Psychology" increased from 9 during the 1960s to 1,395 during the 2000s. But what exactly are these fields of study and practice? The most direct definition of **forensic psychology** is: the study of human behavior in legal settings or relevant legal environments. The most direct definition of **forensic child psychology** is: the study of the behavior of children in legal settings or relevant legal environments. However, there are many nuances to these studies.

Most people have probably heard these terms from their growing utilization in the entertainment media. From these experiences, many people may come to believe that forensic psychology is dedicated to understanding the causes of criminal behavior—and they would not be wrong. However, the field is much broader than this very narrow sliver of interest.

Even the word *forensic* has different implications in various fields. For example, in 1997 this author (Fanetti) was visiting with a law enforcement division that specialized in sex crimes against children. Upon meeting and exchanging introductions, one of the detectives presented a quizzical facial expression when he heard the specialty. After learning what we actually researched, he smiled and said he had thought that "forensic child psychology" meant that we tried to study the behavior of *dead* children. For them, forensics meant *post-mortem*.

Many of the students who use this text may not actually be psychology students. The goal of the text has always been to reach every frontline professional who interacts with children on a daily basis. This includes teachers, counselors, social workers, nurses, law enforcement officers, juvenile officers, direct therapists, court personnel, to name just a few. It is these people who become the first line of intervention when children become part of the legal (i.e., forensic) system. These children may be the victims of crime, witnesses to it, or even the perpetrators of the crime. In these scenarios, the way that professionals interact with children can make the difference between cases that are resolved well and justly, and those in which justice becomes confused or difficult to obtain. For example, when witnesses testify that they saw a specific person at a crime scene, but later details reveal that they were not sure until the person was pointed out by law enforcement, there is a legitimate question to be raised about the accuracy of that identification. Clear and focused understanding of basic psychological principles related to forensic cases (e.g., in this case, memory research) can help professionals to be effective in preventing crimes against children, helping child victims, and creating environments in which children are less likely to become involved in crime.

The remainder of this chapter explores the principles and goals of psychology, the development of forensic psychology as a specific field of inquiry, the many duties of forensic psychologists, the training available to become a forensic psychologist, and some recent examples of cases where forensic child psychology became an important influence.

WHAT IS PSYCHOLOGY—REALLY?

According to the American Psychological Association (APA, 2012), *psychology* is a "profession of scientific research designed to establish basic principles and theories of human behavior, and the subsequent application of those principles and theories to help individuals, organizations and communities." In this sense, psychology is concerned both with the careful and controlled scientific examination of behavior *and* with the use of this knowledge in a variety of applied, beneficial ways.

Modern psychology is a science originating from the same early roots as other sciences, such as physics, mathematics, biology, chemistry, and medicine. Those common roots can be found in the writing of ancient Greek, Persian, Chinese, and Egyptian philosophers. In fact, the evolution of thought from these early roots follows an understandable route. Each science has gradually moved from rational and thought-based explanations for common problems, to more empirical and observation-based answers, and finally to specific methods designed to reduce or remove biases and errors from those systems. This more recent experimental/empirical orientation is considered superior because it requires that ideas (hypotheses) are actually tested against reality (data) to see if the initial ideas are correct. In this way, science is thought to have an error-identifying and error-correcting function (O'Donohue, 2013). All modern sciences can trace their lineages back to the same ancestors. It has only been within the past few centuries that the amount of accumulating knowledge has grown to the point that scientists have found benefit in specializing in one area or another and focusing their attentions on one field of study.

Epistemology

How do you know that something is true? Do you have a preferred way to answer this question or that? If you read about a murder trial in the newspaper or on the web or on television, how is it that you come to your own conclusions about whether the accused is guilty or innocent? We are all tempted to do it. Do you use logic to think through the most probable set of events? Do you rely—only—on such direct evidence as DNA, video, or fingerprints? What if the evidence is eyewitness testimony? Are you willing to rely on the accuracy, honesty, and certainty of others who say they saw a crime? We can use any and all of these methods to come to our own conclusions about the nature of the truth.

Epistemology is the study of *how* we know, or which methods we rely on to come to conclusions about the nature of the world—or the truth of a criminal case. There are many differing *epistemes* (i.e., ways of knowing), but a few are particularly important to the history of the development of the science of psychology. These are rationalism, authority, empiricism, and experimentalism.

Rationalism is the idea that we can gain knowledge from nothing more than thought-based exploration of concepts. Essentially, our sensory observations are thought to be flawed and difficult to interpret within the biases of our environments. Certainly we can at least agree that some concepts we accept every day are not actually observable. Each of us knows that lines, planes, and points exist—but what are they really. By definition, a plane must have two dimensions: two. This means it has *no* depth at all. How can we *observe* something that has *no depth*? What about a line? It is essentially one-dimensional. A point is zero-dimensional. Zero-dimensional? These are concepts that we can represent on paper (e.g., a pencil dot on a piece of paper is a three-dimensional illustration of a zero-dimensional object), but just a little thought makes it clear that they do not exist in *observable* reality. They are truths, but *rational* truths only. The quintessential rationalist, *Socrates*, believed that all knowledge can be derived by simple exploration of our mental faculties and ability to reason. We need not see the truth of nature, because we can reason it out in the absence of observation. Even so, rational explanations (i.e., those that rely on logic) still have a place in modern psychology. Forensic experts still must present their finding to the court in ways that seem to make sense, and are not illogical. Rational explanations have not been replaced, they have been supplemented.

Empiricism is the idea that we can gain knowledge from simple observation. Empiricists, such as *Aristotle*, believed that we are born with a blank slate (i.e., *tabula rasa*) on which our observable sensory experiences will write the truths of the world as we see them. Certainly, we can agree that each of us probably learned about ice and snow from our interactions with them. People may tell you what it means to be cold, but you will not understand the truth of it until you *feel* it. Can you think of a way to rationally explain the experience of being cold to someone who has never felt it? At a concert in Reno (1998), the musical performer Yanni, who was from warm southern Greece, once explained to the audience about his education in "cold." On moving to the United States, his first sensory experience was in Minnesota, in the winter. To him, the realization of what cold meant was shocking, though he had heard and thought about it many times. Simple empirical arguments still play a role in modern forensic settings. For example, many attorneys use reenactments as a way for jurors to feel as though they have experienced a plausible explanation. Seeing an explanation acted out and hearing the attorney's representation remains very important.

The constant companion to both empiricism and rationalism has always been authority. *Authority*, as an *episteme*, is the idea that we gain our own truths about the world from sources or people thought to have the knowledge to be correct, or *authoritative*. During the classical periods of Greek and Roman civilization, there was an accumulating body of knowledge gained through what we might call *early science*. However, a great many problems remained mysterious as they were not yet answerable by rational or empirical inquiry. Thus, powerful governmental and spiritual systems were available to answer questions. Why did a town suffer the plague? According to the ancient Greek philosopher and playwright, Sophocles, the cause for such suffering might be the sins of Oedipus that were illuminated by the Oracle of Delphi. Whether the authoritative source would someday be proven wrong was accepted, but at least an answer was available. Answers are things humans like to have, even if it is known to be just the best one available at that time. Certain witnesses are considered to speak with authority when in court, including expert witnesses. It is assumed that they have accumulated enough knowledge of the issues about which they speak to be given more credence than others. In fact, we are very familiar with using authority as a way of knowing. The concept of textbooks is based on it—even this textbook.

During the medieval era, a new approach to empiricism was developing and formed the seeds of the Enlightenment. This new approach is often called *experimentalism*, an offshoot of empiricism. The problem with simple empiricism, is that while our sensory experiences tend to be vivid and believable, they can also be flawed and lead us to false conclusions. After all, when viewing a straw in a glass of water, your visual experience will tell you that the straw is bent. If you cannot move the straw, you may have trouble refuting that possibility. Experimentalism is the idea that, in order to gain better access to the truth, you must control the possible sources of *bias* in our observations—you must be able to move the straw around to critically evaluate your perceptions. We must be able to test our observations by making predictions about them that would only happen *if* our beliefs were correct. We can also endeavor to demonstrate that our beliefs are, in fact, *not true*—to give our explanations every opportunity to be wrong (perhaps hoping they will be not proven wrong). Sir Karl Popper (1959) believed that this constant striving for falsification of our theories was crucial. Those that could *not* be falsified were simply more *likely* to be true. If a theory failed a test, the choices would be to determine whether the observation was flawed or the theory was flawed. If the latter, then the researcher knows to move onto better explanations—not continue to hang onto untenable beliefs.

This is the *goal* of all modern scientific psychology: to develop explanations for observations that repeatedly withstand critical inquiry. It has been the development of the scientific method that has gradually increased our ability to be systematic and controlled in the way we answer questions. This experimental method is the tool that differentiates a science from a philosophy, or from a mere belief system.

Consider This

Use any recent and well-publicized legal case to examine how rationalism, authority, empiricism, and experimentalism might play a role in how we come to our own personal conclusions.

The Early Scientific Method

Philosophers during medieval and early Enlightenment eras began to consider the ways that our observations (our empirical knowledge) could be incorrectly derived. They sought to explain the various ways that people make observational errors, in the hopes that these could be controlled. *Roger Bacon*, in his *Opus Majus* written in 1269, posited that there were four main causes of error:

1. An unjustified reliance on authority.
2. People become slaves to habit and tradition.
3. People respond quickly to currently popular prejudices.
4. People tend to be arrogant about their own perceived knowledge.

Rather than the correctness of our beliefs or the way that they guide our knowledge, these four tendencies represent a kind of intellectual laziness he believed we experience.

Without critical appraisal of our beliefs, the ease that these four tendencies create will prevent the accumulation of new knowledge or new answers. How many times has each of us been resistant to looking into new things or trying new solutions, simply because they were not how we had done things before?

Francis Bacon (no relation to Roger Bacon) would later provide his own criticism of authority and the overreliance on the "factual" nature of simple empirical observations. He believed scientists should view these sensory observations with moderate skepticism and he suggested four *Idols* or limitations of human thinking:

1. *Idols of the Tribe:* Humans are limited by their own sensory apparatus. Our senses can distort our observations, often in ways outside of our awareness. Our intelligence is great, compared to other animals, but not unlimited. That limit presents the boundary of the things we can understand. The tribe is, roughly, the species.

2. *Idols of the Cave:* Humans develop provincial thinking that represents their own culture, preferences, and prejudices. The cave is our immediate environment.

3. *Idols of the Marketplace:* The terms we use to describe ideas become important in that they begin to define those ideas. How many times do our own politicians race to be the first to label legislation the "(fill in the blank) Bill of Rights"? Once thus labeled, it becomes difficult to argue against the legislation, because it *sounds* like an argument against this or that *right*. No matter what the legislation contains, the label becomes the selling point—because we take these labels too seriously.

4. *Idols of the Theater:* The easiest, most vivid explanations seem to carry their own truth. This is the genesis of fads and faddism. Psychology is replete with examples of therapies that emerged as nothing more than a fad, even when it was potentially dangerous. Rebirthing therapy, thought-field therapy, facilitated communication, and adolescent boot-camps all emerged to some level of acceptance by practicing therapists—even when evidence of actual effectiveness was absent (Lilienfeld, 2007). After all, people had "seen" them working. Only later, when clear evidence emerged that they were ineffective and potentially harmful (Romanczyk, Arnstein, Soorya, & Gillis, 2003) did these practices begin to recede.

Other Biases/Errors in Thought and Observation

The human cognitive process is fraught with tendency toward error and bias. We must process a great deal of information every day and sometimes we create shortcuts, or *heuristics*, to facilitate the process of pragmatic understanding. Conversely, we can work to increase accuracy by using algorithms—comprehensive systems for gathering all important data and fully understanding our experiences. But algorithms are often lengthy and we usually do not have the time to use algorithms everything around us.

Consider the auto mechanic who sees a car being towed into his station as a "no start." He has two courses of action. First, he can pull out his list of every possible cause and slowly go through each until he finds the culprit. Second, he can access his shortcut list of things he has learned are the most-likely causes. When this author was young and naive and working on cars, I once spent an hour trying to diagnose a no-start. Trying this and that, the battery was beginning to suffer from the repeated attempts. After enough time had passed, a friend walked out (smiling) and asked if I had checked the fuel level. This story is done. Heuristics *can* save us time, but can also be flawed and can lead to errors in decision making. The following are just a few well-known biases, heuristics, and cognitive errors. There are many more heuristics that are ready to be studied by eager students of psychology.

Confirmation bias. All undergraduates will at some point be asked to write a term paper for one class or another. What they might not know is that their professor is going to be on the lookout for confirmation bias. Nickerson (1998) describes confirmation as the tendency for humans to find (and pay significant attention to) evidence that tends to support the beliefs we already hold or the points we are trying to make. Conversely, the same bias allows us to easily discredit or find fault with evidence that does not support our positions. This is not to say that this tendency is intentional, but rather insidiously unintentional. When we discredit opposing points of views, we really do think they are flawed and we really do find them to be substandard and unconvincing. However, the same critical eye is not applied as easily to that which supports us.

Think about the way that we view evidence in cases we hear about in the media—especially that concerning celebrities or people we have some information about already. Even worse, think about news pertaining to the politicians we do or do not support. When we hear news or read things from spurious sources on the Internet, confirmation bias will play a large role in the degree to which we say, "Darn right!" or "Internet lies!" In fact, while once watching an ad for a politician (in full agreement), I caught myself abruptly changing my opinion of the information's veracity *when I learned he was from the other political party.* I quickly self-reflected and was privately chagrinned, but we are *all* human.

Are prosecuting attorneys or defense attorneys immune to this influence? The very nature of the adversarial legal system in the United States encourages each side to be more inclusive and careful when they are at the point of making a case. Defense attorneys are likely to pay much more attention to details that confirm their argument that their client is not guilty. Prosecuting attorneys are much more likely to emphasize and focus on the evidence that supports their argument that the defendant is guilty—especially in a system that places the responsibility for highlighting *exculpatory* (i.e., suggesting no guilt) information on the defense attorney.

Availability heuristic. We often answer questions or make decisions based on information that is simply easier to recall (i.e., more available), rather than information based on accuracy. Kahneman, Slovik, and Tversky (1982) explained the availability heuristic as the tendency to estimate the likelihood of an occurrence based on the ease with which it is recalled. Even though airline traffic was and remains the safest way to travel long distances, many people developed anxieties about commercial flight just after the tragic events of September 11, 2001. So many of us watched the dreadful images of two planes flying into the World Trade Center towers—over and over—and it became difficult to *not* think of them. So, when asked if airline travel was safe, many may have tended to doubt. In fact, the Transportation Security Administration (TSA) was created to keep us safe, even though private security had not actually *failed* to do anything they were supposed to be doing.

Hindsight bias. When we examine our past beliefs about the way events will unfold, after they have unfolded, we have a tendency to believe we were more knowledgeable and more prescient than history probably would have recorded. In fact, we have an idiom that describes this very phenomenon, "hindsight is always 20/20." Fischoff (1975) describes hindsight bias as the tendency to *retrospectively* overestimate our *previous* predictive abilities. Think about the number of investigations that went into the reasons our government did not anticipate that members of a terrorist group would fly commercial airplanes into skyscrapers on 9/11. There is no problem with the investigations, but simply concluding that the actions were predictable—after we already know they happened—is likely the result of hindsight bias (and perhaps a little confirmation bias thrown in for good measure).

Representativeness heuristic. Imagine that you began to talk with someone while sitting on a bench at a park. You learn the man is 50 years old and is a university professor. After a brief chat about colleges and majors, you say good-bye and walk to your car. In the lot there are three vehicles—yours, a ratty old pickup truck, and a new Lexus. Which one do you think is owned by the professor? Kahneman et al. (1982) described the representativeness heuristic as the tendency to judge the probability based on its superficial association with a prototype, or stereotype. Walking to the parking lot, many people would probably say that the professor has a nice Lexus. Professors can often communicate well and may seem more cultured or even wealthier than they actually deserve. However, if you *really* knew something about being a professor, you might actually pick the ratty old truck. Lexus vehicles are more expensive than professors can generally afford.

Pseudoscience

All of the biases and frailties of human cognitive decision making create an environment in which it is vital to develop systems which seek to understand and control those known errors. If we know how easy it is for us to derive conclusions which are wrong and we know how they came to be wrong, then we must also be able to design methods to correct these tendencies. Those studies which do not utilize known strategies to control error and which nevertheless yield "factual" conclusions are sometimes known as *pseudoscientific*. Lilienfeld, Ammirati, and David (2012) define **pseudoscience** as that which generates claims that *appear* to be or are touted to be scientific, but really are not.

A good example of this is the recent advancement of the form of psychotherapy known as *Thought Field Therapy* (TFT; Callahan, 2001). The creators of this intervention described the treatment as being more powerful in the treatment of PTSD (i.e., posttraumatic stress disorder) than any other intervention—even claiming 98% effectiveness. To be trained in TFT at the highest level required $100,000 for a week of guidance (as per our last review of its website in 2012). This must be powerful indeed to lure well-trained psychotherapists to part with that much money. In a public debate (SSCP, 2001) the creator, Roger Callahan, was unable to support his claims with any scientific study—*that had been reviewed by peers*.

His claims were thought by members of the debate to be extreme (e.g., curing phobias within minutes by thinking of the feared stimulus and "tapping" on the body in a very important spot), but he assured the group that his results were only not published because they were rejected as contrary to the orthodoxy of the field. In response, he was given unprecedented access to publish any study he wished—without critical scientific screening—in a special edition of a noted journal. The journal was prefaced with the fact that the normal peer-review system was suspended, but critical scientists would also be allowed to publish their critiques. If you wish to read the fascinating episode in the fight between genuine psychological science and (what is believed by many to be) pseudoscience, the journal is *Journal of Clinical Psychology, 57*(10), October 2001, *Special Issue: Thought Field Therapy*.

Bunge (1984) identified seven hallmarks of pseudoscience. These are things that are done by pseudoscientists to prevent actual science from undermining their assertions:

1. Use of ad hoc (as the need arises and convenient) hypotheses to fend off criticism.
2. Heavy use of confirmation strategies, rather than critical challenges.
3. Lack of self-correction.
4. Reversed burden of proof.
5. Reliance on testimonials and anecdotes.

6. Use of obfuscating, scientific-sounding language.
7. Lack of connectivity with other disciplines.

Thus scientific psychology has an important goal to help differentiate knowledge that is generated in controlled and careful processes, from that which is not—whether the latter is due to normal and expected human biases and errors, or due to careless pseudo-scientists in our own field.

Modern Scientific Method

The modern scientific method is designed to provide explanations for observed phenomena that are the most likely to be free from error and systematic bias. The goal of psychology is to explain in a verifiable way how things happen, or why people do what they do, so that we might be able to predict, anticipate, and correct those times when the behavior poses some kind of functional problem. Ultimately, the goal is the development of a sound **theory** for the causes of the observations. Theories are general explanatory mechanisms. They should be useful to understand a behavior or experience and should be open to criticism and the possibility of falsification. A good theory:

- Organizes and explains the known observations about the phenomenon.
- Can be used to generate critical, testable predictions.
- Can be modified to incorporate new observations.

Once a theory has been established, it is most useful if it can be used to generate specific and testable predictions called **hypotheses**. The hypothesis is an extension of the explanatory power of the theory. Essentially, if the theory is correct, then a specific result should occur. More importantly, what if the theory is *not correct*? If a theory can explain any result and no result will provide evidence of theoretical failure, then it is nonscientific. Without the possibility of failure, science cannot address the question. The theory *may* still be correct—it just is not a *scientific* theory.

The third step includes systematic and controlled observations to determine the effect of the manipulations required by the hypotheses. Often experimental steps are used to provide the unbiased control. The variables and terms most associated with experimental manipulations are discussed later. These observations will address the theory in some fashion. If the observations provide evidence that the hypothesis (and thus the theory) was not correct, modifications to the theory can occur, allowing it to produce better future predictions. If the observations do not refute some aspect of the theory, they will be noted as one challenge the theory survived. Good scientists, according to Popper's philosophy of science (1959), will then seek yet another challenge—then another. Good theories are those that survive repeated challenges—though their proponents are always faithfully trying to prove them wrong.

Components in Experimental Studies

In addition to sound theories and hypotheses as discussed earlier, experimental scientific observations often have similar components and features. One of the more important applied aspects of experimental manipulation is the ability of the researcher to reliably measure all of the components of a theory. For example, if a researcher believes that increases in a family's "stress" levels affect a child's academic performance and likelihood of interpersonal aggression, she would first be required to have a stable and reliable measurement of (1) academic performance, (2) interpersonal aggression, and (3) family stress. If we do not have good measures of these things, we will never be able to quantitatively verify that they are changing—at all.

Next, we need to be able to manipulate the variable(s) we believe causes the others to change. In this case, it is not simply good enough to say the variables are "related," for example, that poor performance and school fights tend to occur when there is family stress. This is a merely correlational relationship, and it might just as easily be that the causal arrow goes the other direction, or even that some other unknown influence is causing both things. We need to be able to actively increase or decrease family stress, then measure what happens to school performance and interpersonal aggression. There are many ways to create this manipulation (not simply to "stress out" families and then watch), including some that are statistical or organizational.

The influence that we *believe causes* an effect is often called the *independent variable*, or IV. The presumed effect of changes in the IV is often called the *dependent variable*, or DV. In other words, we presume that the magnitude of the DV will *depend on* the magnitude of the IV. In the example earlier, we would presume that the level of academic performance (i.e., DV-1) and the amount of interpersonal aggression (i.e., DV-2) will depend on the amount of intra-family stress (i.e., IV). If you increase stress, fights should go up and grades should go down. If you decrease stress, fights should go down and grades should go up. (As a point of clarification, we are using this study as a *fictional* example only.)

As a first step this is good, but it is not scientifically sufficient. The other influences that should be controlled or measured are those things that might *also* and reasonably be presumed to influence school performance and fights. What about health? What would you do if you learned that, during the course of the study, the general health status of the school had changed? Perhaps when you began, most of the children had the flu. As the study progressed, they recovered. While you might have been able to decrease family stressors, at the same time the children were just feeling physically better and were less grumpy and found studying to be easier. It is now harder to conclude the stress relief was causative.

Any potential process that might have the power to alter the levels of the DV—but which is not the IV—is considered a potential *confound*. When they exist, a study is considered *confounded* and difficult to interpret. However, simple processes including controlling the confound (when possible) or measuring and recording the levels of the confounding variable (so that their influence can be removed statistically) turn these problems into scientific **controls**. Well-controlled studies are an important part of the scientific method.

Consider This

Take any social problem you may think needs to be fixed and then attempt to broadly design a research project. What is your guiding theory? How are you going to create a specific and testable hypothesis from it? In the design of your experiment, be sure to think through the independent and dependent variables, potential confounds, and controls.

Applying Science to Real-World Child Forensic Interviews

A few years ago a graduate student working in one of our forensic child psychology labs wanted to study the effects of rapport on child interviews (Boles, 2003). The simple idea was that if children were okay with the interviewer and process, they would experience high rapport and if the children did not like what was happening, they would experience low rapport. For many years, every interviewing protocol advocated spending significant time in rapport building. It seemed to make sense, but there was no scientific evidence that it was actually important. The theory (the best it could be specified) was that in conditions of low rapport, children are reluctant to answer and may not provide many details. However, children in conditions of high rapport would be more talkative and provide more details.

All he needed to do was manipulate rapport, right? If the theory was sound, then simply doing this would *cause* a change in the number of spoken details. Children were given math problems to solve after watching a video and before being asked about it. For some children the problems were well above their developmental stage and for others they were easy. Measures of rapport indicated that, yes—the children in the "hard" math group did not want to be there any longer, and those in the "easy" group felt just fine. Those who were experiencing high rapport levels did, in fact, say more things than those experiencing low rapport levels. Though the conclusion is not as important as the way the study was designed, there was some support for the notion that it did impact the number of details they provided.

The benefits of studying such problems using a true scientific method are clear. There are multiple ways that the study can be criticized, but each yields a better study to be run. Arguments about a theory tested this way tend to be data-driven, rather than ideology-driven, or *ad hominem* (i.e., personal attacks against the speakers). Even failures to support a point or nullify a point in a scientific experiment often yield more possibilities for study, rarely fewer. Science becomes a *process* of seeking the truth, rather than a means of convincing others of an arbitrary "fact."

IMPORTANT HISTORICAL DEVELOPMENTS IN THE FIELD OF FORENSIC PSYCHOLOGY

The Case of Daniel M'Naghten

On January 20 in 1843 a man, **Daniel M'Naghten**, who had been lurking in the area of Downing Street in London approached Edward Drummond, the private secretary of British Prime Minister Robert Peel. When M'Naghten was close enough he pulled a pistol from his coat and fired one shot into Mr. Drummond. While trying to produce a second pistol, he was subdued by police constables. Mr. Drummond was able to walk away and received medical treatment and was reported to have been recovering well. He later died, though it eventually became unclear if he actually died from the effects of his wound or the type of subsequent medical treatment he received.

The important question dealt with in his trial was about *why* M'Naghten shot Drummond, not *whether* he shot him. The evidence was clear and observed by constable and other witnesses. He did it. However, he did not seem to intend to assassinate Mr. Drummond. Rather, he was apparently trying to assassinate Mr. Drummond's boss, the Prime Minister, Robert Peel. Was this a cold-blooded politically motivated murder? M'Naghten was known to hold radical political beliefs, which would have made this a feasible motive. He was also known to hold delusional beliefs, especially fears of being persecuted by "the Tories." He had made several complaints to authorities, which were eventually viewed as paranoid and phobic fantasy.

During his trial medical evidence was produced by several physicians, which indicated that M'Naghten was suffering delusions that were so severe that he was not able to tell right from wrong and did not understand the true nature of reality when he acted to assassinate the prime minister, but shot Drummond. The jury was cautioned that they could find him not guilty by reason of insanity if they believed he was not aware of what he was doing—and that he would not be released, but provided medical intervention (e.g., institutionalized). The prosecutors did not push strongly for conviction. The jury quickly returned a verdict of "not guilty by reason of insanity." M'Naghten spent the next two decades in mental health facilities for the criminally insane. He died in custody in 1865.

When Queen Victoria learned of the not guilty verdict, she was incensed and sent a letter to the Prime Minister, demanding an explanation. Subsequently, the House of

Lords sent to the judges of the Court of Common Pleas a set of 12 questions about the case and findings. The answer to one of those questions was:

> To establish a defense on the ground of insanity it must be clearly proved, that, at the time of committing the act, the party accused was laboring under such a defect of reason from disease of the mind, as not to know the nature and quality of the act he was doing, or if he did know it, that he did not know that what he was doing was wrong.

These responses have become known as the M'*Naghten Rules* and continue to be part of the basis for determinations of criminal responsibility in many countries, including most states of the United States and the United Kingdom, though the United Kingdom has subsequently passed rules in 1957 related to homicide, which minimize the M'Naghten standards. Judicial decisions that use these rules and determine reduced responsibility for a crime may still mandate involuntary or voluntary commitments to psychiatric institutions for periods of time that are indeterminate. In other words, those found not guilty by reason of insanity (or guilty, but insane) may actually find themselves in confinement for a longer period of time than those found guilty (and sane). In fact, the confinement may turn out to be for life.

This is certainly not the first case of leniency shown in criminal matters. Such decisions can be found in early Greek, Roman, Norman, and Chinese literature. The notoriety the case was given brought the problems of determining criminal responsibility into public view. Thus, the case was important in the evolution of modern law.

Hugo Munsterberg

The early introduction of psychology to the U.S. legal system was awkward and, at times, bitter. Hugo Munsterberg was a German immigrant and Harvard professor, who had been recruited by William James. Munsterberg believed that psychology had much to offer the judicial system and was somewhat combative about his demand that forensic psychology be considered and utilized (Brigham, 1999). He published a collection of essays on forensic psychology, *On the Witness Stand* (1908). In this collection, he took a strong position that the legal system should be utilizing the forensic psychology literature—and that not doing so was problematic. However, his communication style was widely seen as combative and arrogant and may have backfired. In 1909, John Wigmore authored a rebuttal (in the form of a fictional libel trial against Munsterberg) in which he took the position that psychology did not have enough yet to offer and was guilty of promising things it could not deliver. For the rest of the 20th century, the relationship between the judicial system and the field of forensic psychology was rocky and distant (Brigham, 1999).

Brandeis Briefs, *Muller v. Oregon*

While Hugo Munsterberg was busy arguing with John Wigmore via publications about the role of forensic psychology in the legal system, one of the first widely noted, nonlegal opinions was being offered in a court case by social scientists. An attorney, Louis Brandeis, was presenting a case before the Oregon Supreme Court related to the length of workdays for women (*Muller v. Oregon*, 1908). Brandeis submitted a social science opinion brief that the state's law that limited the length of workdays for women to 10 hours should be upheld. His brief cited social science that he suggested indicated that longer days were shown to be deleterious to women's health. The court upheld the law. Social science opinion briefs that are introduced in legal proceeding are now often referred to as *Brandeis briefs*.

Brown v. Board of Education

In 1954, the U.S. Supreme Court heard a case that challenged the segregation of Caucasian and black children allowed by the much earlier *Plessy v. Ferguson* (1896) decision. *Plessy v. Ferguson* created the "separate but equal" doctrine in the states and was used as justification for racial segregation. During *Brown v. Board of Education*, a legal brief was introduced and endorsed by 35 prominent psychological scholars of the time. The brief outlined the ways that segregation was detrimental to the psychological health of black children and that the earlier *Plessy v. Ferguson* decision should be overturned. Ultimately, the court overturned the separate but equal doctrine and consequently made it illegal to require racial segregation of schools.

Subsequent to this interest in prejudice and racism, which was sparked by *Brown v. Board of Education*, *Gordon Allport* (one of the notable signatories to the social science Brandeis brief introduced in the case) published a (now seminal) book on the psychology of racism and prejudice entitled, *The Nature of Prejudice* (1954). In this pioneering work (which was not specifically forensic), Allport attempted to provide a theoretical basis for understanding how prejudiced views could alter such things as the way that everyday scenes or crime scenes were remembered. Although this book is not often cited as an early forensic psychology tome, these very principles would reemerge later in the 1960s at the beginning of the modern memory research era.

In 1979, **Elizabeth Loftus**, a social psychologist at the University of Washington, authored *Eyewitness Testimony*. This book discussed the memory process and directly challenged the "gold-standard" status of event memory in legal proceedings. Through her elegant work with simple studies, she was able to demonstrate with shocking ease just how fallible memory could be—and how easy it was to corrupt. Though we talk more about her research and memory models later in this book, it is fair to say that her work and the subsequent debates were an important part of the expansion of experimental psychology in the latter half of the 20th century continuing into the 21st century.

This gradually increasing awareness of the value of psychology in legal arenas led to the emergence of professional associations. In 1968, the American Psych-Law Society (aka AP-LS) was founded as the first dedicated professional association of forensic psychologists. In 1977 AP-LS began to publish its forensic psychology journal, *Law and Human Behavior*. Shortly thereafter, the American College of Forensic Psychology was created in 1983 along with its journal, the *American Journal of Forensic Psychology* in 1985. Experimental forensic psychology studies, literature reviews, and forensic conceptual pieces are still published in these journals today. In 1981, the American Psychological Association created its Division 41, *Psychology and Law*, which merged with AP-LS in 1984. In 1995, the APA began to publish *Psychology, Public Policy, and Law*.

Recent Events Relevant to Forensic Psychology

Every day events occur that are relevant to forensic psychology, and for the people involved the consequences are substantial. However, these cases do not often rise to the point of public awareness. When cases arise that capture the attention of the media and the public, the effects of the cases may reach deep into the scholarly activity of social scientists and deep into the actions of government. Though it is difficult to quantify the various impacts of specific cases, some are so well known that they merit special mention as important points in our history. This is not, however, meant to argue that they are the *only* important points.

Serial Murderers

Kenneth Bianchi. In 1977, Yolanda Washington was found dead on a hillside in Los Angeles. Yolanda was a prostitute and it was determined that she has been forcibly raped and murdered. Over the next few months, several more women would be discovered raped, murdered, and placed nude on hillsides in Los Angeles. The murderer became known as the Hillside Strangler. One of the victims was 12 years of age. Later a similar rape and murder of two girls in Bellingham, Washington would lead investigators to Kenneth Bianchi and his cousin, Angelo Buono. Investigators were able to connect both the California and Washington murders to Bianchi—and Bianchi implicated Buono. However, the psychiatrist for the defense soon reported that Kenneth Bianchi was suffering from a disorder known then as *multiple personality disorder*. Today, this is known as dissociative identity disorder. For months psychiatrists debated whether he had this disorder. If he did, he might be found not guilty by reason of insanity and be allowed to be assigned to a forensic mental health center, rather than prison. If this had happened, there was some possibility that he could convince psychiatrists that he was "cured" and perhaps even be released back into society.

Psychiatrists and psychologists disagreed on his state of mind and diagnostic reality, but eventually it was determined that he was *malingering*, faking a mental disorder for functional reasons. In fact, police had discovered numerous and sophisticated textbooks on psychology, psychiatry, and police procedures. In addition to the disagreements about his diagnosis, there were even implications for the use of his testimony against his cousin, Buono. The testimony was collected during hypnosis and afterward. If he has actually been hypnotized, California law would not allow the use of his statements against Buono—because hypnosis had been shown to alter memory, according to Brandeis briefs in other cases.

The court decided eventually that Bianchi did not have multiple personality disorder and that he had never actually been hypnotized. He was sentenced to life in prison and remains there as of publication of this book. While in prison, he had been caught trying to induce women to kill in a copy-cat fashion, to suggest to authorities he was not the guilty party. Forensic psychologists often study his case when researching (1) malingering, (2) psychopathy (which is discussed later), and (3) the processes of expert testimony by mental health professionals.

Jeffrey Dahmer. On July 22, 1991, Jeffrey Dahmer was arrested. Earlier that night he had picked up a young man who was hitchhiking. He brought the man back to his apartment and intended to have sex with him. The man fought back and escaped. He led police to Dahmer's apartment. At the apartment, police first found a human head in Dahmer's refrigerator. They soon found other heads, body parts, and photographs of mutilated bodies. Over the course of their investigation, they were able to determine that Dahmer's behaviors included rape, murder, dismemberment, necrophilia, and cannibalism. In later interviews, Dahmer indicated that he had begun to dissect animals that he had found dead, when he was a young boy, and had escalated to the point that he was experimenting with living humans. He killed 17 young men.

Sentenced in 1992 to 957 years in prison, he was killed while in prison—beaten to death with an iron bar by another inmate. His case remains of interest to forensic psychologists, because (1) he was diagnosed with antisocial personality disorder, borderline personality disorder, and schizotypal personality disorder, (2) he was willing to talk with interviewers about his early life experiences and shed light on the gradual development of his destructive behaviors, and (3) he engaged in particularly unusual behaviors (even for a serial murderer) with his victims.

Dennis Rader. Over the course of two decades in Kansas a serial murderer had killed 10 people while sending letters to police agencies and media outlets, signed BTK (for Bind, Torture, Kill). His murders stopped in the 1990s. In 2004, Rader communicated with police anonymously taking credit for a murder not yet linked to him. Of note, he asked if computer disks could be traced. They told him that they could not be traced. Rader, as BTK, mailed a document in Microsoft Word saved to a floppy disk. Police were able to check the meta-data of the file and trace the disk to a Lutheran church, edited by "Dennis." Police obtained DNA from Rader's daughter and matched it to samples from the fingernails of a known victim. He was arrested and tried for the murders. He eventually pled guilty and discussed his murders in what can be described as a shocking lack of concern or emotion. He was sentenced to 175 years in prison, without the possibility of parole—until 2180.

Dennis Rader's case has been of interest for several reasons. First, he was a deacon at his church and has been known as a family man who was married and raising children. He did not have previous legal difficulties and had worked for the city of Wichita as a dog catcher and as a supervisor for the Compliance Department at Park City—a position that allowed him to roam around looking for small city ordinance violations for which he could issue citations. One female resident reported that he used this position to harass her continually and he eventually had her dog euthanized over violations he stated that he had witnessed.

The other reason his case has been of interest is the very cold manner that he exhibited while discussing with the court his particularly brutal murders. This testimony was videorecorded and was incorporated into several documentaries. As we discuss in a later chapter, one hallmark of antisocial personality disorder is a very low level of sympathetic arousal (i.e., fight or flight response), even in situations that would cause most people to experience high levels of sympathetic arousal.

Day Care Sexual Abuse Scandals

If the above brief accounts of serial murderers shed some light on the behavior of severe psychopaths who murder other humans repeatedly, then what kind of light shines on the cases of large-scale sexual abuse of children that emerged in a rash across the country during the 1980s and early 1990s? For many at the time, it became one more indicator of the depravity that culture had generated. Few societal events generated as much media coverage and sensationalistic coverage as the first of these cases. However, case after case would emerge—each sending the message that children were not safe, even in the very facilities we had to trust to care for them.

McMartin Case, California. In 1983 allegations of brutal sexual abuse occurring at a well-known day care facility owned and managed by Virginia Buckey. Virginia Buckey's daughter, grandson, and granddaughter also worked at the facility. Police investigating the case mailed a letter asking parents to question their children about specific sexual events. When parents became alarmed and reported that they believed their children had, in fact, been abused, police arranged with a private agency to conduct forensic interviews. Ultimately hundreds of interviews were completed and hundreds of allegations were leveled against the Buckey family and others from the facility.

As we discuss in detail in a later chapter, it was soon revealed that the techniques used by the interviewing facility were highly suggestive—and even highly coercive. Pioneering memory research was new to the field of psychology and there was still disagreement about whether children could be led *at all* regarding such events. It took involvement of well-respected psychologists and legal representation to counter allegations that ranged from things that were possible to things that were *fantastical and physically impossible*. Some of these allegations spurred a national fear that some day care facilities were actually engaged in satanic rituals and the sacrificing of human children (Eberle & Eberle, 1993), something most now agree was not actually happening. Raymond Buckey was put through two very long trials, each ending in hung juries (i.e., not acquittals or convictions). Eventually he was released and further charges were not pursued (Eberle & Eberle, 1993).

Rabinowitz (2003) detailed that similar events occurred at about the same time in other places around the country (e.g., Wee Care Case; Fells Acres Case). These cases are considered important because they very openly introduced sexual abuse investigation techniques, and human memory ability to common discussion, to political debate, and to extensive scientific study. Following these cases, there was an increase of dedicated research into children's event recall and the effects of different interviewing techniques. So much research has occurred since the early 1990s that at this point the amount of information psychology has accumulated regarding memory and interviewing is sufficient to answer some questions with a degree of confidence. If you are interested in these issues, stay tuned, because the subsequent memory chapter delves more fully into them.

Children as Perpetrators of Violence

Sometimes children are the perpetrators of violence. Young people are the most common perpetrators of assault against other young people and against adults (FBI, 2010). Cases such as the school shootings that took place at Columbine High School in Colorado in 1999 and Westside Middle School near Jonesboro, Arkansas in 1998 illustrate serious violence against children perpetrated by other children. Both cases involved students who had been able to secure the use of firearms without their parents' knowledge and subsequently use them to commit massacres on the campuses of their schools. The questions raised regarding these events were numerous and varied. To this day the answers are still debated. However, science often begins with difficult questions.

- What was the role of social isolation and depression?
- What was the role of violent video games?
- Were there missed opportunities to intervene and prevent the murders?
- Who or what was responsible for the relative ease with which these children were able to obtain and use firearms?

- How can schools prevent these occurrences?
- How can law enforcement agencies better respond when they arise?

Forensic psychology, criminology, sociology, and other fields continue to study these questions and seek answers. However, as potential answers are crafted, other barriers persist for good reason. If violent video games are shown to play some role in the ability of children to visualize violent behavior, how is it that these can be controlled? If access to firearms plays a role, how can this access be controlled? The line between lawful regulation and unconstitutional infringement on personal rights is sometimes difficult to place—and there are strong and reasonable arguments that are outside the scope of psychology. In essence, psychology may be able to indicate why things happen, but may not have the right or authority to indicate how those circumstances should be changed.

Typical Tasks of Forensic Psychologists

Attempting to specify the duties of a forensic psychologist is a bit like trying to answer the question, "What do physicians do?" Like physicians, each forensic psychologist is trained to perform and understand certain tasks. Their training may be specific and deeply detailed, or generalist and widely varied. During graduate training and subsequent exploration, forensic psychologists largely determine what it is they will do and how specific their research or practice will be. The following are just a few brief descriptions of the many activities that are possible. However, new research emerges every day and new ideas illuminate other needs as of yet unaddressed.

Clinical forensic practice. Many clinically trained psychologists choose to specialize in forensic work. Such things as prisoner rehabilitation, sex offender treatment, and crime victim intervention are common activities. Often these psychologists will work in state or federal correctional environments.

Risk assessment. Forensic psychologists may be asked to provide input into the level of risk in cases of parole, probation, and release from involuntary commitment to psychiatric hospitals. Furthermore, when children are admitted to care facilities and have a history of aggression of assault, the facility may wish to know how to protect the environment. Through batteries of tests and observations, forensic psychologists may be able to inform decision makers, without promising perfect prediction.

Competency. In order to stand trial, defendants must be able to help their attorneys and participate in their own defense. In this respect, forensic psychologists may be able to help the court decide whether a defendant is "competent" enough to communicate with an attorney and the court and understand the procedures and processes with which they are involved.

Sanity determinations. Like competency evaluations, most judicial jurisdictions require (for conviction) that defendants knew what they were doing at the point of the alleged crime and knew that what they were doing was wrong or illegal. Although this is usually the decision of the jury, forensic psychologists are often asked to provide expert opinions on the state of a defendant's awareness at the time of a crime.

Jury selection. Our criminal justice system depends on the consideration of citizens who are asked to decide the verdict of criminal allegations. But who is enlisted to serve on a jury? Before a final set of jurors is selected, both defense and prosecuting attorneys will have opportunities, through a **voir dire** (i.e., questioning) process, to indicate which jurors should be eliminated. Some jurors may be eliminated *for cause*. For example, some jurors may state they are unwilling to consider the full range of potential sanctions, or may show some overt and discernible prejudice about the defendant or the crime. They would likely be eliminated. Some jurors may be eliminated in a *peremptory* fashion. This means they did not show a bias that was obvious enough to be eliminated for cause, but the attorney had other reasons for rejecting them. University professors may be rejected quickly because they may be perceived as opinionated and are used to leading groups of people through debates. Attorneys may worry that they can hijack a deliberation and upset the normal consideration of ideas.

Expert testimony. Forensic psychologists are often called into court to provide expert opinion on issues related to different aspects of a case. These may be the existence of a specific disorder, the possible behaviors associated with a disorder, or the assessment of human behavior. For example, a common modern form of expert testimony involves the frailties of human memory. Some experts may be asked to help a jury understand how a witness can believe they saw an event, but actually be mistaken about the details of the event. With children who have been interviewed about things like sexual abuse, experts may have to help the jury to understand how the interview was conducted and whether the least leading processes were utilized. Once a jury understands the nature of memory and the nature of the process used to collect a specific person's memory, they can make a more informed decision about the weight to place upon that recollection.

Research. A vast majority of forensic psychology still exists in the realm of research—understanding human behavior, crime, memory, and psychopathology. This research is eventually used to assist those that work in the practice world, but the research plays a vital role in the stability of the ideas that are brought into the "real" world. While research may often seem esoteric or academic, it is essential to informing the field. The problem is in how to ensure that (1) researchers remain interested in studying things of practical importance, and (2) practitioners remain interested in using techniques or assessments guided by solid research. Partnerships between the forensic practice world and the academic research world are advantageous to both worlds.

Public affairs/advocacy. There is debate about the degree to which forensic psychologists should become involved in public affairs or public advocacy. Some argue that such advocacy can lead to politics, which can often interfere with the hardnosed neutrality needed in science. However, faithful scientists can always participate in *informing* decision makers, rather than *guiding* them. In much the same way that an expert witness informs a jury (the ultimate decider in a criminal case), there is no reason that forensic psychology cannot provide the best perspectives from the current state of the field to those who are charged with the responsibility to make decisions. The decisions may be right or wrong (from our individual perspectives), but the information provided to them by the field can remain neutral and accurate.

Crime prevention. One area that often remains understudied and underpracticed is crime prevention. If forensic psychology can develop stable theories about the causes of crime, then it seems appropriate to utilize these theories in natural environments to test the degree to which they can help to lower the amount of crime. The barriers to this kind of implementation often involve things such as expense and difficulty (changing things in large environments is tough) and politics. People often have preexisting ideas about important things such as crime and do not wish to try new "experimental" things. Even if old ideas don't seem to be working, there is always a fear that new ideas will make things worse.

Training

Training in forensic psychology usually requires graduate school training in psychology, often a doctoral degree (i.e., PhD or PsyD) or a master's degree (i.e., MA or MS). In most PhD programs, forensic research as a part of the program is the way that graduate students specialize and become forensic psychologists. A few programs, especially clinically oriented programs, seek to specifically train professionals to work in the forensic system. However, these programs are sometimes limited to clinical work and training, rather than experimental.

However, some new programs have begun to offer specialized training in limited aspects of forensic psychology and law for those professionals who (1) do not have formal undergraduate training in psychology and (2) need to understand basic and practical concepts to apply to their own work. For example, police officers would do well to understand some aspects of psychopathology, which may lead people to act in a criminal fashion or respond differently to authority than most other people would respond. Social workers often encounter potential cases of abuse. Understanding how to deal with children in these circumstances in order to minimize damage to the legal case and maximize help to the child are keys to successfully preventing further abuse.

Missouri State University began offering this specialized training in the form of a graduate certificate in forensic child psychology. Those who complete the training gain knowledge in child abuse theory, child abuse assessment, memory, criminal procedure, and other areas relevant to professionals who help children. The program is geared to the working professional. The material is guided by both working academic researchers and working child welfare professionals, which avoids the "ivory tower" phenomenon as well as the "anything goes" mentality. Slowly, other schools are also offering similar programs.

STUDY QUESTIONS

1. Define psychology and forensic psychology.
2. Explain the epistemological concepts of: Rationalism, Empiricism, Authority, and Experimentalism. Provide an example of their use in sides of a common debate.
3. Explain confirmation bias, availability heuristic, hindsight bias, and representativeness heuristic.
4. What is pseudoscience and how can you identify it?
5. What are the different components/variables in an experimental study?
6. Describe the case of Daniel M'Naghten and its impact on legal decisions.
7. What is a Brandeis brief?
8. Describe the contributions of psychology to the Supreme Court case of *Brown v. Board of Education.*
9. What was the impact (on psychology) of the day care sexual abuse scandals of the 1980s and 1990s?
10. Name the nine common tasks of forensic psychologists described in the chapter.

GLOSSARY

availability heuristic The tendency to apply more weight to information that is readily available, perhaps by simple recency or salience.

Brown v. Board of Education An important case in which psychology utilized a Brandeis brief to advocate for the elimination of racial segregation in schools.

confirmation bias The tendency to more readily accept answers or explanations, which tend to reconfirm our already-held opinions or positions.

Daniel M'Naghten A case of a murderer in 19th-century England who was thought to have committed his crime because of mental reasoning difficulties. This case was the impetus for the development of the M'Naghten Rules.

Elizabeth Loftus An early important researcher who successfully incorporated basic memory research into forensic topics such as eyewitness testimony and recollection of childhood experiences.

epistemology The study of differing "ways of knowing, including such things as rationalism, empiricism, experimentalism, and authority."

forensic child psychology The study of the assessments and intervention with children who are thought to have been victims of, witnesses to, or perpetrators of crime.

forensic psychology The study of individual behavior in legal, criminal, or judicial contexts.

hindsight bias The tendency to overestimate (after the conclusion is known) our ability to have answered a problem correctly.

hypothesis A testable prediction derived from the concepts in a theory.

Louis Brandeis Used psychological principle and research in the form of a report to a court in advocacy of a social topic. Now used to advocate a position in legal matters and is referred to as *Brandeis Briefs*.

pseudoscience Conclusion that tends to appear to be scientific, or claim scientific standing, but does not follow the normal conventions of scientific practice.

representativeness heuristic The tendency to more readily accept information when that information fits an already-held stereotype or prototype.

theory A general explanation of a collection of observations. A good theory should incorporate existing data, provide opportunities for testable hypotheses, and be open to adjustment if new data requires.

voir dire Literally "to speak the truth." A process of questioning used to pick reasonable jury members or even to determine the expert status of some expert witnesses.

REFERENCES

American Psychological Association. (2013, June 1). *About APA*. Retrieved from http://www.apa.org/about/index.aspx

Allport, G. (1954). *The nature of prejudice*. Oxford, England: Addison-Wesley.

Boles, R. (2003). *The effects of rapport on forensic interviews of children*. Unpublished thesis submitted to Missouri State University.

Brigham, J. (1999). What is forensic psychology, anyway? *Law and Human Behavior*, *23*(3), 273–298.

Bunge, M. (1984). What is pseudoscience? *Skeptical Inquirer*, *9*, 36–46.

Callahan, R. (2001). The impact of thought field therapy on heart rate variability. *Journal of Clinical Psychology*, *57*(10), 1153–1170.

Eberle, P., & Eberle, S. (1993). *The abuse of innocence: The McMartin preschool trial*. Buffalo, NY: Prometheus.

Federal Bureau of Investigation. (2010). *Uniform crime report: Crime in the United States*.

Fischoff, B. (1975). Hindsight does not equal foresight: The effect of outcome knowledge on judgment under uncertainty. *Journal of Experimental Psychology: Human Perception and Performance*, *1*, 288–299.

Kahneman, D., Slovik, P., & Tversky, A. (1982). *Judgment under uncertainty: Heuristics and biases.* New York, NY: Cambridge University Press.

Lilienfeld, S. (2007). Psychological treatments that cause harm. *Perspectives on Psychological Science, 2*(1), 53–70.

Lilienfeld, S., Ammirati, R., & David, M. (2012, February). Distinguishing science from pseudoscience in school psychology: Science and scientific thinking as safeguards against human error. *Journal of School Psychology, 50*(1), 7–36.

Loftus, E. (1979). *Eyewitness testimony.* Cambridge, MA: Harvard University Press.

Munsterberg, H. (1908). *On the witness stand.* Garden City, NY: Doubleday.

Nickerson, R. (1998). Confirmation bias: A ubiquitous phenomenon in many guises. *Review of General Psychology, 2,* 175–220.

O'Donohue, W. (2013). Errors in psychological practice: Devising a system to improve client safety and well-being. *Professional Psychology: Research and Practice, 45*(5), 314–323.

Popper, K. (1959). *The logic of scientific discovery.* (Translation by author of 1934 edition). Oxford, England: Basic Books.

Rabinowitz, D. (2003). *No crueler tyrannies: Accusation, false witness, and other terrors of our times.* New York, NY: Free Press.

Romanczyk, R., Arnstein, L., Soorya, L., & Gillis, J. (2003). The myriad of controversial treatments for autism: A critical evaluation of efficacy. In S. Lilienfeld, S. Lynn, & J. Lohr (Eds.), *Science and pseudoscience in clinical psychology* (pp. 363–395). New York, NY: Guilford Press.

SSCP. (2001). Online debate of member of the Society for the Science of Clinical Psychology listserv.

Wigmore, J. (1909). Hugo Munsterberg and the psychology of testimony. *Illinois Law Review, 3,* 399–434.

━━━◆━━━

Social and Behavioral Psychology

GOALS OF THIS CHAPTER:

1. To understand the basic social psychology concepts that impact forensic analysis.
2. To understand the basic behavioral concepts that impact forensic analysis.
3. To develop a conceptual method for understanding day-to-day cases.

Research psychologists have been studying the motivation for as long as there have been research psychologists. However, in the past 50 years a great deal of work has been dedicated to understanding both the effects of social environments and the effects of learning processes on human behavior. Students with a background in psychology may be familiar with these concepts, but other students may not be as familiar.

Working with children, families, and the legal system sometimes requires that professionals attempt to explain why individuals or groups of individuals behave in a specific manner. *Some* background in social and behavioral psychology is essential to that explanation, and is the primary goal of this chapter.

SOCIAL PSYCHOLOGY

Mark's wife, Lilli, has noticed that he behaves differently when they are together by themselves than when they are in a large social gathering. She complains that although he is sweet and caring when they are alone, he can be loud and slightly misogynistic when he is around his friends, sometimes making fun of her preferences and abilities. She also recently read some of his anonymous online comments on news stories from the web because he left the computer logged on the page. According to Lilli, his comments were so aggressive and political that they bordered on soliciting violence.

Does Lilli have something to worry about? Are these differences in behavior due to changes in his personality or to the development of a psychological disorder? Or are they the product of different and contrasting social environments? We could not say anything about Mark and Lilli without knowing a lot more of their case. However, both explanations are feasible. It is possible that Mark is suffering from some problems such as stressful events and poor coping, or changes in his physiology or other things. It is also possible that Mark is Mark, another human being whose behavior is elicited not just by his own thoughts and preferences, but also by the restrictions, permissiveness, and perceived consequences of the social environment in which they occur. When Mark is with his wife, the social environment elicits the compassion she admires and reciprocates. When he is with his friends, they may tease him if he appears too sensitive or laugh when he tells those slightly misogynistic jokes—and he knows Lilli will forgive him. When he is on the Internet, he is bombarded by other hostile postings. They make him angry and he can strike out without fear that he will have to explain his expressions (usually). The social environment does not just reinforce specific (to the environment) behaviors; it also provides the cues needed to select which values, thoughts, and judgments will be brought into awareness.

Social psychology is the study of individual behavior when in a group (or social) context. Those working in forensic contexts are wise to consider the effects of social environments on the behaviors, decision making, and problem solving of the people around them. Social psychology has developed some well-known psychological principles that can guide our understanding of problematic personal behavior. We explore just a few of the most important and well understood principles.

OBEDIENCE

What does it take for you to follow the requests or directives of another person? Do the requests need to be sensible, rational behaviors or responses? Do they need to be things you want to do anyway? If asked, what conditions would you place on your own willingness to obey the directives of another person? Would you willingly commit murder or engage in behavior you know causes harm to another person—serious harm? What if you were being asked to punish another adult with consequences so painful that they caused the recipient to scream or pass out and become unconscious? If you caused them to become unconscious, would you continue to punish them if they could not respond to your requests?

I (Fanetti) would posit that most people *believe* they would not engage in such destructive behavior. In fact, it seems quite aggressive when written in black and white text. "Of course not," we might exclaim in defiance. But what if research was able to determine that it was not difficult to make average, decent people do exactly what is described above? Are these average people? Are they decent?

Stanley Milgram (1963) endeavored to discover a basic recipe for obedience to authority. In a classic study of human behavior, he recruited 40 adult males between the ages of 20 and 50. Each participant was paid $4.50. Once the men arrived at the laboratory, they were told they would be allowed to keep the money, no matter what they decided to do in the study. The study, as described to them, was related to the effects of punishment on learning. If they decided to leave at that point, they would still have been given the money, which amounted to about $35 if adjusted to 2013 dollar value. We refer to the men who agreed to be a part of the study as *participants*.

Participants were told that they would be asking questions to another man, whom we call the *learner*. Now here is one thing *you* will be told that the research subjects were *not* told—the learner was always a confederate of the person running the study (aka the *experimenter*). This confederate learner was trained to act out a certain set of answers and responses. So ... the *experimenter* has told the *participant* that he will be asking questions to the *learner* ... follow? The twist of the study was as follows: If the learner answered a question correctly, the participant moved to the next question on the list. If the learner answered the question incorrectly, the participant was instructed to flip a switch. The participant was told that these switches would deliver a jolt of electricity to the learner as a consequence for incorrect responses.

An important addition to this setup was the equipment being used to deliver the jolts of electricity. Essentially, this was a large box with a linear row of toggle switches along the bottom. Above each switch, the "voltage" of the corresponding jolt was listed. After each incorrect response, the participant was told to now utilize the next switch for a subsequence incorrect answer. Switches were labeled from a low of 15 volts or "slight shock" progressively toward 450 volts or "XXX." Remember that the learner was acting out a preplanned script for each switch, crying out with expressions of growing pain. When the participant flipped the "300-volt" switch, the learners pounded and demanded to be let out of room (which appeared to the participant to not happen). The learner answered no more questions, though the participant had every reason to believe he was still connected to the apparatus. When the learner stopped answering questions, the participant was instructed to provide the cues requesting that they continue, and then that they ask the next question and flip the next switch.

The question for Milgram was, "When [where in the switch order] will the participants stop providing shocks to the complaining learners?" Out of the 40 subjects, about 14 (35%) ceased when the participant demanded to be let out and subsequently stopped responding, or shortly after (remember, they had been crying out in pain earlier than that). The majority of participants (i.e., 26, or 65%) continued to follow the command to ask questions and flip switches right to the end of the list, which was marked as "450 volts – XXX." They had shocked a nonresponsive learner 10 times, with increasing severity using switches labeled with strong warnings! They had no way to determine whether they had killed this person. There was no such feedback. That they believed they were doing harm was verified by Milgram's description of the behavior and increasing nervousness of the participants.

Milgram was able to describe four factors that he believed were most responsible for the greatest degree of obedience. These four factors can be found in many cases of obedience to troubling directives, in both actual history (e.g., German compliance with Adolph Hitler's commands in World War II) and in popular fiction (e.g., George Orwell's 1984). The first is the (1) *prestige of the authority figure*. When the authority figure who issues the command appears to have the prestige, rank, or power to issue such commands, people are more likely to obey them. Next is the (2) *proximity of the authority figure*. If the person who issued the command also monitors compliance, people are more likely to obey. Next is the (3) *proximity of the victim*. In Milgram's study, the learner was the victim. If that victim is physically more distant, people are more likely to obey commands which cause harm to the victim. Finally there was the presence or absence of (4) *examples of defiance*. If an example of defiance arises, such as observing another person say no without consequence, then people are *less* likely to obey.

Consider This

If you wish to explore these concepts, take the time read George Orwell's 1984 and see if you can identify each.

CONFORMITY

Social psychologists are not only interested in how people can be made to follow explicit or troubling commands; they have also been interested in how people conform to more subtle social cues. Even if others do not exactly request behavior from you, are there social factors that can increase how likely you are to go along with the prevailing wisdom or the consensus of the group around you? Will this subtle pressure to conform extend to reactions, judgments, or conclusions that you *know are wrong*? In other words, can people be made to agree with something that they would otherwise not endorse?

Solomon Asch (1955) studied this issue to determine if it was possible to (and how to) alter the social context most efficiently to provide the greatest degree of conformity to clearly incorrect conclusions. He asked people to participate in a study of "perceptual judgments." The actual participants entered a room in which other people were already present, presumably also participants. In reality, the other people in the room were only acting as though they were participants. They were actually confederates of the experimenter.

The task was designed to be simple. A card was displayed with three lines, each of different length. Simultaneously another card was displayed with a single line. Participants (real and confederate) were asked to state aloud which line on the first cards (i.e., with three lines) matched the comparison card's line. Participants were arranged so that they had to provide their answers after each of the other people—you know, those pesky confederates. An example of the cards they viewed is provided in Table 2.1.

This is simple, is it not? Certainly the actual participants thought so after the first set of people answered B, leaving our participant to confidently state the same conclusion. However, on some subsequent cards, the confederates confidently stated the wrong answer (i.e., each confederate and the same wrong answer). Then the opportunity to answer falls to the real participant. Imagine the dismay. If the card was as described above, the first people all may have said A. They said that Line A looked like Line X! What would you do—with all attention on you and your desired answer different than everybody else's unanimous response? If you are like the people in this study, 75% of you will (at least once) intentionally state the obviously wrong response. Why?

Reasons for this conformity with incorrect judgments may be numerous. Perhaps the conformers believed they had misunderstood something about the instructions, although the instructions in this example are exceedingly simple. Perhaps the conformers believe that the others in the group have noticed something that the conformer has missed. What exactly could that be, in such a simple task. Perhaps it is a general tendency to not differ from the crowd. Is it better to be incorrect (with company) than take a risk of being incorrect (alone)?

Imagine for a moment the following scenario: You are sitting in class of 20 people and you are paying attention to something you think you know. The professor asks a question and asks for a showing of hands. The choices are A, B, or C, but you know the easy answer is C. When the professor calls out A, the other 19 people in class unanimously raise their hands. The professor calls out B, but nobody raises a hand. Then the professor calls out

Table 2.1 Example of Asch Perceptual Judgment Cards

First Card:

    A: _____

    B: _____

    C: _____

Comparison Card:

    X: _____

C. What would you do? What would you think? You have two choices: Raise your hand or do not. You *know* that C is the correct answer, you are absolutely certain. Solomon Asch's conclusions suggest that most people would either simply keep their hands down, or would have already raised them for A.

There are some other circumstances, however, that affect this tendency. The group (incorrect answer) has to be *unanimous* to produce the strongest conformity. This does not mean that each member must *believe* the group answer is correct, only that they *assert* that it is correct. In this way, a group can come to an incorrect (or otherwise problematic) decision even when a majority of the group's members privately disagree with the decision. If the first assertions were wrong and unanimous we can expect subsequent assertions to simply conform.

In forensically relevant groups, such as youth gangs, this effect, in addition to the Milgram "obedience factors" described earlier, can create conformity to very dangerous group decisions (Uchiyama & Hoshino, 1993). Imagine, the group decision making process deemed as *democratic*, but allowing the group's lead members to voice their opinions first. The next member will have to contend with the push to obey as well as to conform to a unanimous conclusion (so far). It will only get worse for subsequent members.

Asch did provide for alterations to the conformity context, which allowed for change to the tendency to conform. If the previous members did not provide the same answer as the first responders (even if the answers are still wrong), then people are less likely to conform and more likely to provide the answer they believe is correct. Additionally, the conformity effect grows as the size of the preceding group (and the unanimous incorrect decision) grows, until the group size reaches about six. Even larger unanimous groups do have an increasing effect, but the growth in effect diminishes. Essentially, there need be only a handful of people providing the answer before you to create a significant pressure to conform.

Consider This

As one final thought exercise, imagine how the combination of the Asch conformity principle and Milgram obedience principles can have an effect in the social context of a room that is full of deliberating jurors.

DEINDIVIDUATION AND SOCIAL ROLE-PLAYING

During the second Iraq War, a news story flooded the Internet and airwaves. It was a story that brought shock and dismay to many Americans and others throughout the world. Abu Ghraib prison was a facility in Baghdad predominantly administered by U.S. forces holding Iraqi prisoners. What emerged from the news stories was an image of guards forcing prisoners to engage in brutal and humiliating behavior—and the guards seemed to be enjoying the enterprise, often posing for photos with their prisoners in the middle of the acts. Although there is no evidence that this was widespread abusive behavior, there was significant evidence that it did happen with a handful of guards.

Explanations for why it happened included suggestions that the guards were psychopathic in some fashion and/or that there was a dereliction of training and supervision over the facility. Ignoring the personal assessments of the guards involved in the Abu Ghraib fiasco, it is interesting for forensic social psychologists to examine the effect of a lack of supervision on people poorly trained for a task. The problem at Abu Ghraib need not have been a surprise. The very type of behavior (absent the sexual assault) displayed by these guards had already been displayed by a set of untrained guards who had been given little supervision. Furthermore, this previous experience was well recorded, well analyzed, and very well studied because it was the basis of a 1970s psychological study of prisoner and guard behavior. It was a study in which guards (who knew they were being studied) became so abusive that the experiment had to be ended early.

Haney, Banks, and Zimbardo (1973) recruited participants to be a part of a "psychological study of prison life." These people were to be randomly assigned to play either the role of a prisoner or a guard. A well-simulated prison was constructed on the lower level of the Stanford psychology department, complete with realistic jail cells. Prisoners and guards were given role-appropriate clothes to wear. The prisoners were mock-arrested by actual police officers and brought to the jail. From that point they were referred to by number, not name. Individuality was de-emphasized at all opportunities.

Though this was supposed to be a 2-week study, the guards became aggressive on the very first day. Soon after, the prisoners tried a revolt, which was harshly ended by the guards. Before the experiment was ended early, the guards had engaged in some of the very behavior that guards at Abu Ghraib displayed. They placed bags over the prisoner's head, forced them into nudity, forced them to simulate sex act with inanimate objects, and made them engage in painful punishments. The guards were reported to be disappointed at the early end, but the prisoners were reported to be thankful.

Although this has been interpreted by some to suggest that trouble brews in all of us, a better interpretation is that when we are given to a task for which we have been poorly trained, and when we are given the freedom of relative anonymity, we may begin to respond in a stereotyped fashion. We may exaggerate the problems of the stereotype and begin to minimize the individual problem solving we use in familiar tasks. In other words, if you do not really know how to direct prisoners you are more likely to "do what guards do," even if that means to be brutal. If supervisory intervention is limited, and your personal identity is relatively removed from what you are doing, your behavior may become extreme.

Groupthink is related to deindividuation (as well as to the concept of conformity). **Groupthink** happens when like-minded people come to a common conclusion, but fail to consider alternative information. If all members of a jury already basically believe that a defendant is guilty, how likely is it that they will be forced to thoroughly review exculpatory evidence during deliberations? The quick conclusion may be, "We are all in basic agreement here, let's take a vote." They still have the duty to examine all of the evidence, but they may fail to do so. You can then understand why a defense attorney tries so hard to place the kernel of doubt in at least one juror's mind.

Consider This

If this is true, what would you suggest to prevent or minimize these problematic and exaggerated responses? How do you think the conformity and obedience concepts interacted with the social role playing and deindividuation concepts in the Stanford study or at Abu Ghraib?

GROUP POLARIZATION

What happens when a group of like-minded people discuss a problem, for the purposes of coming to a conclusion or solving a problem? For example, why do Democrats and Republicans in Washington, DC rarely show the willingness to come to consensus decisions? (By the way, I (Fanetti) am not suggesting that they *should*—just that they do not). Perhaps the problem is in the way that they develop their answers to problems they are being asked to address. One potential explanatory mechanism is called *group polarization*. **Group polarization** (Moscovici, Zavalloni, & Louis-Guerin, 1972) is the tendency for groups of like-minded people who are discussing a problem to generate solutions that tend to be both more uniform (i.e., less intragroup dissent) and more extreme than the original positions held by its members.

Now imagine our representatives in Washington. If they face a big problem (let us say it is one that they actually have to solve), they may first caucus independently. That is, the Republicans will talk to other Republicans and the Democrats will talk to other Democrats. Only later will they bring their general approaches to a solution before the larger, combined group. Do we expect that these answers will be *closer* to each than they were before the caucusing? No. Group polarization predicts that each group will emerge with a proposal that is farther from the other side and that the members will be more uniformly in support of their side's proposal. Coming to a consensus decision then becomes a protracted melee to determine which side can leverage the most support for their solution. Sound familiar?

✍ Consider This

Think about the way that advocacy groups come to decisions about how to influence public policy. How might group polarization impact this process?

Think of the ways that groupthink, group polarization, conformity, and obedience might affect the decision making that happens when a group of youths is deciding how to respond to a perceived threat.

SOCIAL LOAFING AND NONRESPONDERS

Have you ever been part of a group effort to move a heavy piece of furniture? Did you give it your best effort? Personally, I (Fanetti) can remember doing so and also knowing that I was not giving it my all, but nevertheless providing the appropriate amount of grunting sounds to sell the effort. This tendency to decrease effort, intentionally or unintentionally, when participating in a group effort is known as **social loafing.** Athletic coaches often work against this tendency in their teams, especially teams of young and inexperienced players. A 1913 study of players of a game of tug-of-war (Kravitz & Martin, 1986; Ringelmann, 1913) found that players exerted less pulling force when pulling as a group than they did when they were pulling alone. This effect increased as the size of the cooperating group increased. Additionally, some critics suggested that the real culprit was a lack of communication, so Ingham et al. (1974) replicated Ringelmann's study, but also utilized a group with one real puller and confederate sham puller (i.e., who exerted no genuine force). The results of both supported the conclusion that the reason for the decreased amount of effort used in group setting was *the existence of the cooperating group.*

Why do we do this? Explanations for this include the concept of **diffusion of responsibility**—the idea that when other people of presumed competence are present some of the responsibility for the action or the response is removed and placed on others. If one person is present to see another person fall and become unconscious, then we might assume we have all of the responsibility to help. This does not mean that the observer will *choose* to help. If two people are present to see the other fall and become unconscious, then the amount of responsibility to act might be halved. Thus, a failure to help is not *solely* our fault. "But, I was not the only one." Imagine the effect if 12 people are in view, or 30.

A famous case of social loafing and diffusion of responsibility occurred in 1964. Kitty Genovese was a young woman living in New York City. At about 3:15 A.M., she was returning home from work as a bar manager and was approaching the door of her apartment, located in the back alley of her apartment building. She was approached by Winston Moseley and began to run to her door. He overtook her and stabbed her. When she cried out a neighbor yelled at him to leave her alone. Moseley left. However, he returned later to search the parking lot, stab her again, and rape her. The troubling part of the story involves the reaction of the neighbors. Though details are hotly debated and not well established, reports indicate that between 6 and 30 people were, at some level, aware that the attack was occurring—yet police were not called and given details until much later. Though we cannot fully understand the actions or motivations of the neighbors in this case, it is an important opportunity to consider the impact of diffusion of responsibility on this, a possible example of the **bystander effect** (Darley & Latane, 1968). Research has replicated this nonresponse effect in many contexts (Fischer et al., 2011).

◢◤ Consider This

Why do you think most CPR guides recommend that the first responder point to a specific person and direct them to "call 911"? Think how would you respond in two scenarios: (1) on campus during the noon rush, you see a person lying face down on the grass of the quad, (2) you see the same thing—but at late at night when nobody else is around.

ATTRIBUTION

What do you say to yourself after you receive a test score? Does it matter if you did well, or poorly? How do you explain your test performances? Perhaps you received a low score and said, "Good grief, I'm stupid." (*Aside: If you are in a college class, you are intellectually functional*). Perhaps you said, "That professor is a real %&#!" On the other hand, if the score was high perhaps you said, "Man, I rock. I *aced* it!" Or maybe you said, "That professor gives easy tests." What about the people sitting near to you? You know you should not be looking, but you did. They did really well, or really poorly. How do you explain *their* performance?

By this point, you are familiar with the experience described earlier. You have been through it many times. Understanding how you answered the above questions is a small part of a field of psychology known as *attribution theory*. **Attribution theory** is used to explain the causes for others' behavior, as well as our own. It is not restricted to explaining test performance, but instead is a central part of the daily lives of human beings, especially when in a social or comparative context.

Attribution processes even work their way into the forensic world, especially when we are part of or observing behaviors that are on the border between acceptable behaviors and unacceptable behaviors. Jurors are often asked to make a decision about why a potentially criminal behavior occurred.

One way that attributions can be described is whether the "cause" found in the attribution is internal to the person or external. *Internal attributions* are those that posit a cause for people's behavior that the people take with them whereever they go. External attributions are those that posit that the cause for a behavior as contextual, or "other than" a personal attribute of the person who exhibited the behavior. In other words, internal attributions assign blame to the person and external attributions assign blame to the context or at least to someone else.

For example, if you hear that John and Dave were in a physically combative altercation you might say, "John is always looking for a fight." You have clearly decided that the cause for the fight is (predominantly) *inside* of John—the ultimate cause for the fight was John's hostility or anger. If you conclude that John must have been "egged on," you are making an external attribution—the ultimate cause for the fight was the situation or the aggression by the other person.

Attributions are generally made only for behaviors that are unusual or salient to us in some fashion. We do not spend much time assigning a cause for a squirrel's behavior as we walk across campus. It is unimportant to us, unless that squirrel does something unusual or important. What if that squirrel starts barking and threatening you? Very quickly, we would seek an explanation. Did I encroach into its territory—if squirrels have territory they feel needs to be defended from humans? This is an external attribution for the squirrel's behavior and it does impact the remedies we generate. First on the list? Walk away. What if we draw in internal attribution? "That squirrel has rabies!" If we walk away, do we think we will be left alone? Probably not. Therefore, other or additional options may be selected (e.g., *run* away). Whatever we do, the process of making an attribution has affected our analysis of the problem.

Think through examples of the attributions we might make when watching children play outside our own homes, especially if they are playing in a fashion we think is disruptive or destructive. What kinds of things might people say to themselves, or others, about the causes of the child's behavior?

Researchers have tried to identify tendencies in the process of the formation of attributions. One tendency is called the **fundamental attribution error** (Sicoly & Ross, 1977). The fundamental attribution error involves overestimating the importance of *internal factors* for the behavior of *other people*. When we see other people engaging in problematic behavior, we are likely to avow that we would never do the same thing, even if we were to find ourselves in the same situation. How many times have you yelled at the screen during a horror movie, "Don't go there! What? Are you an idiot?"

In a classic study of the fundamental attribution error concept (Jones & Harris, 1967), researched asked students to read aloud speeches from a debate regarding controversial national leader, Fidel Castro. They simply had to read the speech and no mention was made that they actually endorsed the speech in any way. Later others (who knew they were just reading) were asked to rate the degree to which they agreed with the speech they read. Results suggest that having read the speech made others believe you personally agreed with it. In other words, the fundamental attribution error was at work. They assigned a cause for the words you read—your belief system, not the assignment.

Consider This

Why do we think we know things about celebrities from the movies they complete? What role would the fundamental attribution error play in a juror's decision about a trial?

PREJUDICE AND DISCRIMINATION

As the name implies, a *prejudice* is a prejudgment. The concept of *adaptive conservatism* (Henderson, 1985) holds that there is a certain adaptive value to holding a more favorable attitude toward those things with which we are familiar, those people we know or those behaviors we have observed. If this is a relative favoritism, then the contrasting perspective is that we hold less favorable attitudes about unfamiliar people, things, or actions. While the term *prejudice* implies a negativistic tendency, especially when applied to other people, it is simply a heuristic, a shortcut we use to be efficient in making choices through our lives. Prejudices will be adaptive in the long run, provided they do not ignore actual evidence or experience. Ultimately a prejudice is a judgment *before the facts*. If you avoid a person because their skin color is different than yours, this is a prejudice. If you continue to avoid or dislike this person after they have demonstrated good character, you have allowed your prejudice to be more important than your observations.

Prejudiced *in-group* bias involves treating members of your specific group favorably. *Out-group homogeneity* (Park & Rothbart, 1982) involves viewing all those who are not in your group, even if these "others" come from disparate groups themselves, as uniformly less favorable. We may develop mental stereotypes to represent a generalized member of other groups. A *stereotype* is a representative model of the qualities of others. Once again, stereotypes are nearly unavoidable when our experience is limited. They are not indicators of flawed thinking, but rather tools our perceptual processes utilize to make decisions in new environments. These stereotypes may be *implicit*, meaning that we are unaware that we hold them. They may also be *explicit*, meaning that we know we hold them. If your prejudices are explicit, this does not mean they are maladaptive. It means that you have a better opportunity to compare the model to your experiences. Essentially, you can challenge that stereotypic belief. Implicit stereotypes may be more difficult to change, because we do not know we hold them and may be less likely to challenge them, or even admit they exist. Prejudices and stereotypes are not automatically destructive. They only become problematic when they persist, despite contrary evidence.

When we allow our attitudes about others to evolve into specific actions against those others, we have begun *discrimination*. Although it is difficult to codify laws against prejudice, most jurisdictions have specific laws regarding *actions* based on those beliefs. Law enforcement officers in high-crime areas may have numerous interactions with youths who are part of organized and illegal gang activity. Those gang members may have specific prejudices about the officers and the officers may have prejudices about the youths. Those prejudices will undoubtedly lead to stereotypes for both. However, we know that not all law enforcement officers are similar and not all gang members are similar.

Consider This

Think about and discuss how prejudices and stereotypes held by youths about officers and officers about youths might disrupt the peacekeeping mission of a police force. Think through what things might be done to minimize this and what difficulties this would entail.

LEARNING AND BEHAVIOR

Social psychologists examine the effects of groups or group membership on the expression of individual behavior. **Behavioral** psychologists examine the effects of contextual events on individual behavior. Behavioral psychologists look to the immediate environment for causal influences to behavior. While the field of behavioral psychology is large and diverse, there remain two predominant behavioral theories to explain why living organisms exhibit behavior.

"Classical" Conditioning

During the 16th century a school of thought known as *associationism*, or British associationism, emerged that suggested (among other things) that organisms learn by forming associations between objects or events that occur closely together in time. The philosophers David Hartley and John Stuart Mill believed that we develop complex ideas and concepts about the world by creating patterns of smaller associations. Later, Ivan Pavlov would provide the empirical evidence that these association concepts might actually be true.

Ivan Pavlov was a Russian physiologist whose primary research interest was digestion, a pursuit for which he won the 1904 Nobel Prize. During his research into salivary reflexes he ran into a problem. He was attempting to study how dogs salivate when a meat powder is fed to them. To do this he attached a cannula (i.e., a graduated vial into which saliva flows directly) to the dog. However, as the study progressed, he found that the animal began to salivate *before* it received the food. Even the sound of the approaching researchers would cause salivation. This was a problem for his digestive research because it made distinguishing the independent effect of the meat powders impossible.

To understand this, imagine that you are trying to decide which hamburgers make you salivate more (pick your favorite and think about it). If you are hungry, then you might already be salivating. In fact, if you carefully measured your actual saliva output (rather than perceived output), you might be surprised at how quickly it changed. To what were you measuring salivation—the hamburger or to your thoughts of the hamburger? If you never knew what you were going to eat, but a dinner bell always preceded your meal (and you were hungry), you would automatically begin to salivate.

Pavlov then studied how he could replicate this result. He believed that he could use a stimulus that did not elicit salivation (i.e., a neutral stimulus) and associate it with a stimulus that always elicits salivation (i.e., unconditional stimulus or US). After this association, the previously neutral stimulus would begin to elicit salivation even when the US was absent. In other words, with proper association, the animal would begin to predict the arrival of the US by the mere occurrence of the neutral stimulus. If the neutral stimulus did, in fact, elicit salivation (all by itself) after the association, then it could no longer be called *neutral*. In this case, it had become a *conditional* stimulus. In other words, under some condition it could elicit salivation and the *condition* was the prior association.

Pavlov used a metronome as the neutral stimulus. He verified that it was neutral by observing the animal's salivary response to it clicking sounds. His dogs did not salivate to the metronome. He knew that an unlearned reflex did exist for salivation; if you place food in a dog's mouth, it will salivate. There are no conditions that must be met (other than the health of the dog and its state of hydration)—it is an unconditional reflex. The dog's mother did not have to teach it to salivate to the presence of food. Nature took care of that response.

Next, he began to pair the metronome and the food. First he started the clicking metronome and then he gave the food. The dogs salivated—food was in the mix. Was something else also happening? Was some sort of internal or neural association being created? He would soon find out. After repeated pairing of the clicks and the food, he changed the routine. He started the clicks, but did not immediately produce the food. The last time he had done this, the clicks produce nothing other than mild interest (i.e., the orienting response). However, this time the animal salivated.

There was not food around, just the clicking metronome. Since the metronome now could produce salivation, it could not be *neutral* to salivation. Instead, he referred to the clicks (if the cause salivation) now as *conditional stimuli*, or CSs. The salivation that was produced by the clicks only was referred to as a *conditional response*, or CR.

Examine the words *stimulus* and *response*. These are terms that must be used together, because each implies the existence of the other. For example, if I were to tell you that I saw a squirrel respond by jumping in a backward flip, you should be wondering something. Hopefully, you are wondering just what caused such a response—what event *stimulated* it? Conversely, if I state that I honked my car horn at a pedestrian and add, "That sure was a stimulus," you should be wondering about the actions that the car horn caused the pedestrian to exhibit—what was the *response* to that stimulus? Here's why we have to be so careful. If I ask you, "In Pavlov's experiment, salivation was which of the following: NS, US, UR, CS, or CR?" What would you answer? If you are tempted to pick one, you will be potentially wrong. We can presume that salivation is a response (though in odd cases it can also be a stimulus). But how do we know if it is an unconditional or conditional response? We know only by knowing the event that caused it. If food caused it, then salivation is a UR. If the clicks caused it, then salivation is a CR. We cannot know whether a response is learned or instinctive without first knowing the events that primarily caused it.

Can we *unlearn* associations already formed? Pavlov also studied the effects of postassociation exposure to the CS, in the absence of the US. What this means is that he used the clicks of the metronome repeatedly to elicit salivation, but did not allow it to precede the introduction of the food. Eventually, the dogs began to salivate less and less to the clicks, until the clicks caused no further measureable salivary response. At first glance it may it appear that the subsequent presentations of the click (*sans* food) erased the associations formed earlier. However, we need to do only one thing to see a different result: wait. If we put the metronome away for a time but pull it out later and let it click to see the dog's response, we will see that the dog once again salivates. Why? We did not again associate the metronome click and the food.

These results are referred to as *spontaneous recovery* (Hovland, 1937), the reappearance of an extinguished conditioned response following a time lag. Spontaneous recovery of the CR suggests that the association which was formed during acquisition period (i.e., the pairing of the food and sound) was not actually erased during the extinction period (i.e., sound presented by itself). Instead, the CR was suppressed. More specifically, the extinction period only taught the animal that the sound no longer predicted food. It had not erased the prior learning—that is, clicks precede food. When the clicks make their return, the animal retrieves both experiences. Thus, the (anthropomorphized) lesson learned is something like, "Clicks sometime predict food—and sometimes they do not. I will be best served by producing some saliva in case food will show up, but not so much as to waste the fluid if food does not show up. I will hedge my bet."

How is this relevant to human behavior—behavior that seems so voluntary? People who are in romantic relationships that end sometimes experience a common delayed effect. If they are still unattached after a month, they begin thinking about their ex. To do so seems foolish. After all, they left that person for a reason. If you consider spontaneous recovery as an explanatory mechanism (which is arguable), we might understand. During the relationship, there were at least two learning experiences: (1) I really dig this person (early), and (2) I want to leave this person (later). At the end of the relationship, we are responding to the most recent learning experience. After a time lag (that pesky month), we are better able to integrate both experiences into our responses to the stimulus (i.e., the ex). Essentially, associations tend to exert their influence long after they have ceased to be valid, especially strongly formed associations.

Consider This

A person's first experience with police officers involves their coming aggressively into his house to arrest his father. Even if he later has more positive experiences with police officers, how can spontaneous recovery play a role in future interactions?

What are some solutions to minimize the effect of this early negative event?

"Operant" Conditioning

Pavlov's learning theory maintains that the important association to be formed during a learning experience is between two stimuli that occur together closely in time. Other theorists have proposed that these associations need not be between *stimuli*, but instead between specific *behaviors* we might exhibit and *the consequences* for having done them. Edward Thorndike, proposed the **law of effect** (1927), which states that the frequency of a behavior is functionally related to the effects that the behavior has on our environment. If the effects are pleasant, we will engage the behavior more often. If the effects are unpleasant, we will engage the behavior less often. This idea is often referred to as *instrumental conditioning*.

Burrhus Frederic (B.F.) Skinner proposed a refinement of the Law of Effect, in *operant conditioning*. He identified the types of effects or "contingencies" that a behavior might create as either reinforcing or punishing (or no effect). A contingency is any postbehavior change in the environment, which can be (causally) associated with the behavior, a kind of consequence for having done the behavior. The cause-effect mechanism need not be real, but simply perceived as real. Thus, we engage the behavior and we experience the contingency. If the effect is not neutral, then we will expect the future frequency of the behavior to either increase or decrease. A contingency is considered *reinforcement* if the future frequency of the behavior increases. In this case, the consequence strengthened the behavior—reinforced it. A contingency is considered *punishment* if the future frequency of the behavior decreases. In fact, a contingency can *only* be labeled as reinforcement or punishment *after* the effect has been measured. We will see how important this is a bit later.

Contingencies can also be labeled as *positive* or *negative* yielding positive reinforcement, negative reinforcement, positive punishment, and negative punishment. Unfortunately, this latter labeling distinction creates more problems in understanding operant learning that would be hoped. The reason for this confusion is that the words *positive* and *negative* already have a strong semantic value in the English language. We quickly think of the concept *pleasant* when we hear *positive* and *unpleasant* when we hear *negative*—which is not how these terms are used in operant theory. For our uses, positive is really an arithmetic term, meaning something akin to *added*, and *negative* means something like *subtracted* or *removed*.

Let us examine the practical definitions of all four contingencies in very specific language.

1. *Positive reinforcement.* A behavioral contingency that causes an increase in frequency of the preceding (or causally associated) behavior, by adding a contextual article or event.
2. *Negative reinforcement.* A behavioral contingency that causes an increase in frequency of the preceding (or causally associated) behavior, by removing a contextual article or event.
3. *Positive punishment.* A behavioral contingency that causes a decrease in frequency of the preceding (or causally associated) behavior, by adding a contextual article or event.
4. *Negative punishment.* A behavioral contingency that causes a decrease in frequency of the preceding (or causally associated) behavior, by removing a contextual article or event.

Now examine what these mean and the implications of the chosen words. You notice that the same basic sentence is used for each definition, with only two words varied between them. These two words are the key to truly understanding the concepts: "increase versus decrease" and "adding versus removing." Reinforcers always increase the frequency of behavior. Punishers always decrease the frequency of behavior. Positive contingencies are not "nice" contingencies; they simply involve the introduction of some new thing (i.e., added). Negative contingencies are not necessarily "bad"; they simply involve the removal of something that was already there or expected.

Try to answer this question: Is a candy bar a reinforcer or a punisher?

Answer: We don't know (yet). The reason we do not know is that we have not observed or been informed of any change to behavioral frequency. Although we might agree that a candy bar is generally a good thing, this does not mean it is a reinforcer. It is possible (perhaps not likely) that it will cause behavioral frequency to plummet. Furthermore, because we cannot determine the degree to which the receiver likes the candy bar (it is a highly internal and personal experience), we cannot use this goodness to define the consequence. The only thing we can measure reliably is resultant behavior frequency. So we will not know with certainty that the candy bar was a reinforcer until later—guess all you want, but call it a guess or hypothesis.

To complete the definition, we must determine if the effect was for the addition of something or the removal of something. It seems easy in the case, but that is deceiving. We certainly added a new candy bar, so is the contingency positive? At the same time we may have also removed hunger. It can be very difficult to determine the positive or negative aspect of the contingency, but it is fairly straightforward to determine whether it is reinforcing or punishing.

In an episode of *The Big Bang Theory* ("The Gothowitz Deviation" 2009), two characters, Leonard and Sheldon, are discussing the possibility of using operant conditioning principles to shape Leonard's girlfriend's behaviors into more appealing social manners using chocolates as positive reinforcement. Because they seem to be changing the behaviors as expected and seem to be the addition of something, they are correct. However, the writers soon make a common mistake. When the characters disagree on another point, Sheldon sprays Leonard with a bottle and says, "Bad Leonard," hoping to make him stop disagreeing. Sheldon then calls this *negative reinforcement*. Why is this wrong? Why do you think this mistake is so common? (An argument could be made that this would be negative reinforcement *if* the spraying only stopped when Leonard agreed—*and then he continued to agree*).

DUAL-PROCESS THEORY

Dual-process theory mechanisms are usually used in discussions of habituation and sensitization to stimuli. However, the concept can be applied to operant principles as well. A behavior need not create one, and only one, contingency. Rather, a behavior can create a large variety of contingencies. Some of these contingencies may be reinforcing and some may be punishing. Each will exert its effect on the same associated behavior. What we will finally observe is the net result of these various effects. Think about driving with one foot on the accelerator and one on the brake. Your net speed is the combined effect of the force of the brakes compared to the force of accelerator. When observing the speed of the car we might ask, "Why are they moving so slowly?" We may think they are only using the accelerator, but mildly. Knowing that to be false, we can generate two solutions to make the car go faster, lessen the braking force or maximize the acceleration force. Either will change the net speed of the car.

Consider This

Working with victims of ongoing abuse in long-term relationships can be difficult. Therapists may fail to understand why a victim continues to return to a relationship that is so obviously filled with punishment. Can you use dual-process mechanisms in an attempt to explain why people return to abusive relationships?

SCHEDULES OF REINFORCEMENT

Up to this point we have discussed contingencies as though they are always provided after a behavior and then affect the probability of the next occurrence. This is what is often referred to as a *continuous reinforcement schedule*, or CRF. However, this may not be the most effective way to deliver contingencies for several reasons. First, it can become time consuming and expensive. To use a CRF schedule you must actually be watching each behavior and you must have a reinforcing event ready to provide. Second, the CRF may actually decrease the reinforcing value of your contingency through satiation. Finally, the CRF schedule may actually slow the frequency of the behavior if the receiver must spend time to consume it.

The *partial reinforcement effect* or PRE (Crum, Brown, & Bitterman, 1951) describes that behavioral probability may increase when the amount of reinforcement is reduced by the use of a reinforcement *schedule*. Schedules of reinforcement may be described as placing the reinforcement on either a *fixed* rate of reinforcement or a *variable* rate of reinforcement; and as placing the reinforcement either on a *ratio* (e.g., number of behaviors per reinforcement) or an *interval* (e.g., reinforcement made available after a period of time has passed since the last reinforcement).

Fixed ratio schedules are those that allocate a specific amount of reinforcement to be delivered precisely after a specific number of behaviors has been performed. These schedules are often abbreviated FR. Following the FR will be the value of the ratio (e.g., 3 behaviors to 1 reinforcement or 3:1). Because the normal convention is to count behaviors for each reinforcement, the one can be omitted. In this case the schedule would be labeled as FR(3). The CRF schedules we mentioned earlier can also be labeled FR(1). *Variable ratio* schedules are similar to fixed ratio, except that the number of behaviors needed to receive the reinforcement varies around an average, or mean. Thus, a variable ratio schedule in which reinforcement is provided about every 20th behavior would be labeled VR(20). If you are thinking about measures of central tendency, you may notice that VR schedules provide two ways to alter the delivery of reinforcement; through changes of the mean number of behaviors and through changes to the variance, or standard deviation.

🔊 Consider This

If you are given one dime for each time you tap a button, but you receive that reinforcement on an FR(1) schedule, what impact would the schedule have on how long it takes to tap the button 100 times and earn 10 dollars? Now change to a fixed ratio schedule of FR(10), but keep the per tap reinforcement the same. This means reinforcement will be provided at the rate of one dollar for 10 taps. What effect does this have on the rate of tapping? (By the way, we can even decrease the per tap value, but the rate will still increase.)

Fixed interval schedules are those in which reinforcement is provided only after a time interval has elapsed and the behavior is displayed. In other words, the reinforcement is unavailable until the interval has elapsed. At that point the contingency is *available* but not delivered until the behavior is completed. Fixed interval schedules will be labeled FI, followed by the length of the interval—including unit of time. A fixed interval of 1 hour will be labeled FI(1h). *Variable interval* schedules are similar, but the length of time noted only reflects the average interval length and will be labeled something like VI(1h). Once again variable interval schedules can be changed by altering either the interval length or the standard deviation of the intervals.

Effect of Schedules on Acquisition and Extinction

We already know that a ratio schedule other than FR(1) can increase behavior frequency. However, there is a relationship between rate of acquisition and rate of extinction that must be considered. Ratio schedules, especially those with low ratio values, can help achieve a rapid rate of acquisition (i.e., the behavior is learned quickly). However, these FR schedules can also experience rapid extinction (i.e., the behavior is stopped rapidly after reinforcement stops). Conversely, interval schedules typically experience very low rates of acquisition, but enjoy slow rates of extinction.

Behavioral perseveration (i.e., slow rate of extinction; Crum et al., 1951; Lewis & Duncan, 1956) can be thought of as the result of unpredictability in the delivery of reinforcement. Reinforcement in an FR(1) schedule is very predictable, thus we know accurately when it has ended. However, reinforcement in a VR(100) schedule with a standard deviation of 50 is fairly unpredictable. It is hard to keep track of when we are going to be reinforced. Therefore we will keep displaying the behavior until we are convinced that no reward is coming. Interval schedules can create significant behavioral perseveration, especially if those intervals are long and the standard deviation is high.

Experienced behavior planners working with children know how to utilize many schedules in order to maximize rapid acquisition as well as maximizing perseveration. Although there are many ways to organize a multiple schedule plan, here is one to think about:

- Start with FR(1).
- When the behavior is competently completed, gradually increase the FR *ratio*.
- When the ratio is sufficiently high that its completion is not positively known, move to a VR schedule with a small standard deviation.
- Gradually increase the standard deviation.
- Use the time to complete the average deviation to adjust the schedule to a VI schedule and gradually increase both the length and variance.

 Consider This

Discuss the usage of multiple schedules of reinforcement as a way to increase the prosocial behaviors of children who are having social difficulties. Do not forget to consider the impact of reinforcing behaviors you want to increase, rather than punishing behaviors you want to decrease.

Differential Reinforcement

There is more than one way to affect the frequency of a behavior than by providing direct contingencies. You can cause the decrease in frequency of a behavior, without using punishment and without simply removing reinforcement for the behavior (which may not always be possible anyway). In order to understand this, you have to view the availability of behaviors as finite. We cannot engage in an infinite variety of behaviors, because we do not have infinite time to do them. Furthermore, we are creatures who like to maximize the reinforcement we receive. An *operant baseline* (Burnstein, 1971) is a measurement of the amount of time spent in specific behaviors throughout a specified time period. The **matching law** (Herrnstein, 1961) specifies that the relative rate or frequency of a behavior will match the relative rate of reinforcement. Thus, by looking at the operant baseline we can find the most and least preferred behavior and infer how much reinforcement is available for each.

In addition, the graphic depiction of the data allows an interesting analysis. If you provided additional reinforcement for one "slice" of the pie chart, for example, homework, what would happen to the size of the corresponding slice? (Answer: It would grow.) If the time period for these behaviors is finite, what would necessarily happen to the other slices? (Answer: They would have to shrink.) Finally, if we provided collectively a bit more reinforcement for each of the behaviors we prefer, we would expect those left alone to shrink even more rapidly. Eventually, the growing slices might be able to force out the others. Thus, we have decreased the frequency of an unwanted behavior without resorting to direct punishment of it. This procedure is called *Differential Reinforcement of Other Behavior* (DRO), sometimes referred to as omission training (Uhl & Garcia, 1969).

DRO routines are preferred over direct punishment for several reasons. First, punishment can have a problematic effect on the nature of the relationship between the giver and receiver. Second, if we simply reinforce the unwanted behavior and leave the wanted behaviors alone, we may find that the receivers simply replace that behavior with a similar behavior—and we have to start again. After all, they are already getting the "right" amount of reinforcement from the wanted behaviors—and there was some kind of reinforcement available for the problem behaviors. If we have instead maximized the *wanted* behaviors they will have increased in frequency. Thus, the missing problem behavior does not leave a hole to be filled.

A related procedure, *Differential Reinforcement of Alternate Behavior* (DRA), uses the same basic reinforcement principles, but instead relies on providing reinforcement for a specific behavior, which, when done, prevents the unwanted behavior. If your children have behavioral problems at bedtime, such as whining and arguing, you can positively punish those behaviors if you wish, but think about the problems we have discussed. Instead, you can begin to reinforce appropriate bedtime behaviors. They cannot do both. In using DRA, you get to use two contingencies simultaneously: positive reinforcement for wanted behavior and negative punishment (i.e., no reinforcement) for unwanted behaviors.

Extinction Bursts

One predictable effect of the removal of reinforcement (i.e., operant extinction) is called an **extinction burst** (Ratner, 1956). When a behavior has been reinforced (remember that every behavior that exists has been reinforced to some extent), the removal of the reinforcing contingencies can cause a temporary *increase* in the frequency of the behavior. At first, this may sound counterintuitive: You remove the reinforcer (which supposedly increases the behavior) and the behavior frequency increases even more. How can this be?

Extinction bursts are believed to be related to temporary frustration experienced when a behavior, which predictably receives a reward, suddenly fails to work properly.

For example, watch people respond to a computer that stops responding to their input. At first, there may be a simple repetition of the behavior. However, for many people that simple repetition will soon be followed by a more aggressive tapping (dare I say pounding) on the keyboard. However, this more aggressive pursuit of the anticipated reinforce (i.e., the functioning computer) is usually short lived. The frustration may be palpable. If the anticipated reinforcer was going to be very large, the resulting frustration at its loss may be proportionally large. I have heard a roommate yell, beat his keyboard, and threaten to throw a computer out of our window when it froze right after he completed a difficult task (in a role-playing game)—*but before he saved.*

Why is this important in psychology, other than the simple understanding of trends in operant contingencies? Extinction bursts may be the cause of many misunderstandings in the attempts to decrease the frequency of troublesome behavior.

Consider the problem of toddlers or infants who begin screaming or crying at bedtime. The behavior is common and can create tremendous emotional stress for parents. Most parents can properly analyze the cause of the screaming behavior—reinforcement for returning to the room when the child cries. These parents may create their own behavior change plan, which primarily includes no longer going to the room after the bedtime rituals are complete. They may have even visited a counselor who advised this plan. However, failing to properly prepare for extinction bursts can problematic. What will we expect to happen when the parents stop coming in because the child is crying (knowing what we know about extinction bursts)? Correct! We expect the cries to intensify, to become louder, or to become even more insistent and demanding. If this has not been considered, parents may misinterpret the burst.

As the screams of a child experiencing an extinction burst grow, they may completely change in nature. Parents may think, "Oh, I wonder if she has hurt herself," or "There's something really wrong in there." At the same time, the screams are particularly aversive to the parents. They are used to being able to do something that quieted the aversion—going into the room. This effectively negatively reinforced the *parents* for engaging the behavior, which reinforces the child's screams. The bidirectional reinforcement becomes a kind of armed truce.

Child: I'll stop screaming if you visit me.

Parent: I'll come visit you if you stop screaming.

(Everybody is temporarily relieved.)

If unprepared parents hear the intensified screaming and now come in to soothe the child, they may inadvertently have reinforced *louder* screaming and made the problem worse than it was before the intervention was attempted. Essentially, the child may have just learned, "If help does not arrive as expected, get louder. It will come eventually." I (Fanetti) have seen cases where the parents attempted to utilize ignoring the behavior but failed each time it got worse, resulting in children who were screaming in a near panic state for more than an hour and 30 minutes. If it was a therapist or counselor who failed to prepare the parents for this and had not warned them to wait out the fit, we might even call this *iatrogenic* harm, harm *caused by the doctor*.

Consider This

Discuss the impact of extinction bursts on bullies. What problems might emerge? For what outcomes must people be prepared?

STUDY QUESTIONS

1. Explain the obedience study conducted by Stanley Milgram, including the factors that he believed generated the greatest obedience.

2. Explain the conformity study conducted by Solomon Asch, including the factors that he believed generated the greatest conformity.

3. Explain each of the following terms and provide an example of how they might affect the behavior of children in gang-related groups: Groupthink, group polarization, social loafing, diffusion of responsibility, and the bystander effect.

4. Explain the concept of attributions.

5. Explain the study conducted by Haney, Banks, and Zimbardo (1973) and how it might have been somewhat predictive of the Abu Ghraib incident.

6. What is the difference between prejudice and discrimination?

7. Explain the differences between Pavlovian classical conditioning and Skinnerian operant conditioning.

8. Define: positive reinforcement, negative reinforcement, positive punishment, and negative punishment.

9. How can the dual-process concept help to explain complex responses to operant contingencies?

10. What is the matching law? How might it help to understand available reinforcement?

11. What is differential reinforcement and how can it help to reduce reliance on punishment?

12. What is an extinction burst and why does it cause the failure of some behavior programs?

GLOSSARY

attribution theory The tendency to seek causal explanations for others' behaviors (and our own), when that behavior is salient in some fashion.

behavioral psychology The use of learning theory, including Pavlovian and operant conditioning, to explain behavior.

bystander effect Like diffusion of responsibility, the tendency to be less likely to offer aid in social situations where others are present.

classical conditioning Learning that occurs due to the association of two stimuli that co-occur closely in time.

conformity The tendency to behave in a way that is consistent with others in a social comparison, even if endorsing details viewed as incorrect.

diffusion of responsibility The tendency to view personal responsibility for responding to a situation as decreased by the presence of other observers.

extinction burst A rapid, but brief, increase in behavior, which predictably follows the termination of reinforcement for the behavior.

fundamental attribution error In attributions, the overestimate of the impact of internal variables for behavior of others that we are observing, as well as external variables for our own behavior.

group polarization The tendency for more extreme and less varied opinions to emerge after group discussions in which the group was already in basic agreement about a topic.

groupthink Setting aside one's personal values in favor of those espoused by a larger group. Allowing the group opinion to direct personal behavior, even when the two beliefs are in conflict.

law of effect Behaviors will increase or decrease in frequency based on the nature of the effect of the behavior on a organism's environment.

matching law The relative frequency of behaviors will match the relative reinforcement available for those behaviors.

obedience The tendency to follow directive commands, even when they are inconsistent with personal beliefs.

operant conditioning Learning that occurs because certain behaviors are followed by important consequences or contingencies.

social loafing The tendency to exert less effort on a shared goal when others are participating cooperatively.

social psychology The study of individual behavior when in social situations.

REFERENCES

Burnstein, D. (1971). Development of a conditioned reinforcer. *Psychological Reports, 29*(3), 1170.

Crum, J., Brown, W., & Bitterman, M. (1951). The effect of partial and delayed reinforcement on resistance to extinction. *American Journal of Psychology, 64,* 228–237.

Darley, J., & Latane, B. (1968). Bystander intervention in emergencies: Diffusion of responsibility. *Journal of Personality and Social Psychology, 8*(4), 377–383.

Fischer, P., Krueger, J., Greitemeyer, T., Vogrincic, C., Kastenmüller, A., Frey, D., ... Kainbacher, M. (2011). The bystander-effect: A meta-analytic review on bystander intervention in dangerous and non-dangerous emergencies. *Psychological Bulletin, 137*(4), 517–537.

The Gothowitz Deviation. (2009, October 5). *The Big Bang Theory,* [Television series].

Haney, C., Banks, C., & Zimbardo, P. (1973). Interpersonal dynamics in a simulated prison. *International Journal of Criminology and Penology, 1*(1), 69–97.

Henderson, R. (1985). Fearful memories: The motivational significance of forgetting. In F. R. Brush & J. B. Overmier (Eds.), *Affect, conditioning and cognition: Essays on the determinants of behavior* (pp. 43–53). Hillsdale, NJ: Erlbaum.

Herrnstein, R. (1961). Relative and absolute strength of response as a function of frequency of reinforcement. *Journal of the Experimental Analysis of Behavior, 4,* 267–272.

Hovland, C. (1937). The generalization of conditioned responses. III. Extinction, spontaneous recovery, and disinhibition of conditioned and of generalized responses. *Journal of Experimental Psychology, 21*(1), 47–62.

Ingham, A., Levinger, G., Graves, J., & Peckham, V. (1974). The Ringelmann effect: Studies of group size and group performance. *Journal of Experimental Social Psychology, 10,* 371–384.

Jones, E., & Harris, V. (1967). The attribution of attitudes. *Journal of Experimental Social Psychology, 3*(1), 1–24.

Kravitz, D., & Martin, B. (1986). Ringelmann rediscovered: The original article. *Journal of Personality and Social Psychology, 50*(5), 936–941.

Lewis, D., & Duncan, C. (1956). The effect of partial reinforcement and length of acquisition-series upon resistance to extinction of a motor and a verbal response. *American Journal of Psychology, 69,* 644–646.

Moscovici, S., Zavalloni, M., & Louis-Guerin, C. (1972). Studies on polarizations of judgments. *European Journal of Social Psychology, 2*(1), 87–91.

Park, B., & Rothbart, M. (1982). Perception of out-group homogeneity and levels of social categorization: Memory for the subordinate attributes of in-group and out-group members. *Journal of Personality and Social Psychology, 42*(6), 1051–1068.

Ratner, S. (1956). Effect of extinction of dipper-approaching on subsequent extinction of bar-pressing and dipper-approaching. *Journal of Comparative and Physiological Psychology, 49*(6), 576–581.

Ringelmann, M. (1913). Recherches sur les moteurs animes: Travail de l'homme [Research on animate sources of power: The work of man]. *Annales de l'Institut National Agronomique, 2*(12), 1–40.

Sicoly, F., & Ross, M. (1977). Facilitation of ego-biased attributions by means of self-serving observer feedback. *Journal of Personality and Social Psychology, 35*(10), 734–741.

Thorndike, E. (1927). The law of effect. *American Journal of Psychology, 39*, 212–222.

Uchiyama, A., & Hoshino, K. (1993). A study on the conformity of Boryokudan members to the Boryokudan subculture. *Reports of the National Research Institute of Police Science, 34*(2), 113–121.

Uhl, C., & Garcia, E. (1969). Comparison of omission with extinction in response elimination in rats. *Journal of Comparative and Physiological Psychology, 69*(3), 554–562.

CHAPTER

3

───────◆◆◆───────

Understanding Psychopathology
and Disruptive Behavior

GOALS OF THIS CHAPTER:

1. To understand the concept of psychopathology.
2. To understand the developmental influences on psychopathology.
3. To understand disruptive behavior disorders.

WHAT IS A PSYCHOLOGICAL DISORDER?

Throughout history humans have attempted to understand the causes of behaviors that seem to be unusual or dysfunctional. Humans seem to have both an ability to allow a wide variety of responses to any one event (without assuming something is "wrong") and to identify when behavior becomes worrisome. We give others space to behave in normal, predictable ways or even in odd and unpredictable ways. But there is also a limit, a line that people or societies may draw to differentiate the range of normal behavior from behavior that is substantially *ab*normal.

Greek and Roman medicine sought to understand human behavior from a very biological perspective. The Greek scientist and physician *Hippocrates* (often considered the founder of Western medicine, and the namesake for the Hippocratic Oath) believed that human health was importantly related to the balance of four "humors" in the body: phlegm, yellow bile, black bile, and blood. Imbalances in these liquids would affect not only people's physical health, but also their behavior. Hippocrates also worked to begin a system to classify emotional disorders, using terms still popular today, including *mania*, *melancholia*, and *paranoia*. There is a long and evolving tradition for natural science in the investigation of human behavior.

There is also a long history of looking to the supernatural for causal explanations of unusual behavior. The ancient *Persians* believed that many of the stresses of life could be tied to the actions of demons and *demonism* including two especially important gods, Angro-Mainyus (the malicious actor) and Ahura-Mazda (the benevolent actor). Exceedingly unusual behaviors could be seen as the direct influence of malevolent demons and intervention or treatment could be sought by appeal to Ahura-Mazda. This demonism, however, is not confined to ancient Persia, but also is a part of many more modern religions. Jewish, Christian, and Islamic lore or belief continues to hold that demons exist and exert influence over human life—or even occasionally "possess" certain humans. Although no evidence exists to disconfirm existence of these supernatural beings, dealing with them will remain a clerical or spiritual duty. Sciences such as psychology must attempt to study observable causes of mental distress of dysfunctional behavior.

The fifth edition of the *Diagnostic and Statistical Manual of Mental Disorders* (DSM-5; American Psychiatric Association [APA], 2013) defines a mental disorder as a pattern of behavior that affects a person's ability to be successful in social, occupational, or other environments and causes distress. A mental disorder is often reflective of a difficulty in regulating emotions, thoughts, or behaviors caused by problems in psychological, biological, or developmental functioning. Behaviors, even dysfunctional behaviors, that are part of a normal response to significant stressors or are only viewed as deviant from society, but create no other major distress or dysfunction are not disorders (APA, 2013, p. 20).

What this definition means is that, according to the *DSM-5*, a pattern of behavior must have certain characteristics in order for it to be identified as "disordered." Generally, all three must be present to qualify as a mental disorder. Specifically, they are:

1. *Abnormality*. One basic idea of psychopathology is that the disorder is somehow different from the norm, that the behaviors represent some deviance from "normal" behaviors. After all, what would it mean to label a set of behaviors as a mental disorder when they represent behaviors exhibited by *most* children? But even common behaviors can be dysfunctional or distressing. Some classes in university psychology departments are entitled "Abnormal Psychology." Is this all we are looking for—behavior that is not normal—or is there something else involved in the classification of mental disorders? Students in those classes will soon learn that abnormality is only part of the picture, and perhaps not even the most important part.

2. *Distress*. If behaviors cause no distress to the child, to the child's caregivers, nor to the child's important environments, it might be inappropriate to diagnose the child with a mental disorder. Furthermore, distress (in and of itself) caused by one's own behavior is

not sufficient to qualify the behavior as disordered. Many common and necessary behaviors are also distressing. However, behaviors that cause chronic distress do add to the difficulties in life and may even contribute to more serious illnesses including physical health. Distress is a subjective, but important, consideration in mental illness.

3. *Adaptive functioning.* Not all behavior is useful. In fact, some might be considered useless. However, some behaviors may actually impede the ability of an individual to successfully navigate the many challenges of their life. Drinking alcohol is not necessarily a problem until the consumption of it becomes great enough to interfere with a person's ability to remain employed, pay bills, maintain interpersonal relationships, or succeed in school. When a behavior begins to decrease one's ability to succeed in important duties, it is considered maladaptive. Childhood aggression and defiance might begin to interfere with learning social and academic skills. In this sense, the aggression begins to decrease the child's ability to learn and succeed in other areas. On the other hand, a child may seem to others to be excitable and even a bit hyperactive. However, if the child remains adaptive, succeeds in school, and maintains good peer friendships, is it important to label the behaviors?

Consider This

Spend some time thinking of behaviors that might meet one or two of the above features of a disorder—but not all three. Think about if, how, and why these behaviors might be addressed by professionals.

In addition to the earlier features of mental disorders, other considerations must be taken, including *alternative explanations* for the behaviors. If a set of behaviors has been found to be significantly abnormal, to cause significant distress, and to impede the adaptive functioning of a child, does this mean that it is appropriate to classify it as a mental disorder? Perhaps. To make this determination, it is also important to consider other possible explanations that are more mundane and not necessarily psychological. Things such as nutrition, biomedical conditions, medications, and sleep problems can result in behavior that is less than adaptive or even that appear to be a part of a mental disorder—especially in children. Before a psychological disorder is diagnosed, it is imperative that these nonpsychological problems be assessed and ruled out. Treating a child for the symptoms of ADHD (attention-deficit/hyperactivity disorder) when they are actually just sleep-deprived can create unnecessary complications, or even mask a serious medical condition such as sleep apnea (i.e., the interruption of respirations during sleep).

Consider This

What are the common signs that someone is sleep deprived? Have you ever been deprived of sleep for more than 24 hours? As the time progressed, how did you feel? How do you think you appeared to others?

Social relevance. Thomas Szasz (1960) suggested that it may be difficult to understand the nature of mental illnesses without a full understanding of the *social circumstances* under which the symptoms of mental illness emerge. For example, some Native American cultures place value on experiences (e.g., visions) that other cultures might consider symptomatic. They are not necessarily considered a problem based only on the sensory or perceptual nature of the experience. In this way, social pressures can create different probabilities that we will perceive or report our experiences in the same way. While working as a psychiatric aide as a young man, I (Fanetti) tried to remember this when dealing with people who were hearing voices. The question for me was not totally focused on the *pathology of hearing voices.* After all, I could not *prove* they were not real (think back to the Chapter 1 discussion of epistemology and the limits of proof). If that was my goal, all I could actually do was determine if anybody *else* was hearing them. Instead, my focus was on whether those voices were causing a functional problem. Were they causing distraction or fear? Were they asking the person to do something problematic? Remember, at no point did we prove that we were able to stop the voices; we were only able to demonstrate they the clients stopped responding to them. Maintaining a humble perspective on my own perspective has helped to differentiate troublesome pathology from nonproblematic experiences that just happened to be different than mine.

If you sat next to a man on the subway and he said (during the course of a conversation), "God just told me you are special to him," what would you think? What would you do? Would you stop the conversation? Would you move? Now answer this: Why or why not?

POTENTIAL CAUSES OF MENTAL DISORDERS

If we remove supernatural causes of mental disorders from our discussion (e.g., demonism, divine intervention or retribution), then we are left only natural causes to explore. This does not rule out the supernatural as possible, only as scientifically unobservable. Natural causes for mental disorders can be boiled down to three broad categories: biological, behavioral (contextual), or cognitive.

Biological Causation

There is a great deal of research to suggest that changes in physiology can have an impact on behavior, beginning with the case of Phineas Gage (Kotowicz, 2007). Gage was a mid-19th-century railroad construction foreman who experienced a serious accident. While handling explosives in preparation to excavate a pass, the material detonated and drove an iron bar through his head and out the top of his cranium, destroying a large part of the left hemisphere of his brain. Though he eventually recovered, friends and family later reported that his behavior had changed and that he was "no longer Gage." Though actual details are sometimes hard to find, the case provided early support for the notion that brain changes and brain damage could have an impact not only on your intellectual and cognitive abilities, but also on your *personality*. This focus on the functioning of the brain in the display of personality has persisted in the medical community.

Parents of children who are going through the biological changes associated with puberty are also quick to identify the ways that their child's behavior has changed. When we suffer injury and pain, become intoxicated, experience hormone level changes, become fatigued, or fail to drink our morning coffee, we *know* our behavior changes. Part of the process of getting to know people is understanding how these things affect ourselves and those around us and beginning to be able to subsequently predict behavioral changes based on their physiological status.

Thus, it is not hard to understand why some professionals focus on physiology and biology to explain and intervene in cases of mental dysfunction. If depression becomes a problem, those who rely on biology will seek to change that biology in some fashion. The wide diversity and availability of pharmaceutical interventions is a good example. Many people can quickly name several medications thought to impact behavioral functioning, including Ritalin and Prozac. Do you know which disorders these drugs are designed to treat?

Cognitive Causation

The word *cognition* is derived from the Latin *cogitere*, which means "to think." Cognitive theories of mental disorders often posit that more than the actual world and more than our own biology, the way we *think about* the world is an important factor in how we respond to it (Beck, 1970). In this way, the first line of intervention should be assessing and then changing thought patterns.

This perspective is not new. In fact, we can find traces of this in the way that ancient Persian physicians sometimes dealt with mental disorders to challenge the thought, or force the client to take the thought to its extreme (ostensibly to demonstrate the irrational nature of the thought). For example, the Persian physician Avicenna is said to have once dealt with a client who believed he was a cow. Viewing this not as a medical problem, but as a thought problem, Avicenna then proceeded to bring the "cow" to a place of slaughter. Shortly after, the client became rational and (reportedly) never had such delusions again. Although included in jest (it is a real story, though unverifiable), it nevertheless illustrates the causative thinking that Avicenna was using. The delusion was not demonic, it was not biological, it was thought-based. An argument can also be made that it was contextual, but we see that later.

The most well-known modern model of cognitive intervention was developed by Aaron Beck (1973). Beck proposed that people become depressed when they develop a pervasive set of negative beliefs about themselves and the world. Essentially, these beliefs begin to add a depressive hue to all things a person experiences, like a depressive lens through which they see the world. As they see the world to be more and more hostile, more and more defeating, they begin to retreat from it. They become depressed.

Internal Belief Systems

Core beliefs. These are our global and rigid beliefs about ourselves. Are we good or bad, attractive or ugly, wanted or unwanted, intelligent or incapable, etc.? These tend to be the products of the way we were raised, how we learned to handle barriers and the actual nature of the world as our context. That is, people who were verbally abused as children, who tend to avoid challenges (and thus successes), and live in a materially or socially impoverished environment tend to have negative views of themselves. It is difficult to change these beliefs as they are based on many years of collected experiences. Even though the experiences may be biased (e.g., we see ourselves as incapable of success even though we give ourselves little chance of success), they tend to carry heavy weight and are viewed as confirmatory. Ultimately, changing negative core beliefs into positive core beliefs is the goal of most cognitive therapies, but this is often a time-consuming enterprise.

Intermediate beliefs/thoughts. Intermediate beliefs are the predictive statements we make about the probabilities of our future experiences. They are based on our core beliefs and tend to set a kind of interpretation in motion that reflects these core beliefs, and it does not matter if the nature of the actual experience is different. One common type of intermediate belief is an if/then statement. *"If I ask that girl out on a date, she will say, 'no,' because I am undesirable."* This kind of self-statement or belief tends to lower the probability of actually engaging in behavior challenges. After all, why would he ask her out if she is only going to say no and prove that you are unlikable? Most of us are not gluttons for punishment.

Automatic thoughts. Automatic thoughts are the immediate statements we make to ourselves upon encountering a challenge, or experiencing a failure or success. They are based on our core beliefs in that they reflect our self-concept. They are often the product of the interpretive biases created by those if/then intermediate thoughts we had earlier.

So if the above man was negative about asking a girl out on a date, what would happen if he did? If she said yes, he may be likely to think (i.e., automatically and to himself), "Well she sure is *charitable*. She must be to say yes to me." If she says no, he may be likely to think, "That's what I thought. I don't blame her. Why would she want to go out with me?" In either case, the man's immediate thoughts tend to support his core beliefs and the predictions made in his intermediate beliefs. Whether he got the date or did not, his automatic thoughts are likely to reflect his core beliefs. Cognitive theorists would say that this individual is likely to be or become depressed over time.

 Consider This

> Discuss the possibility of these types of thoughts in teenagers when they decide if the hard work of academic success is worth the effort. Explore each of the types of thoughts.

Contextual/Behavioral Explanations

As discussed in Chapter 2, contextual explanations for behavior focus on environmental conditions that serve to encourage or support behavior. Children may learn behavior patterns observationally, by watching how parents, teachers, and friends conduct themselves. If this behavior also is followed by sufficient reinforcement, then it will continue. According to operant conditioning theory, any behavior that exists or continues to exist is being reinforced in some fashion (Skinner, 1938; Thorndike, 1913). The goal of the behavioral interventionist is to identify the ways that a behavior is being supported (or not supported) by contingencies and then make changes to the environment or context that support the most appropriate behaviors.

Chapter 2 discussed the processes of operant conditioning in some detail. These principles are thought to impact all living creatures. This means that even if a person is experiencing a serious mental disorder, they are still bound to the Law of Effect. Their behavior is still supported by reinforcers that exist in the environment. Children with autistic disorder may experience a great deal of difficulty with learning and social interaction. There is little doubt that the causes for the disorder are neurological. However, the best interventions remain behavioral and focused on providing sufficient reinforcement to support adaptive behaviors (Lovaas, 1987).

DIAGNOSTIC SYSTEMS AND METHODS

Categorical and dimensional methods. What makes a child's behaviors diagnosable? Perhaps the child's behaviors are just very unusual and rarely seen in normal child development. This is certainly possible and would support the notion that some disorders should be considered as categorically different than other behaviors. In fact, this **categorical** approach is the dominant perspective in most diagnostic labeling systems. These systems attempt to identify the most common behaviors associated with a specific disorder and then group (i.e., categorize) those individuals. Thus, you may hear people discuss *the disorder*, rather than the person. For example, once a person says, "John has ADHD," the term ADHD begins to exert a definitional pressure on John. For conversational purposes, this may be acceptable because it abbreviates the discussion. However, professionals who need to understand or help John will have a much greater need for information than is provided in the label. As we see when we investigate the DSM and ADHD, the label says little about the specific problems John faces, because there are many different patterns of behavior that can each yield a diagnosis of ADHD, and many different severities.

Conversely, many psychologists advocate using a **dimensional** approach to diagnosis. A dimensional approach assumes that behavior can be understood in terms of its probability or frequency. Furthermore, it assumes that the existence of a behavior is not automatically problematic. Instead, problems arise when the behavior becomes too frequent or too severe. Have you ever been working on a task, surrounded by noise, and "heard" someone call your name or ask a question only to be told nobody said anything? Is this a normal experience? No real data exists on how frequently this actually happens, but it is assumed that most people have had the experience. Technically, it might be considered a hallucination (i.e., a sensory or perceptual experience without environmental cause). However, hallucinations only become diagnosable when they are frequent enough and severe enough to cause difficulty in adjustment. One extreme of the quantitative dimension for hallucinations is the observation that they are completely *nonexistent* (i.e., a zero-percent frequency). This is probably rare. The other extreme is that the experience of hallucinations is so severe in terms of frequency or magnitude that they are highly disruptive to everyday functioning. This is also probably rare. Most people will fall somewhere between those two extremes—somewhere along that *dimension*. Many psychologists are primarily interested in a simple assessment of frequency and severity of a hallucination, rather than dichotomous statements about its presence. These frequencies can then be compared to normalized distributions of the same behavior for other children of the same age, to determine if they are more frequent for a particular child.

However, it is difficult to use a dimensional system of diagnosis when behavioral measurements are elusive or when the normalized base rates of behaviors are unavailable. Furthermore, these dimensions do not necessarily preclude the ultimate use of a categorical diagnostic system. However, thinking dimensionally when considering the occurrences of problematic behavior can help any professional to avoid automatically pathologizing a child that would better benefit from a focus on specific behaviors.

THE DSM SYSTEM

The most ubiquitous tool in psychology or psychiatry for psychopathological diagnosis is the *Diagnostic and Statistical Manual of Mental Disorders*, usually abbreviated as the *DSM*. The first *DSM* (*DSM-I*) was published in 1952, followed by revisions in 1968 (*DSM-II*), 1980 (*DSM-III*), 1987 (*DSM-III-R*), and 1994 (*DSM-IV*). A slight set of modifications to the supporting text, but not the diagnostic criteria, yielded the *DSM-IV-TR* in 2000. In 2013, the *DSM-5* was released.

The *DSM* was designed to be a system for aggregating patterns of behavior into diagnostic categories. Most diagnostic categories in the *DSM* are assigned by comparing the symptoms exhibited by an individual to lists of potential symptoms, described by "working group" panels of experts. These experts decide which symptoms are required for each diagnostic category. If the symptoms of the individual match the lists provided by the *DSM*, the diagnosis can be assigned.

Well … almost. Because most (but not all) symptoms are actually expressions of normal behaviors that have become maladaptive in some fashion (e.g., intensity, duration, contextual appropriateness, or distress), the *DSM* usually requires the diagnosing professional to assess the degree to which the behaviors are maladaptive and cause significant distress. That Goth or Punk teenager who lives down the street may seem odd to some people. He or she may engage in behaviors that are outside the norm, like wearing vampire makeup or sporting spiked hair. These teens may also seem more withdrawn than other students, or more ill-tempered and suspicious. However, if they have no problems with social, academic, or occupational functioning that are outside the norm (remember that many young people have trouble learning to adapt in adolescence), if they are not in distress about their own behaviors and are not causing significant distress to others (e.g., thinking that they are strange is not distress), then they can usually *not* be classified as having a psychological disorder. Essentially, we are all allowed to be eccentric without the worry of having others label our behavior in ways that carry legal and social consequences.

DEVELOPMENTAL PATHWAYS

Finality. Another difficulty for understanding the causes of problematic behaviors in childhood stems from the various developmental effects that rearing environments can exert. Cicchetti and Rogosch (2002) describe two different developmental pathways that make causal statements in child psychodiagnosis particularly difficult.

Multifinality. Single events that are thought to be problematic do not always lead predictably to the same outcome. In fact, traumatic events, abusive experiences, and harsh environments can lead to one of many different types of behavioral outcomes. There is not one certain pathway between an event and its outcome.

Equifinality. If multifinality was not enough of a problem, there is more. Equifinality is the idea that similar problematic behaviors do not always arise from a specific causal events. In fact, many different types of problematic events can lead to the same set of behaviors. So we cannot reason backward from a set of behaviors to identify their cause.

VIOLENT AND DISRUPTIVE BEHAVIOR IN CHILDREN

Elliott and Tolan (1998) attempted to provide a categorization of violent behaviors, especially those seen in groups of young people. Though all violence is a concern, their idea was to differentiate the least and most worrisome types of violence.

Situational violence. Situational violence is often reactive. Sometimes people find themselves or place themselves in environments where they encounter threats. Normally they may be calm and peaceful, but in these environments they resort to physicality to respond to perceived threats. Interventions with reactive, situational violence are straightforward: Remove the individuals from the situation and help them better understand the consequences for being in that context. Additionally, help them learn new skills that can defuse, rather than escalate, situations and thus avoid the anger and violent responding.

Relationship violence. Relationship violence is that which arises as a function of long-term relationships. Sometimes nonviolent people remain in interpersonal relationships that they find frustrating and anger-provoking. Difficulty with effective problem solving and communication complicates this problem. Intervention in this type of violence requires either an improvement in the communication between the individuals (so that the frustration subsides enough to prevent violence) or to remove the people from the relationship. However, it may be preferable to improve communication skills in either solution, because new relationships may suffer from the same dysfunction if communication remains troubled.

Predatory violence. Predatory violence is violence used to affect some goal or gain. These goals can be either material (e.g., money or goods) or they can be interpersonal (e.g., to intimidate others into compliance, or bullying). Unlike situational and relationship violence, predatory violence is usually a *planned choice.* That is, it is used as a tool rather than as an automatic reply or response. This planfulness makes this kind of violence particularly worrisome to others, including law enforcement agencies. However, because the violence has a functional goal, then the intervention simply requires an alteration of the effectiveness of the behavior. In other words, if the violence no longer creates the intimidation or the cost of the violence is sufficiently high, then the individual will seek other (hopefully nonviolent) means to affect that goal. Education and skills training are useful tools to help these people learn alternative strategies while also maintaining the high cost of the violence for them.

Psychopathological violence. Psychopathological violence is the most worrisome because it involves violence as a self-rewarding behavior. The pleasure or satisfaction of the violence becomes the goal. It is self-reinforcing. Individuals who engage in psychopathological violence do so because they enjoy the process. It may be that they enjoy the experience of frightening others, or actually harming them. In either case, it will be difficult to intervene in a way that changes this dynamic. Although the predator may use violence as a means to an end, for the psychopath, violence *is* the end.

Consider This

Sometimes youth gangs exhibit violence from all four categories mentioned earlier. Try to imagine and discuss how each of these may emerge in the context of such a gang. Which kind of person is likely to emerge as a gang leader, and why?

Types of Legal Violations

Status violations. Status crimes are those that are illegal only for people of, or without, a certain status. For example, many behaviors are legal only for adults, including drinking alcohol, smoking cigarettes, failing to attend school, or adult sexual entertainment. Any child who voluntarily engages in these activities is committing a status offense. Because they are allowable for some people (e.g., adults) they are often viewed as less serious. Many times the limitation is placed simply for the well-being of the child. Even so, commission of many or repeated status offenses can be an indicator of more serious problems and may eventually lead to more serious types of offenses.

Index violations. Index crimes are those that are illegal for any person. For example, there are no circumstances under which crimes such as vandalism, stealing, assault, rape, or murder are legal. Although there is a range of severity that needs to be considered, index offenses are generally of more concern than status offenses. In the expected progression of conduct problems, those children who have started to commit index offenses are more likely to progress into more serious offenses unless intervention is offered and is effective.

DIMENSIONS OF DISRUPTIVE BEHAVIOR

Externalizing behaviors can be understood when viewed on one of several dimensions of behavior. Each of these dimensions is used to place the behavior in relative comparison to other behaviors.

Delinquent versus aggressive (Achenbach, 1991). For example, the first dimension often used is delinquent versus aggressive behavior. On this dimension, behaviors to one extreme are highly aggressive and are actively encroaching on others' rights. Behaviors existing on the other side of this dimension are called *delinquent*. Delinquent behaviors are those that are somewhat passive and usually involve a failure to meet some obligation. Assault is aggressive, while skipping school is delinquent.

Overt versus covert (Frick et al., 1993). The overt versus covert dimension is used to identify how visible the problem behaviors are. Behaviors such as lying and stealing are more covert. Children engaging in these behaviors are often trying to hide them from others. In contrast, bullying and assault are overt behaviors. Little to no effort may be made to hide these behaviors from others, unless those others are authority figures with the power to intervene.

Destructive versus nondestructive (Frick et al., 1993). Another acknowledged dimension of conduct disordered behavior involves the amount of damage the behavior creates. Although the damage does have to be real (e.g., vandalizing a building), it does not have to be material. For example, spreading rumors about another person to cause them social harm or damage can be considered a destructive behavior.

Though children's behaviors often start with those that are delinquent, covert, and nondestructive, it can be expected that they will gradually become more overt, aggressive, and destructive if intervention does not happen. How far and for how long they are allowed to progress into these more serious behaviors is indicative of prognosis.

PATTERSON'S EARLY STARTER MODEL

Many children exhibit some conduct problems during adolescence. Many children also stop those behaviors when they become an adult. Sometimes intervention is necessary, but often the cessation of these behaviors seems almost spontaneous. On the other hand, some children will continue to display these problem behaviors well into their adulthood, perhaps even escalating the severity of their behaviors. Recovery may be unlikely for some and require significant intervention for others.

Gerald Patterson, Capaldi, and Bank (1980) attempted to determine if there was a way to differentiate these generally difficult or persistent cases from the less worrisome cases. This determination can be made *post hoc* (i.e., after the conclusion) but that offers little insight into how to help children before they have traveled too far down the road to ruin.

Patterson et al. (1980) were able to determine and empirically demonstrate that many of these cases can be differentiated based on when the earliest signs of trouble began to be noticed. They were able to show that some children only began to display serious conduct problem during adolescence. They were often noted to have had normal early childhoods, normal academic experiences, and fewer difficulties in family life. They also typically had a better prognosis and tended to limit their problem behaviors to less catastrophic varieties, often staying with more serious status offenses and avoiding more serious index offenses.

On the other hand some children began having conduct problems very early, sometimes in early elementary school or even earlier. In their histories was more indication of conflict, family discord, and academic difficulty. These *early starters* were more likely to commit more serious offenses and were also more likely to continue having trouble into adulthood.

Interventions With Patterson's Model

Behaviorists believe that nearly every behavior can be understood in terms of the environmental context in which it occurs. In this case, the reinforcers for behavior are relevant. The idea is that making sure that a child's choices are guided by reinforcers (or punishers) that are effective is useful. If we know the benefits and costs of our choices and those attributes are well known, then behavior should conform to that plan. Perhaps we can just create a more structured and predictable environment. Well, it turns out that this is fairly effective with late starters, but less effective with early starters. On reflection, the reasons may be easy to understand.

Late starters often have a childhood in which they were successful at acquiring and using skills: social skills, family skills, and academic skills. However, when they arrived at adolescence, the consequences that support the use of those skills changed and began to support more problematic behaviors. Consequently, if we effectively alter the environment to once again support positive skills and behaviors, then the child should have the abilities needed to exhibit those behaviors and change is more likely.

Those early starters may not be so easy. During their more tumultuous childhood, they may not have acquired those skills or developed any proficiency with them. It is difficult to develop academic skill when much of your time is spent in the principal's office or in the hallway. It is hard to develop positive social skills when your family has relied on coercive behavior and you have relied on coercive behaviors to deal with your peers. So, simply changing consequences will not work. If you told a person who has never seen an engine, "I'll give you $1,000 if you replace this engine," would you expect them to be able to do it? Probably not. They do not know how. In order for that car repair to happen, we will need to offer both an incentive (e.g., the money), but we will also need to teach them how to do it (e.g., the steps of the skill). This is how to view intervention with early starters. It will require a careful examination of the contingencies in the child's life, as would an intervention with a late starter. But in addition, the early starters will need various skills training. They will need to learn how to study, how to withhold angry responses, how to resist illegal behaviors, how to understand other people's perspectives, and so on. This is a much more complex task. Professionals who are first learning about a child who is engaging in illegal or conduct disordered behaviors will often find valuable information in determining when these things started, using that information to assess the contextual environment as well as the child's knowledge and usage of social and academic skills. This assessment offers the best opportunity to help both groups.

RISK AND RESILIENCE

Why is it that some children emerge from impoverished and difficult childhoods to become productive and well-adjusted adults, while other children from the same environments do not? We can even imagine two neighbors, both with similar family financial status and both with similar family supervision. These neighbors go to the same schools and graduate at the same time. In every externally observable way they led similar lives. However, one goes on to higher education and one becomes a prison inmate.

All of those externally observable barriers are known as *risk factors*. Risk factors are general variables that are known to be associated with poor outcomes. For example, low socioeconomic status (i.e., SES) is known to be associated with a host of problematic outcomes that range from health problems to legal problems. We may sometimes be tempted to believe that the risk factor is the problem. After all, if we can eliminate poverty, would we not also eliminate the host of associated problems? Eliminating risk factors is either a hugely difficult endeavor or it is impossible. Instead, some researchers suggest that we look not at the risk factors (though efforts to reduce poverty remain worthy), but we instead examine the factors that produce positive outcomes—*even when risk factors are present*. In the earlier example about neighbors, we can look at the effects of risk factors on the boy who went to prison or we can try to determine why the other boy was able to rise above the risk.

Michael Rutter (1987) suggested that instead of examining risk with a singular focus, health professionals should examine the experiences that either make the risk produce negative outcomes or the factors that shield us from the risk to produce positive outcomes. *In other words, why do good things happen in bad places?* If we can figure this out, then perhaps we can repeat the process. For Rutter, there are at least four important concepts which can help us to understand why some do better and some do worse: risk, resilience, protective factors, and vulnerability mechanisms.

Risk is the presence of problematic environmental, personal, or inter-personal experiences. Risk is known to be associated with poor outcome. **Resilience** is the experience of positive outcomes, in spite of the presence of risk factors. It does not explain why the individual experienced the positive outcome—just that he or she did. *Protective factors* are those experiences that appear to increase resistance to risk and provide for resilient outcomes. For example, parents who insist on effort in school work may provide for their children a mechanism by which they can escape poverty in the future. *Vulnerability mechanisms* are those experiences that tend to increase the power of the risk factors. For example, children who endure impoverished environments may also be burdened with parents who are addicted to alcohol or other substances. This addiction may cause a greater void in parental supervision or may increase the probability of the extra burden of abuse. In addition to the barriers presented by the primary risk factor, vulnerability mechanisms make resilience less likely.

ECOLOGICAL SYSTEMS THEORY

Why is it that some children can seem to follow the rules while in school or while at their family home, but exhibit more problematic behavior when away from those environments with their friends and peers? Most parents, professionals, and adults already understand that the rules seem (to these children) to be different in each environment. Behavior that is acceptable in the family environment may be not be appreciated by peers, when the peers are away from family and school. For example, children quickly learn how to use slang or foul language when with peers, but refrain from its use at home or school. Then how do we change problematic behavior, if it will be supported in a different environment as soon as the child leaves the therapeutic environment?

For Urie Bronfenbrenner (1986), the answer first lies in the way that we understand the influences that are being exerted in each environment. Bronfenbrenner developed the Family Ecological Systems theory to explain the divergent patterns of support that exist in different aspects of a child's life. In this theory we must first understand the concept of systems and how they operate together and independently, before we can apply an appropriate style of intervention for disruptive behaviors.

A **system** is an environment in which the rules for behavior are defined by a single context, such as the family system, the school system, or the peer system. In each of these systems, an individual comes to understand which behaviors will be supported and which will not be supported. Their behaviors begin to conform to the rules set up by the players in that environment. This can be referred to as a microsystem, as it is often the most basic level system.

These systems are not usually completely independent, especially in young childhood. Children of preschool age rarely have friends with whom they interact when their parents are not present. Therefore, for them the peer system and family systems are highly overlapping. Furthermore, when children do first attend kindergarten, parents are often communicative with the teacher and somewhat involved in the child's education. In addition, while a child's peer group may expand during this time, it remains highly overlapping with both the family system (e.g., parents attend other children's birthday parties) and the school system (e.g., elementary school teachers are almost always monitoring children during the day). This overlapping of systems in which the rules for two or three systems comingle are called *mesosystems*.

Other systems also affect a child's life and behavior. *Exosystems* are those systems that affect the major rule setters in a microsystem but are not always observable to the child. Parents' bad days at work may affect the way they support certain behaviors at home. Although the child may not be privy to this bad day for the parent, they indirectly feel the effects of it. For the child, the parent's external experiences create an exosystem.

Macrosystems are those that surround and set the stage for all other systems for the child. Macrosystems can be things such as culture, community, and poverty. These systems have a general effect on other systems. Alterations to culture or community (e.g., the rapid changes created by the terrorist attacks in New York City in 2001) can significantly change the behaviors that are deemed appropriate or inappropriate.

Changes in Systems as Children Mature

As discussed earlier, the mesosystem status of young children tends to be highly overlapping. As children develop, these systems may begin to pull apart and separate. As children age, they may be given more opportunity to play with friends without direct supervision. As that happens, there may be more "pure" peer system influence. Consider the young teenager who first attends high school. Here there is less teacher supervision (e.g., teens tend to be responsible for getting themselves to classes) and more independent peer interaction. Adults are not listening all that closely to the conversations occurring in the hallways. After school, there are more opportunities to interact with peers outside of school and home (e.g., an afternoon at the mall). As children mature, they spend more time with their peers and in more environments with less oversight by parents and teachers. Overall, the peer system begins to grow in *size* and *independence*—and thus influence. If this peer system is functional and reasonable then the influence is not problematic. However, when this peer system includes dysfunctional peer group members, the newly found power of the peer system may begin to exert greater influence or carry over into the child's general behavioral dispositions. Normally, this growing independence is a healthy part of development.

Figures 3.1 to 3.3 illustrate the relative size and overlap of the three major microsystems in a child's life during three distinct developmental periods. Figure 3.1 emphasizes the kindergarten period. During this period, the family system remains most influential, but the school system gains considerable influence. The peer system exists (usually) completely within the family and/or school systems. That is, interactions with friends are normally also observed and guided by parents and/or teachers. Rare is the opportunity for children to interact completely outside of the observations of adults.

Figure 3.2 represents possible systemic balances as children develop through elementary school. Family and school systems remain influential, but the child may build a

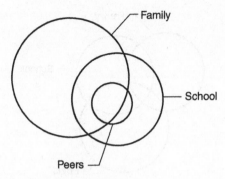

Figure 3.1 The Child's Systems During Kindergarten

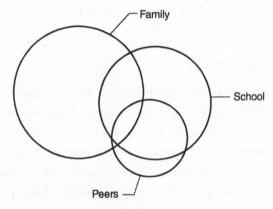

Figure 3.2 The Child's Systems During Elementary School

larger network of peers. In addition, they may be able to interact with these peers more frequently outside of the observations of adults. On the playground, teachers may not be hovering and may only observe from afar. At home, parents may be more willing to let children play by themselves outside or otherwise away from direct supervision. This newly growing peer group, which is also gaining some independence, may begin to exert greater influence on the child's behavior. Here they begin to learn words they did not learn at home or school and may pick up mannerisms from friends.

Figure 3.3 represents a possible balance of systems for a child during high school. Notice that the power of the peer system has grown in comparison to the family and school systems. It has also gained considerable independence. Now children spend a good deal of time with peers and not within observation of parent and teachers. In some cases, this peer group may become more influential than the family or school system. At this point, parental or school influence becomes difficult. In essence, these systems may no longer be capable of exerting enough influence to overcome the power of the peer system. If the peer system is working in ways that are at odds with the goals of the

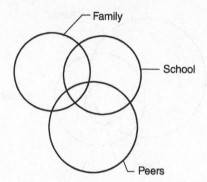

Figure 3.3 The Child's Systems During High School

family system or school system, then parents and teachers may experience frustration as their influence wanes.

Multisystemic Therapy (MST)

Multisystemic therapy (MST) is a multifaceted form of intervention for children who are at risk in several systems and have become disruptive or violent. Of primary importance in this therapy approach is Bronfenbrenner's conceptualizations of systemic interdependence. Primarily, MST requires one therapist to enter into each of the primary systems of the child and help to create a similar set of rules and skills in each system. Specifically, the therapist will engage in family therapy to help ensure that the child's parents are able to provide stability, and can help to model and support the appropriate behaviors. Additionally, the therapist will also work with the child's school environment to help teachers and administrators understand how to help the child stay in the social school environment and succeed in both behavioral disposition as well as academic competence. Finally, the peer system remains. If the peer system continues to support problematic behaviors, then it will work against the progress that is possible in the other systems. Therefore, it becomes necessary (especially when the children's behaviors are serious and illegal) to restructure the children's peer environment, to change their peers. MST often accomplishes this through the use of after-school centers monitored by staff members who also serve as tutors and social skills trainers.

In this way, MST has been effective at reducing *recidivism*, the tendency to reoffend after intervention, even in more violent youth offenders (Henggeler, 2011; Klietz, Borduin, & Schaeffer, 2010; Sawyer & Borduin, 2011). However, while formal MST is the most supported intervention for serious and violent offenders, the same principles apply to all children and can be used to understand why some attempts at intervention fail. Therefore, understanding MST and Bronfenbrenner's systems theory are good places to start when conceptualizing any specific case.

Father Flanagan's Girls and Boys Home (i.e., Girls and Boystown USA) in Omaha, Nebraska uses a modified version of this idea (Dowd & Tierney, 2005), which even pre-dates the development of MST. When children are admitted to the facility they stay in homes run by family teachers. These teachers are married and often have children of their own staying in the home. They live at this home permanently. They become the well-trained authorities in the new family system. Additionally, every child attends schools run by the facility. These teachers are trained in the same model of intervention as the family teachers. Finally, the campus is a large facility with more than 500 children. These children range from new admits to experienced attendees who can serve as proxy authorities. The peer environment is supportive, rather than destructive. With three well-designed systems that communicate regularly, Father Flanagan's is the best example of an effective MST or Bronfenbrenner application.

DISORDERS OF INTEREST TO FORENSIC PROFESSIONALS WHO WORK WITH CHILDREN

Attention-Deficit/Hyperactivity Disorder (ADHD)

Children can be energetic, especially when viewed through the lenses of the adult parents. Excitement and anticipation can sometimes be more than a child's self-control can tolerate and the result is behavior that would be excessive for older individuals. Often while walking with my 6-year-old daughter to the store, she will … prance. She may even sing a song while hopping along and holding my hand. Nobody even gives a second glance. It is normal. It is cute. However, when Dad decides to play along and we both skip along the sidewalk, people look. I suspect nobody wants to see a 45-year-old man skipping—though I get enough leeway when I'm with my daughter. (I have not yet tried it without her.) Most adults look at such displays as unusual, because it requires so much energy. It is fine for kids who have bundles of energy, but strange for adults who are assumed to have less.

However, there is some limit to the allowable excessive behavior of children that people will tolerate. In fact, Western society has been attempting to understand the difference between youthful exuberance and dysfunctional overactivity for many decades, or even millennia. The genesis of the diagnostic category we now refer to as attention-deficit/hyperactivity disorder, ADHD, can be found in research dating to the early part of the 20th century. In 1902, George Still described overactive behaviors found in children as the result of low "inhibitory volition," suggesting that they suffered from a lack of ability to voluntarily stop themselves from acting out. Furthermore, and as a reflection of the late Victorian culture, he also described the behaviors as reflecting "defective moral control." Victorianism often combined the concepts of inhibition and morality, thus conflating immorality or amorality with excessive behavior.

A series of encephalitis epidemics in the late 1910s began to lead researchers toward a more biological explanation of hyperactive behavior. These children, who had suffered objective brain injury as a result of encephalitis or other traumas, often exhibited behaviors such as hyperactivity, impulsivity, and an irritable interactional style. Within two decades researchers began to believe that children with these behaviors, but no obvious source of brain trauma, must nevertheless also be suffering from neurological brain damage. This led to the introduction of the label *minimal brain dysfunction* (MBD) as a way to categorize children with hyperactive and impulsive symptoms, but no obvious cause (Strauss & Lehtinen, 1947).

In the 1970s, researchers began to suggest that hyperactivity and impulsivity were not the only symptoms related to each other in overactive children, but that inattention was also a part of the mix (Douglas, 1972), which led to the "dual symptom" categories of ADHD that we use today. At the same time, a theory was developing that the cause for these symptoms, while still brain-related, was in fact systemic autonomic underarousal. The resultant behaviors were a direct result of the brain attempting to correct for this by autostimulating. In the same way that others can become agitated, fidgety, and inattentive when we are very fatigued, it was thought that children with hyperactive and inattentive symptoms in fact needed stimulating intervention. Early work with stimulants including *Ritalin* ensued (Sykes & Douglas, 1972).

The most modern (biological) ideas about the causes of ADHD do not focus on autonomic stimulation, but rather on prefrontal cortical stimulation (Barkley, 1996). It is thought that the prefrontal cortex (i.e., the area of your brain roughly in your forehead) is responsible for inhibiting behaviors momentarily as we apply memory and planning. This is called *executive function*. Without this ability, we are often left to react impulsively with responses that are automatically reinforcing, but carry long-term disadvantages. It becomes difficult to screen out novel or interesting stimuli and makes it difficult to concentrate on more difficult tasks, such as listening to lectures or reading a textbook. Interestingly, stimulant medications are also thought to work by increasing neural activity in the brain, but the presumed primary locus of that effect has simply moved.

The diagnostic criteria for ADHD (APA, 2013) describe two primary types of symptoms that are important to diagnosis: symptoms of inattention and symptoms of hyperactivity/impulsivity (p. 59). An example of one of the nine potential symptoms of *inattention* is, "Often has difficulty sustaining attention in tasks or play activities" (p. 59). Eight of the nine symptoms are quantified by the word *often*. The goal is to identify children who seem to have more trouble than other children in focusing on tasks that are difficult or nonrewarding.

Hyperactivity and impulsivity is characterized by children's difficulty in regulating their behavioral responses at appropriate levels or a difficulty in inhibiting responses to situations in which the response might be viewed as inappropriate. An example of a symptom of hyperactivity in the DSM (2013) is, "Often talks excessively" (p. 60). Again, all nine of the DSM symptoms of hyperactivity or impulsivity are quantified using the word *often*.

The DSM also provides for a specification of whether the child's symptoms are mostly from one category (i.e., "predominantly hyperactive/impulsive" or "predominantly inattentive," p. 60) or are more evenly distributed across the categories (i.e., "combined," p. 60).

Criticisms of the ADHD category include the difficulty in implementing the word *often* in normal practice to differentiate problematic childhood behaviors from those that are a part of the spectrum of normal child behaviors. In essence: What is "often"? Other criticisms are related to the focus on neurology as the primary facilitator of hyperactive behaviors, which may lead to an undervaluing of environmental factors as causal ingredients or intervention possibilities.

The DSM-5 (2013) organizes other childhood behavior disorders as "disruptive." The first is oppositional defiant disorder, that is, ODD (p. 462). According to the DSM, ODD is characterized by a mood state that is often angry and behaviors that are defiant and confrontational (p. 462). Children with ODD cause disruption in educational and family environments. They may begin to create (or be the product of) hostile environments, which ultimately provide more reinforcement and support for coercive behaviors than cooperative behaviors (Patterson, 2002). If these behaviors begin to generalize to peer relationships and the general community, the child may be at risk for the more serious behaviors associated with conduct disorder.

Conduct Disorder

Conduct disorder (CD) is a serious disorder of childhood and adolescence that typically includes behaviors that violate the rights of others or violated the rules, laws, and expectations of society in such a way as to make community response necessary. Many times these behaviors include forms of violence discussed earlier in this chapter or true index violations (things that are illegal for people of any age). An example of the symptoms reflected in the DSM-5 (2013) criteria include, "Often bullies, threatens, or intimidates others" (p. 468). Although these behaviors also sometimes rely on the quantifier *often*, it might be argued that the behaviors themselves are so much more aggressive and unusual that those of ADHD or ODD that they become easier to identify. A second example that reflects the greater severity of these criteria is, "Has forced someone into sexual activity" (p. 470).

According to Patterson's coercive systems model (Patterson, 2002), these behaviors, if left unchecked, may put the child at risk to continue the disruption into adulthood, and into more serious interactions with society. Some may develop adult antisocial personality disorder (APD), which is characterized impulsive behavior, habitual lying, violating others' rights, and a lack of remorse for transgressions. Prison populations are often heavily populated by adults with diagnosable APD (Hare, 1983). But what differentiates those adolescents at greatest risk for continuing problems from those who are more likely to eventually cease the behavior or respond favorably to intervention? Evidence is not yet clear on the answer to this question.

STUDY QUESTIONS

1. Explain the three features of behavior that usually must be present to diagnose a mental disorder.

2. Explain the differences among the ideas of biological, cognitive, and behavioral causation.

3. In the cognitive model, explain core beliefs, intermediate beliefs, and automatic thoughts.

4. What is the difference between a categorical and a dimensional model of psychopathology?

5. Explain multifinality and equifinality.

6. Describe the four classifications of violence offered by Elliott and Tolan (1998).

7. Describe the three "dimensions" of conduct problems.

8. Explain the concepts of risk, resilience, protective factors, and vulnerability mechanisms.

9. According to Bronfenbrenner, what are systems? Next, explain microsystems, mesosystems, exosystems, and macrosystems.

10. Without memorizing the symptoms, describe the disorders of ADHD, ODD, and CD.

GLOSSARY

abnormality The degree to which a behavior is different from that which is expected by a society or group of people.

adaptive functioning The degree to which a behavior does or does not prevent behavior functioning that allows a person to successfully navigate the necessities of daily life.

behavioral explanations The degree to which learning processes can be used to explain behavior.

biological causation The degree to which biological factors can be used to explain behavior.

categorical models Models used to diagnose mental illness, which rely primarily on group assignment.

cognitive causation The degree to which thought-based processes, especially in humans, can be used to explain behavior.

dimensional models Models used to diagnose mental illness, which rely primarily on the severity, magnitude, or frequency of behaviors compared to norms.

distress The degree to which a behavior causes psychological pain or difficulty to the person or his/her significant others.

early starters/late starters A prognostic indicator for children who are diagnosed with conduct disorder. Early starters tend to have a worse prognosis than late starters.

equifinality Similar problematic behaviors do not always arise from a specific causal events.

multifinality Single events that are thought to be problematic do not always lead predictably to the same outcome.

risk/resilience The idea that some children emerge from difficult environments (risk) with productive healthy lives (resilience).

social relevance The degree to which a behavior is reflective of the motivations and support of a person's social environment.

systems Bronfenbrenners's idea that behavior can be affected by differing factors across situations. For example, children may behave differently when with peers, family, or at school.

REFERENCES

Achenbach, T. (1991). The Child Behavior Checklist and related instruments. In M. Maruish (Ed.), *The use of psychological testing for treatment planning and outcomes assessment* (2nd ed., pp. 429–466). Hillsdale, NJ: Erlbaum.

American Psychiatric Association. (2013). *Diagnostic and statistical manual of mental disorders* (5th ed.). Arlington, VA: American Psychiatric Publishing.

Barkley, R. (1996). Linkages between attention and executive functions. In G. Lyon & N. Krasnegor (Eds.), *Attention, memory, and executive function*. Baltimore, MD: Paul H. Brookes.

Beck, A. (1970). Cognitive therapy: Nature and relation to behavior therapy. *Behavior Therapy*, *1*(2), 184–200.

Beck, A. (1973). *The diagnosis and management of depression*. Oxford, England: University of Pennsylvania Press.

Bronfenbrenner, U. (1986). Ecology of the family as a context for human development: Research perspectives. *Developmental Psychology*, *22*(6), 723–742.

Cicchetti, D., & Rogosch, F. (2002). A developmental psychopathology perspective on adolescence. *Journal of Consulting and Clinical Psychology*, *70*(1), 6–20.

Douglas, V. (1972). Stop, look and listen: The problem of sustained attention and impulse control in hyperactive and normal children. *Canadian Journal of Behavioural Science*, *4*(4), 259–282.

Dowd, T., & Tierney, J. (2005). *Teaching social skills to youth* (2nd ed.). Omaha, NE: Boys Town Press.

Elliott, D., & Tolan, P. (1998). Youth violence prevention, intervention, and social policy: An overview. In D. Flannery & C. Huff (Eds.), *Youth violence: Prevention, intervention, and social policy*. Washington, DC: American Psychiatric Publishing.

Frick, P., Lahey, B., Loeber, R., Tannenbaum, I., Van Horn, Y., Christ, M., … Hanson, K. (1993). Oppositional defiant disorder and conduct disorder: A meta-analytic review of factor analyses and cross-validation in a clinical sample. *Clinical Psychology Review*, *13*, 319–340.

Hare, R. (1983). Diagnosis of antisocial personality disorder in two prison populations. *American Journal of Psychiatry*, *140*(7), 887–890.

Henggeler, S. (2011). Efficacy studies to large-scale transport: The development and validation of multisystemic therapy programs. *Annual Review of Clinical Psychology*, *7*, 351–381.

Klietz, S., Borduin, C., & Schaeffer, C. (2010). Cost–benefit analysis of multisystemic therapy with serious and violent juvenile offenders. *Journal of Family Psychology*, *24*(5), 657–666.

Kotowicz, Z. (2007). The strange case of Phineas Gage. *History of the Human Sciences*, *20*(1), 115–131.

Lovaas, I. (1987). Behavioral treatment and normal educational and intellectual functioning in young autistic children. *Journal of Consulting and Clinical Psychology*, *55*(1), 3–9.

Patterson, G. (1982). *Coercive family practices*. Eugene, OR: Castalia.

Patterson, G. (2002). The early development of coercive family process. In J. Reid & G. Patterson (Eds.), *Antisocial behavior in children and adolescents: A developmental analysis and model for intervention*. Washington, DC: American Psychological Association.

Patterson, G., Capaldi, D., & Bank, L. (1980). An early starter model for predicting delinquency. In D. Pepler & K. Rubin (Eds.), *The development and treatment of childhood aggression* (pp. 139–168). Hillsdale, NJ: Erlbaum.

Rutter, M. (1987). Psychosocial resilience and protective mechanisms. *American Journal of Orthopsychiatry*, *57*(3), 316–331.

Sawyer, A., & Borduin, C. (2011). Effects of multisystemic therapy through midlife: A 21.9-year follow-up to a randomized clinical trial with serious and violent juvenile offenders. *Journal of Consulting and Clinical Psychology*, *79*(5), 643–652.

Skinner, B. F. (1938). *The behavior of organisms: An experimental analysis*. Oxford, England: Appleton-Century.

Strauss, A., & Lehtinen, L. (1947). *Psychopathology and education of the brain-injured child.* Oxford, England: Grune & Stratton.

Sykes, D., & Douglas, V. (1972). The effect of methylphenidate (ritalin) on sustained attention in hyperactive children. *Psychopharmacologia, 25*(3), 262–274.

Szasz, T. (1960). The myth of mental illness. In B. Gentile & B. Miller (Eds.), *Foundations of psychological thought: A history of psychology.* (pp. 113–118). Thousand Oaks, CA: Sage.

Thorndike, E. (1913). Associative learning in man. In E. Thorndike (Ed.), *Educational psychology: The psychology of learning* (pp. 138–152). New York, NY: Teachers College Press.

CHAPTER
4

Memory

GOALS OF THIS CHAPTER:

1. To understand the basic structure and organization of memory.
2. To understand how memory can be accurate or inaccurate.
3. To become familiar with some of the most famous studies of memory.

"No. The kid with the bat came from the back of the truck. I remember it clearly. He jumped out of the truck bed with the bat in his hand and started to run towards us," the witness said in disagreement with his girlfriend. She, however, clearly remembered that the kid who jumped from the back of the truck had *run away* and the *driver* had stepped out with the bat. The problem is common. Two people have differing memories of the same event and both had been equally present when it happened. The man had his memory and it was clear. He could close his eyes and *see* events exactly as he had recalled. His friend remembered something fairly different. She could see her version just as strongly and swore that she was correct. How can this be? One must be correct. One must be wrong.

This mismatching memory experience is common and can sometimes be the foundation of serious arguments. When we can imagine a visual image of our memory, it seems so real. Yet we know that our memories can be wrong because we have been in the position of admitting it. We know that memory can fail us and that memory can convince us of things that are not true. However, memory is also the important glue that binds our lives together. It is what allows us to adapt and learn from past experiences. It must have its strengths as well as weaknesses.

One of the most important fields in forensic psychology is the study of memory. Most crime occurs without being recorded in any way. Rarely is there a security video to capture the details of a child being abused. Even when cameras are available, they do not always capture enough of the context to fully understand what was happening. Quite often witnesses or victims are asked to describe events and this is the only account of the details of a crime. Sometimes they are asked to simply fill in details left unknown by a recording device. In almost every forensic case, people are involved and how they remember their experiences is vital. In cases of child abuse, especially sexual abuse, the children's report of their experiences (i.e., their event memory) is often the most important or only source of information.

For many decades, researchers have been working to better understand what memory is, how memory operates, and how it can be made more or less accurate. As with most knowledge in science memory research is still theoretical, but the theories are becoming more helpful. We are now gaining enough of an understanding of the processes of memory to be able to predict how some events or experiences will alter them. In this chapter, we endeavor to understand what memory is, how it operates, how it is affected by circumstances, and how children's memory abilities compare to those of adults. Though memory research is a large and complex field, important aspects can be learned that will help us to work more effectively with children whose memories are so important.

WHAT IS MEMORY?

Memory is commonly thought of as *our ability to create a mental record of our experiences and then later recall them, or think about them again.* How this happens (i.e., how we are able to create this permanent or semipermanent mental record of our experiences) is still a matter of scientific study and research. We can go back to early Greek philosophers such as Plato to see models of memory being formulated. Plato saw memory as a kind of *wax slate* on which our experiences draw indentations. Over time those waxy indentations fade (or melt) away. Other examples of the same interesting discussions can be found in all cultures and from even earlier eras. You might think that 2,000-plus years of study would yield some finality. Not yet. In fact, the very models we use to describe memory are still in flux.

INFORMATION PROCESSING MODEL

One often-used memory model is known as the *information processing model*. It lists five stages through which information is filtered in order for it to be experienced and then recalled at a later point: sensation, perception, encoding, storage, and retrieval.

Sensation

Sensation is the process by which our physical sensory receptors interact with the environment and produce action potentials (i.e., nerve impulses). The most-strict definitions of sensation require only the formation of these action potentials, not the recognition of them. What this means is that we can sense environmental events on a regular basis without awareness. While we sleep we sense an immense variety of events, though we will never know. A breeze may disturb the air of the room or a gentle rain may tap on our window sill for just a few moments. Our tactile and auditory neurons are active, but we have no awareness. Nor will we have memory of these events.

During recent brain surgery on this author (Fanetti), surgeons monitored auditory sensory activity to a specific clicking sound, but not my recognition of it—I was under general anesthesia. They simply monitored the action potentials moving through these areas of the brain. I did sense the events (as I was later told), but that is all.

Perception

Perception is the process by which our brain organizes some sensory information into meaningful experiences. This meaning can be very simple. When we are walking on a sidewalk, the light reflected off a person who is approaching enters our eyes (sensation). Your brain will analyze the patterns of that reflected light—the colors, shapes, contours, and contrasts—and assign a meaning, such as "person." That can be the limit of perception; the recognition that the patterns of our sensations reflect a unified whole, an object. Perception can also include such information as distance, orientation, and size, but does not usually involve any specific labeling or naming.

Encoding

Encoding is the process by which our brain takes information that has been first sensed and perceived, and assigns a meaningful label—a way to understand what we are experiencing and make predictions about it. This is the first stage at which our human strengths (to make cognitive associations and interpret our experiences) begin to differentiate our abilities from most other animals. Think of this stage as the point at which we name the event or at least classify it as in some way similar to other events.

Storage

Storage is the process by which sensed and perceived (and sometimes encoded) information is represented in our minds for an amount of time without being actively manipulated or considered. Atkinson and Shiffrin (1968; and Shiffrin & Atkinson, 1969) proposed that storage occurs in three stages: sensory memory, short-term memory, and long-term memory. Their idea was that rehearsal (repeating or rethinking an idea) is the primary mechanism by which we make storage more permanent.

Sensory memory is a neurological aftereffect of sensation. After our sensory neurons have fired action potentials, there is a brief moment during which the conductivity of the neuron is reduced. This is called the *refractory period*. If the sensation was visual, the visual field will contain an iconic sensory memory. Try this: Draw a dot in the center of an image of a flag, then stare *at the dot* without looking around for 30 seconds. Next, quickly look at a blank, white page. You will see the reverse afterimage of the flag. Its duration is roughly equivalent to your iconic or visual sensory memory. The activation is a real and measurable effect, though its duration may be very short (i.e., less than a second or two). We normally do not notice any lingering of this effect because we are usually refilling the same sense with new stimuli. However, if we are ill or dehydrated or intoxicated the effect may be noticeable because these neural systems recover from activation more slowly. Sensory memory exists for all five senses.

Short-term memory (STM) is our working memory. It is active whenever you are thinking about something. Furthermore, things that we experience once but stop thinking about may stay in short-term memory for around 20 seconds, as long as you do not then think of something else. However, if you continually repeat the information (i.e., **rehearsal**) you may be able to keep it in STM indefinitely. If you are trying to remember a license plate number long enough to jot it down, what do you do? You repeat it over and over again. In fact, Atkinson and Shiffrin (1968) suggest that this rehearsal is the prime mechanism to move information from STM to **long-term memory** (LTM). Even so, the amount of information that we can keep in STM is limited. Most estimates suggest that the average person can keep five to nine items in STM at once. This is why most phone numbers (setting aside area and country codes) are about seven numbers long and license plates tend to be seven symbols or fewer.

Long-term memory (LTM) is the part of our memory experience that is the most long-lasting. In fact, science has not been able to establish the true limits of human memory, though to suggest it has no limit is probably inaccurate. What we know is that people who are elderly can have vivid and accurate memories of things that happened when they were children. My great-grandmother died when she was 104 years of age. To her last day she remembered verifiable childhood experiences, such as the aftermath of a tornado, with great clarity. Also, when there is no identifiable disease process, we remain able to form new memories for our entire lives. So we might say that LTM has no "functional" limit on capacity or duration.

Retrieval

Retrieval is the process by which we attempt to pull previously experienced information back into our conscious awareness. This is often the first stage at which we are able to determine the success or failure of our entire memory process with regard to specific events. Although we may be tempted to assign blame for a "memory failure" on our inability to "pull up" supposedly experienced events, failures in recall can be attributed to many things, including problems or failures in each of the prior information processing stages.

Sensation failures. If events did not actually occur, then those events did not enter our information processing system and we will not have direct memory of them. In the same fashion, if we had some sensory deficit that prevented our sensory experience, we will have no memory of those specific events. An example might be physical sensory loss or sensory overloading, such as very loud or very dark environments.

Perception failures or errors. If you are walking through a busy shopping mall during the holidays, your senses will be filled with an unimaginable variety of activity. You will select a very small portion of it to consider—the people right in front of you or the sale in the store to your left. In fact, you may walk past and never notice friends waving at you, simply because you were trying to wind your way through the crowd without being pushed around. The people may have been sensed (e.g., the images ran across your retinas), but your attention was elsewhere. Thus, you have no chance of retrieving the experience later. Similarly, if you are under the influence of sleeping medication, your senses are active, but not your perceptual ability. You will not likely be able to recall any events that occurred while in that condition.

Encoding failures or errors. Labeling can be automatic or it can require great effort. Automatic encoding is that which normally is utilized while experiencing the events of everyday life, such as going to the store, interacting at work, studying at school, or talking with friends. We have a running script for our days into which we try to place each event, so that we might easily understand it. If we experience unusual things, we may try to understand it in terms of our normal expectations. A child who experiences molestation from an adult they normally play with might at first think the experience is strange. But they may conclude it is part of a "tickling" game, perhaps because they were told this by the adult. If the explanation is sufficient for them, that is how the experience will be encoded. If later asked about "bad things" or "bad touches," they may retrieve no memory. However, if asked open-ended questions about how people play, the details may emerge very easily.

Storage failures or errors. Finally, memory failures can also be related to problems in storage processes. Memory decay and memory interference can either prevent access to our stored memories or can allow access to the wrong memories.

Memory decay is the process by which the integrity of our memory is gradually lost over time. While the decay process of sensory memory and short-term memory is quick, easy to witness, and easy to understand, the longer decay process in long-term memory is also evident and potentially problematic. Sensory memories decay and are nearly 100% gone in just a few seconds. Short-term memories, if not maintained or overwritten, are likely to be gone in about 20 to 30 seconds. Long-term memories may have greater longevity, but most will be gone in a week. Those that remain longer than 1 week are likely to remain for a much longer time, perhaps indefinitely.

The decay process is not maladaptive. Imagine if you actually remembered each and every experience that you had during your life. The number of these memories would likely be immense and probably burdensome. The decay process might be the best way to automatically clean your storage capacity of the events that are "not needed." The problem may only be that your brain might make mistakes in the determination of need.

What are the things your brain uses to decide which memories are strong enough to be saved? The most likely explanation for the length of these memories is the strength of the processing steps that preceded them.

Consider This

Think back to any occasion when you were unable to recall information that others seemed to remember. Go through each of the stages of memory (i.e., sensation, perception, encoding, storage, and retrieval) and use each to create an explanation of how that stage could cause such a memory failure.

DEPTH OF PROCESSING MODEL OF MEMORY

One problem with the Atkinson and Shiffrin (1968) model is that we experience things and remember them for long periods of time even when we have not gone through lengthy or elaborate repetitions or rehearsals. Thus, experiences can make it to LTM without rehearsal.

The explanation for this that has been most widely accepted is called the **depth-of-processing model** (e.g., Craik & Lockhart, 1972). The main idea of this model is that, rather than simple rehearsal, the feature of our experiences that is most important in determining how well we will remember them is how deeply we think about them—how many associations and connections we make. Essentially, this refers to how well we understand them.

Deeper processing can also occur when an experience is **salient** in some way. Salient experiences are in some fashion novel or easily attract our awareness. The event may be unusual in intensity or in simple probability. A salient event is not a common occurrence, but is different enough from the norm to draw our attention. Thus depth of processing is aided by both deeper understanding and by novelty or salience—*in addition to rehearsal.*

An experienced security guard may be assigned to monitor a video feed of shoppers navigating a mall during the holiday seasons. This guard may know how people usually move through the stores and how traffic flows. He may be able to write essays for new officers on what to watch for and how to monitor. But these shoppers are normal in every way. He is unlikely to remember what he sees here because there is nothing to require special thought or deeper processing—*unless something unusual happens*. If a child stops in the middle of the pathway without looking here or there, without an adult nearby and while traffic parts around her (for a long enough period of time), the guard's attention is likely to be quickly drawn. It is unusual. The guard will think about this and try to decide what is happening. He may think of different possibilities and search the area to decide which is valid. He may even decide to intervene. Even if a parent then shows up, the amount of processing and thought that was used will ensure the guard remembers this for some time.

As we see later in this chapter, depth-of-processing is also particularly helpful in explaining why children's memory differs from that of adults in some important ways.

THE RECONSTRUCTIVE MODEL OF MEMORY

When you take the time to reminisce, you will probably try to re-experience things as they happened. Your experience of the memory often seems to emerge in much the same serial fashion as the original events. Think back to the day that you graduated from high school, the first date with your current romantic partner, or any other important day in your life. We remember in images, smells, and sometimes even in sounds. All of our senses can contribute to the memory.

If you are a child that is coming home from school, only to be attacked by bullies just a block from your home, you will likely think about the attack again—probably many times.

But where are those things coming from? Do we have a place in our brain labeled, "First Date" or "Disneyland Visit," or "Punched by Bullies"? It sure seems that way. Our impression of memory can be like we have pressed the "play" button on that single event and we passively sit and watch it unfold in our mind's eye. Memory can seem so much like a recording that we often believe that it is truer than it is. After all, if I am watching a video of my first date then what I see has to be what happened. Videos do not lie.

The problem is that we know our memories are fallible. Furthermore, we also know that we can remember some things about our experiences, but have no recall about others. Even worse, sometimes our memories for details of a specific event can seem clearer and sometimes later they can seem fuzzier. What causes these variations? Do we have any models that help to explain them? Yes.

Early models of **reconstructive memory** (Braine, 1965; Pollio & Foote, 1971) suggested that it is more helpful to envision memory not as a "finite state" associative process (where memories exist in unitary wholes held together by webs of associations), but rather as a reconstructive process. The reconstructive model was further refined by Hasher and Griffin (1978) and Elizabeth Loftus in many venues.

In the reconstructive model there may still be associations between details, but more importantly there is a script of events and how they occurred. Think of a script as a kind of assembly instructions for your memories. When you recall an event, you first access the script of the event. Then you bit by bit assemble the details to fit the instructions, but automatically and without awareness. With a clear and comprehensive set of instructions, the final product (the memory) will be complete and accurate.

But what happens to that memory if the script is not so complete? Have you ever tried to assemble a child's toy only to find that the instructions had left out a step or two? The end product does not look the way it was intended. If you are resourceful, you may be able to figure out what was missing and fix it—or you may just figure out a *new* way for the toy to work.

If you are going about your day, walking through the city and suddenly loud and frightening events begin to occur around you (e.g., a gunshot, a scream, a tire squeal, people running), those details will probably be well-stored because they were very salient. However, the relationships between them may not yet be understood at all. Later when you think about the scene, you begin to form a script. Perhaps you form this script from your experiences, perhaps from your logical conclusions, and perhaps from what other people have said about what happened.

In any case, the script becomes the glue to tie these details together into a memory. The script tells your mind which details go where and in what order. If the script is particularly powerful (you watch the news and now really have a strong idea about the scene), the script may actually begin to *change the details*—emphasizing some and altering others.

You may also find that there are blank spots in those scripts. You may not notice them for long, because you will attempt to fill them in automatically. The "filler" may come from simple probabilistic expectation—what we think might have happened or what normally happens in such experiences. The filler may also come from the suggestions of others who either should know or seem to be authorities on the subject. In any case, your mind will search through the possibilities and test-fit them. You may grudgingly accept them at first, but as you continue to work with the memories you will gradually *lose the skepticism* you originally felt.

Eventually, the filler becomes the substance and is remembered in much the same fashion as any other experienced memory. In the end, you may have a solid and serial recollection, but it was pieced together from somewhat random details and a logical explanation (the script), which glued them together (or at least stuck them together).

Scripts can serve helpful purposes as well. Adults who watch a production of *Hamlet* may have already seen other productions or at least know of the story. When they watch, they will automatically compare this version to the ones that are stored in their memory as scripts. Bits and pieces that are similar to their own script will be simply stored as "as expected." Bits and pieces that are different from their expectations may be more closely attended to: "Why did they do it that way"? The salience of this alteration is the result of knowledge and experience. When asked about the play, the adult may accurately describe the play by pulling up the "as expected" information in addition to the small number of alterations. The well-constructed premade script reduced the number of things that must be attended to, and then *all* things are remembered more easily.

Children, on the other hand, do not always have a full understanding of the events that unfold around them. They do not always have established "scripts" for the things they experience. Thus, the advantage of the "as expected" details disappears. More things will need to be encoded with effort. The greater number of things to be encoded means that only the most salient of them are likely to make it to the child's long-term memory. Upon recall, children will similarly pull up the as-expected details, but there are fewer of them (because the script is less complete). Then they will fill in the rest of the story with the new details that they can remember. These new details may contain mostly things salient to the child, not necessarily things other people might consider important. For example, children may have great memory for shoes or clothes, but not facial details or body posture. Fewer *as expected* details plus more selective *other* details may yield fewer forensically relevant memories.

 Consider This

> Some child sexual abusers use descriptions of their behaviors such as "playing a game" or "loving." Think about how this can create difficulties in recall later for a child, and about how the age of the child might compound this problem.

CONTEXT AND STATE EFFECTS ON MEMORY

Your ability to recall experienced events can be affected by the degree to which the context of your experience is similar to the context in which you are recalling the events. This process is called *context-dependent retrieval*. Sometimes the phrase *state dependent* retrieval is also used, but as a reference to a more specific and personal physiological context, such as fatigue or illness.

A classic and oft-cited example of this context effect was conducted by Godden and Baddeley in 1975. They asked divers to learn and recall lists of words both underwater and out of the water. Their results indicate that memory is significantly improved when the learning and recall contexts are the same. Specifically, when divers learned a list while underwater, they recalled that list more accurately and completely underwater, rather than out of the water. Conversely, the lists learned out of the water were more accurately and completely recalled when the diver was out of the water.

When people are asked about events that they have experienced, the same effect operates on them. If asked about your memories, but in a different place or with many other differing contextual variables, your ability to recall them accurately and completely will diminish to some degree. If you wished to be as accurate as possible, then returning to the original context (or reimagining it) will likely improve the accuracy of your memory.

Think about the implications of this for the standard forensic interview of children who are alleged to be the victims of or witnesses to crimes. Often, these interviews are conducted in facilities designed to create the greatest impression of comfort and safety possible. However, these facilities rarely reflect the same context in which the child experienced the events in question (not that this is even possible). Thus consider the effects of these controlled environments on the results of these interviews. What can be done?

Geiselman (1984) developed the *cognitive interview* as a way to improve the accuracy of details provided by eyewitnesses to crimes. Part of this interview involves "context reinstatement," a method for allowing the witness to mentally re-create the environment in which the events originally occurred. Results have consistently demonstrated that overall recall improves with this technique. The problems that have been suggested are that the interview itself is cumbersome for frontline professionals and that *improperly* administered context reinstatement may increase the dangers associated with memory contamination. Even so, the cognitive interview does demonstrate the validity of context considerations in forensic interviews.

Consider This

Using this idea of context-dependent retrieval, explain why the place of a forensic interview is important to collecting information from children about their potential abuse experiences.

INTERFERENCE

Interference occurs when one memory is accidentally retrieved while we are attempting to gain access to another memory. Details of the incorrect memory can contaminate the sought memory. Sometimes this is obvious, like talking about a spouse and pulling up details of a date with an old boyfriend or girlfriend. Sometimes these errors are insidious, like trying to remember the face of a mugger and accidentally recalling the face of another witness.

Interference is usually defined by the directionality of the erroneous memory. *Retroactive interference* is when a newer memory is pulled up as a component of an older experience. Forensic interviewers who ask questions that contain important details may cause unintentional problems. If the child subsequently uses the detail, it may be difficult to determine whether the child said this as the result of true experience, or as the result of retroactive interference. Is the detail originally stored from the interview, but now emerging as part of the forensic event? Thus has this newer memory of the detail from the interview moved backward to contaminate an older memory.

Proactive interference is when an older memory is accidentally pulled up while discussing a later event. A child who is answering questions about occurrences between her mother and father may recall some earlier fights where hostile things were said, but recall them as part of a later event (where the hostility was actually absent or markedly decreased). Thus, this older memory of hostility has incorrectly moved forward to contaminate a newer memory.

MEMORY ACCURACY AND DEVELOPMENTAL DIFFERENCES

What does it mean to have an accurate memory of something you experienced? Does this mean that you recall everything about the time, place, and events? Probably not. We accept that our memories are limited to the things we were paying attention to. We also accept some degree of error, without assuming our memory is "faulty." In fact, even with these well-known limitations, eyewitness memory is not only used but also *valued* in judicial environments. Yet, we rarely have information about just how flawed a *particular* witness's memory is for a *particular* set of events. We will probably never have that specific ability to judge *current* accuracy, but we do have information about general memory accuracy and how that of adults compares to that of children.

To understand the meaning of *accuracy* in memory research, let us first examine four possible memory interview outcomes. *First*, an event or detail can be iterated and also be correct. This is known as a *hit*, or *correct detail*. *Second*, an event or detail can be iterated but also be incorrect. This is known as a *miss*, or *error of commission*. *Third*, an event or detail can be not-iterated, even though it did occur (and was important or forensically relevant). This is known as an *error of omission*. *Fourth*, a detail can be not-iterated and did not actually occur. This is known as a *correct rejection*.

For pure memory research, the fourth category (i.e., correct rejections) represents an infinite category and this is often not included in estimates of accuracy. After all, there are an infinite number of things that *did not happen* and it is correct to not mention each of them (and impossible). The remaining three categories are the basis for most definitions of accuracy. Primarily, accuracy is defined as the *ratio of hits to misses*, or correct details to errors of commission. Alternatively and equivalently, this ratio can be expressed as the *percentage of hits in the total number of detail iterations*. Over several decades of research, the ratio that continuously emerges for human free-recall (e.g., open-ended questions and nonleading interviews) is approximately 3:1, or three accurate details for every error of commission. This rate is also expressed as 75% accuracy.

Interestingly, Steven Ceci and Maggie Bruck (1993; Bruck and Ceci, 1999) demonstrated that this ratio holds for adults, children, and adolescents. What this means is that, in true free recall, children and adolescents commit the same percentage of errors as adults—*not more*. But this is only part of the child-recall picture. Unfortunately, a difference between adults and children does emerge. This difference is in the number of omissions—important things that are left unsaid or unrecalled.

These errors of omission decrease as age increases. Young children tend to leave more out than do older children. Older children leave more out than do adolescents. Adolescents leave more out than do adults. Why this happens is an important, but as of yet unresolved, question. Most likely, this greater rate of omissions is the result of a less-sophisticated understanding of events and thus a less-complete framework for encoding and storing memories of them (i.e., less complete scripts). Furthermore, the things children find salient may differ from the events adults later *wish children had found salient.*

Children may also not feel as comfortable providing a conversational style of recall to an adult. That conversational or *narrative* style may engender greater contextual recall and thus fewer omissions. In other words, as adults recall they are more likely to tell a story about the events, and the story helps flesh-out the script used to access the actual details. Children, when talking with adults, may do less of this.

Regardless of the reasons for the increased number of omissions, details are the things from which cases are made. These omissions pose a special problem for forensic interviewers: Is the omission due to an error (an alleged event happened but the child is not stating it) or a "correct rejection" (an alleged event did not in fact happen and the child is correct in failing to mention it). If an interviewer personally believes that an allegation is true, they may *perceive* the omission as an error.

In most cases, forensic interviews are conducted because authorities believe there is a likelihood that the child did experience a forensic event. They may then believe certain omissions are in error. The next steps the interviewers take are important. If an interviewer leaves the omissions to stand, then there will be no child report to support the case and often the case will end. However, if the interviewer chooses to follow up with more specific questions, the child's report may become more full. However, these specific questions may introduce commission errors through "contamination." If a child provides an affirmative response to a direct question that contains details, the accuracy of that response is still open to analysis. In fact, this new iterated detail can be either a hit or a miss (error of commission) and we may never truly know which.

While self-generated commission errors happen with predictable frequency in free recall, we are also interested in commission errors that occur as the result of information provided in the interview, because this information may be more relevant (the interviewer knows what details are needed) and may also reflect the interviewer's beliefs. If the information *first* came from the interviewer (even if in the form of a question), we call it *contamination*. *Suggestibility* is the degree to which a person is susceptible to the inclusion of contaminating information in memories.

There is a great deal of debate about suggestibility. Debate focuses on the degree to which children and adults are different, on the degree to which the type of events alter suggestibility, the degree to which trauma affects suggestibility, and many other problems. However, there is agreement in the field that memory can be suggestible and that children may have more difficulty filtering out contaminating influences than adults. The final portion of this chapter examines several classic and seminal studies of both adult and children's memory. Do not be fooled into believing, though, that this issue has been settled.

SEMINAL STUDIES OF SUGGESTIBILITY IN CHILD EVENT MEMORY

A great deal of debate and effort has gone into understanding the reliability of children's memory in forensic settings. The problem emerges when juries or prosecutorial decision makers listen to the testimony of a child and wonder if it should be used as evidence. They may wonder if children are reliable enough to be used as witnesses. Actually, the debate should not be about whether children can or cannot be accurate, but whether children can be *as accurate as adults*.

As discussed earlier, adults accept the less-than-perfect qualities of their own memories. Even so, we utilize adult eyewitness testimony easily with only mild skepticism. For four decades, Elizabeth Loftus has engaged in a program of research that examines the memory abilities of both adults and children. It can be argued that she has been a driving influence in the development of our understanding of memory.

If you were to see an automobile accident, do you think your memory would guide your report strongly enough to be a witness—even in the face of incorrect information being hinted at by others? What if that hinted information was so subtle that you did not notice it? What if that incorrect information was only to be found in the semantic *implications* of the words people used to ask you questions?

Loftus and Palmer (1974) examined just that: Was it possible to make people remember things differently simply by asking a question with one suggestive word? They asked subjects to view short film clips depicting mild automobile accidents. After each clip, participants were asked to write a short description of what they had seen. Next, they were asked several specific questions. Among those questions was the crucial question for the study: "About how fast were the cars going when they hit each other?" Their response was to be a speed in MPH. However, the word *hit* was replaced in some conditions with the words, *bumped, contacted, collided,* or *smashed.* They found that the alteration of that one word resulted in significantly different average estimates of speed:

Smashed 40.8 MPH
Collided 39.3 MPH
Bumped 38.1 MPH
Hit 34.0 MPH
Contacted 31.8 MPH

These results indicate that one subtly suggestive word in a question can influence the *way that people remember the event.* Furthermore, if this seems inconsequential there is more. In a follow-up study, Loftus and Palmer (1974) allowed participants to view another accident, then asked them the same question about speed. This time they only altered it with the words *hit* and *smashed.* A control group was not asked about speed. One week later participants were brought back and asked if they had seen any *broken glass* (there had been none). Those that been asked the smashed question were subsequently more likely to remember *seeing broken glass.*

Explanations for this can vary, but it seems to indicate that participants were influenced in speed judgments by the question wording—and then remembered details that would correspond more accurately with the suggestion, than with reality. They were remembering things that did not happen.

Dale, Loftus, and Rathburn (1978). If the 1974 study was useful in establishing that subtle verbal differences can affect an adult's memory, do these same verbal influences exist with children? They studied this with school children and utilized even more subtle verbal suggestion. They allowed children to watch short film clips and then asked a series of questions. They varied the form of the questions in several ways, including using indicators *a* versus *the.* For example, "Did you see a bridge?" or "Did you see the bridge?"

When the object did exist in the films, the children were fairly accurate with any question form. When the object was *not* in the films, children's answered the different questions with different accuracy. In this case, 56% answered *yes* to the question with the word *the*, and 22% answered *yes* to the question with the word *a. No was the correct answer.* According to the 3:1 ratio discussed earlier, we *expect* about 25% to get it wrong. However, the 56% error rate suggests the wording of the question implied something to the children.

These results suggest that children may use conversational information to answer questions when they do not have a direct memory. In this case, the implication of the word *the* (as a specifier) is that the *interviewer* believes that one (i.e., a bridge) was present. Ask those questions to yourself again to understand the effect.

It may be that children are used to memories that are riddled with omissions. They may then not assume that the lack of a memory is due to a lack of actual events, but rather due to their own memory failings. This is not to say that they are lying, but that they are quick to automatically fill in perceived memory holes as they detect them, especially if they believe an authority figure has the answer.

At this point, we have some evidence that memories can be influenced by subtle question semantics. But what about memories for experiences that should have been somewhat frightening or psychologically traumatic (not subtle at all)? Is there a special strength that these memories garner, a strength caused by the attention that must have been paid when the memory was created? Furthermore, are we able to detect a suggested memory by the *lack* of this special strength? While the answer to these questions is not settled, there is some research evidence to suggest that even these memories can be falsely created and believed, and even by adults.

Loftus and Pickrell (1995). Do you think you would remember clearly whether you had been lost in a mall as a child? Assuming you were old enough to form other memories that you clearly remember from the same era, do you think this is the kind of memory that you will keep or that you would *know* if you had in fact *not* been lost? Loftus and Pickrell (1995) studied this with college-aged students. They talked with an older relative of the students and learned of three events that each student had actually experienced, but added one to the list—being lost in a mall.

When talking with subjects, researchers strongly suggested that all four had happened and they even had details to go with the mall story, because it was certain that the subjects would have none of their own. Later, subjects were asked about the confidence they had in the memories of each of the four events. Although not all of the subjects "remembered" being lost in a mall, about 29% did. About 3 in 10 subjects could be convinced at some level that something traumatic had happened to them and would report being able to *remember* the events. In fact, some even clung to the memories when skepticism was introduced. The researchers point out that this kind of direct false memory creation is possible, not that it is easy to create and/or reliable.

Leichtman and Ceci (1995). What would happen to the way that people remember your actions if another person told them that you were sneaky or had nefarious motivations? Would they remember your actions as accurately as they had before or do you think some of those stereotypes might put new spins on their memories? Leichtman and Ceci (1995) wanted to study this with children. Could they use questions that imply stereotypic information about a person and alter the way that children remember them?

In their study, Sam Stone came to visit classroom. For some children, his clumsy behavior was described before he came. This was called *stereotype induction*.

The stereotypes described were about the personality of a man who was "well-meaning," but "very clumsy."

For some children, there was no stereotype induction, but they were asked suggestive questions about him afterward. These suggestive questions included details such as that Sam Stone had "soiled a teddy bear" or "ripped a book," neither of which happened.

For some children, both the pre-event stereotype induction and the postevent suggestions were used. Finally, a group of students were controls for whom neither manipulation was used.

Researchers found that the children in the control group answered questions as accurately as normal. But children in both the stereotype induction group and the suggestive questions group showed a significant number of inaccuracies in line with the manipulations. Furthermore, the group with both manipulations showed a very high number of inaccuracies.

What this means is that the effect of suggestive questions with children can be amplified when used in conjunction with other problematic influences. If you ask mildly suggestive questions about a person's behavior while also implying that the person is "bad," or that the interviewer is not going to let the person "hurt" them (an understandable temptation for an interviewer), you may experience an inflated set of details in line with the suggestions and implications—even if those details are inaccurate. You can understand how this stereotype induction might serve to create *new* parts of the child's schema, parts that will affect later memory.

Thompson, Clarke-Stewart, and Lepore (1997) wanted to know if they could utilize fairly coercive questioning styles to get children to report something exactly opposite from what they had seen. Children were left alone (for a few moments) in a laboratory room. During that time Chester, a janitor, entered the room and either played with toys or cleaned them. Chester was, in fact, a confederate of the experimenter and was playing out a role. Later, children were interviewed by Chester's "boss," sometimes suggesting strongly that Chester had been doing the opposite of what the children actually witnessed. Children's reports strongly favored the suggestions made by the boss, even when it was different from their own observations.

More interestingly, parents were not informed of actual events but were directed to ask specific, nonleading questions to learn what happened. Children's reports to their parents still reflected the suggestions of the boss, rather than their own observations. If children were simply and voluntarily yielding to the coercion of the boss they might have been expected to report their own observations to their parent. They might have even been likely to tell their parents about the boss's behavior. Their report indicates that their own memory of events may have been altered, rather than just their *reports* of it.

Consider This

Some advocates in the field of child forensics make statements such as, "children never lie about abuse," or "children's memories of abuse are less fallible than other memories" (due to their traumatic nature), in order to support the verbalizations children make in forensic interviews. Although these statements are certainly well intentioned, think about the way that memory research and forensic interviewing experts would respond to such statements. This is a difficult question and can be used to stimulate class discussion.

SUMMARY THOUGHTS ABOUT CHILDREN'S MEMORY OF FORENSIC EVENTS

So, what do we take from children's memory research? At this point in memory research, some general conclusions can be drawn. First, all memory is less than perfect. However, it also has points of incredible accuracy and strength. This strength may be related to how well we understood the original experiences *while experiencing them*.

Second, children have the capacity to be as accurate as adults. This, however, depends on the way that their memories are elicited, with free-recall and narrative styles of recall being the most productive. However, this accuracy only applies to the things they say, not to the things they do not say. Children are prone to omission errors, which often prompts professionals to ask specific questions.

Finally, both children and adults can be the victims of contamination created in problematic questions or requests for recall. It may be that children are more vulnerable to this effect when either they did not have a good understanding of the things that were happening to them, or when they were being asked detailed questions about things that did not happen to them. Thus, the way that an interviewer (or any person) asks questions to a child can alter the way that the child (yes, adults as well) remember the events. Training in controlled forensic interviewing is vital to ensure that these influences do not occur and that children's memories are protected. After all, in many cases that child's memory *is the crime scene* and should be treated as such, with caution and concern for contamination.

REVIEW QUESTIONS

1. Define memory.
2. Discuss the information-processing model of human memory. Specifically define and differentiate each of the five steps.

3. Discuss the three stages of the Atkinson and Shiffrin model of storage, including the special role of rehearsal.

4. Describe the advantages and disadvantages of memory decay.

5. What does the Depth-of-Processing Model of memory tell us about the way that memories are formed and how they gain strength?

6. Define *salience* and how it affects the formation of memories.

7. What is a memory script?

8. Discuss the Reconstructive Model of human memory, including the way that *details* and *scripts* are used.

9. Discuss the following terms:
   a. Context effects
   b. Context reinstatement
   c. Interference, retroactive, and proactive

10. Define:
   a. Errors of commission
   b. Errors of omission
   c. Hits
   d. Correct rejections

11. How can you use the above (#10) terms to describe the accuracy of human memory? How are children's memory and adult's memory the same and how are they different?

12. Describe the basic methods and findings of each of the following seminal studies:
   a. Loftus and Palmer (1974)
   b. Dale, Loftus, and Rathburn (1978)
   c. Loftus and Pickrell (1995)
   d. Leichtman and Ceci (1995)
   e. Thompson, Clarke-Stewart, and Lepore (1997)

GLOSSARY

depth-of-processing model The idea that, rather than simple rehearsal, memories can be moved into longer-term storage based on the level at which we understand an experience, or how salient it is.

encoding The "labeling" of perceptions, which serves to better identify and recall experiences after long-term storage.

interference The process by which, during recall, details of one event can mistakenly become involved in the recall of another event.

long-term memory The process by which more salient or important memories are saved for longer periods of time. Long-term storage can be *functionally* unlimited in both duration and capacity.

memory Our ability to create a mental record of our experiences and then later recall them, or think about them again.

perception The interpretation of sensations into sensible wholes.

reconstructive model A model of memory that suggests memories are not stored as integrated units (e.g., video recordings), but rather as independent details loosely connected by associations and scripts. It is used as a basis for suggestibility literature.

rehearsal The process of repeating or thinking an idea in order to move it into long-term storage.

retrieval The reutilization of sensory/perceptual information that was previously stored.

salience The degree to which an experience is viewed as important, unusual, novel, or attention-grabbing.

sensation The collection of environmental stimulus energies by the sensory organs.

sensory memory The neural aftereffects of stimulus energies in the sensory systems. This often lasts only seconds, or fractions of a second.

short-term memory Working memory that serves to monitor and guide the contents of current consciousness. This tends to be short in capacity and duration.

storage The long-term retention of experience's sensory/perceptual information.

REFERENCES

Atkinson, R., & Shiffrin, R. (1968). Human memory: A proposed system and its control processes. In K. W. Spence & J. T. Spence (Eds.), *The psychology of learning and motivation* (Vol. 2, pp. 89–195). New York, NY: Academic Press.

Braine, M. (1965). The insufficiency of a finite state model for verbal reconstructive memory. *Psychonomic Science, 2*(10), 291–292.

Bruck, M., & Ceci, S. (1999). The suggestibility of children's memory. *Annual Review of Psychology, 50,* 419–439.

Ceci, S., & Bruck, M. (1993). Suggestibility of the child witness: A historical review and synthesis. *Psychological Bulletin, 113*(3), 403–439.

Craik, F., & Lockhart, R. (1972). Level of processing: A framework for memory research. *Journal of Verbal Learning and Verbal Behavior, 11*(6), 671–684.

Dale, P., Loftus, E., & Rathburn, L. (1978). The influence of the form of the question on the eyewitness testimony of preschool children. *Journal of Psycholinguistic Research, 7*(4), 269–277.

Geiselman, R. (1984). Enhancement of eyewitness memory: An empirical evaluation of the cognitive interview. *Journal of Police Science and Administration, 12*(1), 74–80.

Godden, D., & Baddeley, A. (1975). Context-dependent memory in two natural environments: On land and underwater. *British Journal of Psychology, 66*(3), 325–331.

Hasher, L., & Griffin, M. (1978). Reconstructive and reproductive processes in memory. *Journal of Experimental Psychology, 4*(4), 318–330.

Leichtman, M., & Ceci, S. (1995). The effects of stereotypes and suggestions on preschoolers' reports. *Developmental Psychology, 31*(4), 568–578.

Loftus, E., & Palmer, J. (1974). Reconstruction of automobile destruction: An example of the interaction between language and memory. *Journal of Verbal Learning and Verbal Behavior, 13*, 585–589.

Loftus, E., & Pickrell, J. (1995). The formation of false memories. *Psychiatric Annals, 25*(12), 720–725.

Pollio, H., & Foote, R. (1971). Memory as a reconstructive process. *British Journal of Psychology, 62*(1), 53–58.

Shiffrin, R., & Atkinson, R. (1969). Storage and retrieval processes in long-term memory. *Psychological Review, 76*(2), 179–193.

Thompson, W., Clarke-Stewart, K., & Lepore, S. (1997). What did the janitor do? Suggestive interviewing and the accuracy of children's accounts. *Law and Human Behavior, 21*(4), 405–426.

—◆—

Applied Principles in Child Abuse

CHAPTER

5

Child Abuse and Neglect

GOALS OF THIS CHAPTER:

1. Readers will understand the different types of child abuse and neglect and their characteristics.
2. Readers will learn statistics and other considerations associated with child abuse and neglect.
3. Readers will recognize victim and offender characteristics related to child abuse and neglect.

*I*t was the third time this month that Billy* came to school with a bruise on his face or neck. Mrs. Jones didn't know what to do; she was worried about Billy, but every time she asked about what happened, Billy would always have a story to describe what had happened to him. Mrs. Jones didn't always think the story Billy gave sounded credible, but she didn't know what else to do. Mrs. Jones decided to seek guidance from a colleague, who suggested she call Child Protective Services (or CPS) in their area. Mrs. Jones was concerned she didn't have enough information to make a hotline call; in fact, she had heard of hotlines before, but never made a call to one. Mrs. Jones didn't know if something really was happening to hurt Billy or who was hurting Billy and Mrs. Jones's colleague explained that an investigation would help find these things out—she didn't have to have any proof, just reasonable concern. Mrs. Jones decided to make the hotline call during her lunch break.

Billy grabbed his coat to take to lunch and then recess and Mrs. Jones noticed several bruises on Billy's arms. She asked Billy what happened and he angrily said, "Nothing, I just fell, okay?" Mrs. Jones didn't have a good feeling about this and decided to make the hotline call about her concerns. The hotline was taken from the central call center and routed to the local county office for further investigation.

---

*This is a fictional depiction of a child physical abuse case for illustrative purposes only. Any similarity to real individuals or cases is by chance and is unintended.

Billy's stepfather, Jay, had been physically abusing Billy for several months. Jay was typically pretty good at covering up any evidence of marks or bruises, but had gotten sloppy over the last several weeks. He threatened Billy and explained that if Billy told anyone about the hitting, he would kill Billy's whole family. Plus, his mom had seen Jay hit him before and never stopped it or said anything. Fortunately, Mrs. Jones contacted local authorities and Billy and his siblings were able to be protected. Because Billy's mom needed help for domestic violence concerns as well, which Billy often witnessed, Billy and his siblings were taken into foster care and placed with a nice family just outside of their hometown. Billy's mom plans to leave Jay and to work hard to get her children back, but it will take significant effort on her part and the state needs to see it before the boys can be returned home. A very detailed treatment plan was written so all parties know what their responsibilities are in the situation. The children's safety comes first and the state will ensure all decisions made for the boys are in their best interest. Billy was very thankful Mrs. Jones had stepped in and gotten him the help he couldn't ask for himself.

INTRODUCTION TO CHILD ABUSE AND NEGLECT

Regrettably, the scenario depicted earlier is not uncommon; children are abused and neglected every day. Child abuse is an unfortunate occurrence that impacts hundreds of thousands of children in the United States each year. According to the U.S. Department of Health and Human Services (2011), 676,569 victims of child abuse and neglect were reported in fiscal year (FY) 2011. Some of these victims may have been subject to more than one report and when examining those numbers, more than 3.7 million children were subject to at least one report in the same fiscal year. These numbers suggest there are approximately 9 reported victims for every 1,000 children in the United States, which is a devastating number considering the data suggesting many child abuse incidents are never reported to authorities (DHHS, 2011).

When examining child abuse victim characteristics further, children under the age of 1 were the most represented age group in the statistics reported above. Typically, victimization in this age group is most closely associated with neglect versus abuse (Children's Bureau, 2011). **Neglect** is an act of omission (not giving the children something they need like food, water, shelter, or medical care), whereas **abuse** is an act of commission (doing something to a child that is in excess of what is appropriate). Neglect is actually the most common form of reported abuse, although it is not discussed as frequently as other types of abuse.

Gender is equally distributed in the statistics in this report and in general, the rate of abuse and/or neglect decreased with age. It is possible that older children may come to the attention of authorities sooner (remember Billy's scenario) because they are more visible (in school, etc.) and more verbal and able to communicate concerns more easily than older children.

As you will learn in Chapter 12, a big responsibility of professionals is mandated reporting. Mandated reporting laws vary by state, but in general, they require certain individuals or professionals to report concerns of child abuse and neglect. If these professionals do not appropriately follow these laws, criminal charges are possible. Through mandated reporting, many concerns of child abuse are brought to light. People do not have to be required by law to contact their state's child abuse and neglect hotline or local authorities. Essentially, making a report, or calling a hotline, begins an investigative process when concerns, like the ones you learn about in this chapter, are present. People do not have to have proof of their concerns to make a hotline call, as you learn in Chapter 12; in fact, a reasonable suspicion is all that is required and the investigation of the concerns should be left to the professionals. As you read through this chapter and the various scenarios presented, consider if you believe the situation warrants additional investigation.

 Consider This

> Try to imagine that you have become aware of a child who may have been abused or neglected. What if this were the child of a friend, or neighbor, or family member? Think through the concerns, barriers, and consequences for deciding to report the abuse or neglect. Also take time to consider the consequences for not reporting the abuse.

NEGLECT

As was mentioned earlier, neglect is an act of omission, where people, typically caregivers, fail to provide adequate care to another person dependent on them. There are various forms of neglect including physical, medical, emotional, and educational. According to Gaudin (1993), defining neglect includes analysis of the following items:

- Minimally adequate types of care that are required by children.
- Actions that would constitute neglectful behavior.
- Intent of the action (or lack of action).
- Effects or potential effects on the child's health, safety, well-being, development, and so on.
- Situational factors (poverty, etc.).

Like other forms of abuse, each state defines and delivers consequences for neglect differently. In general, the definitions for each state follow Gaudin's criteria when considering whether neglect, an act, or failure to act causes harm, exploitation, or death or a risk of such consequences. In general, the four most common forms of neglect are defined as follows, according to American Humane Society (n.d.).

Physical Neglect

Physical neglect accounts for the majority of cases of neglect that are reported. Physical neglect generally involves the parent(s) or caregiver(s) not providing the child with basic provisions needed for survival such as adequate food, clothing, supervision, and/or shelter. Because these are important to our survival, failure to provide these necessities can have long-term consequences including developmental concerns, cognitive deficits, and/or mental health issues. For example, a father who eats all of the food in the household and does not provide food for his children may be neglecting a need related to physical neglect.

Medical Neglect

Medical neglect is the failure to provide suitable health care for a child when the means exist to provide such care. Said another way, financially, a person is able to provide access to health care services and does not do so. This is an important distinction because the law may view a lack of medical care due to poverty in a different way than a lack of medical care due to a motivation issue. If a child breaks his arm and his parents refuse to take him to the doctor because of inconvenience, this would be viewed differently than a family who does not seek medical services due to financial concerns and lack of access. Lower-income families may have difficulty gaining access to the medical services they need—some families may be placed on significant waiting lists to see physicians, including psychiatrists, due to the type of insurance they have. They may not be able to seek alternate care because the psychiatrist contacted is the only person in their region who accepts their insurance. Authorities would not necessarily look at this delay in care as neglect, but a lack of available resources. The delay in care may have deleterious effects, however, as waiting many months to address a problem that is currently an issue is unacceptable.

A lack of access to appropriate health care can have serious consequences, including lifelong medical concerns or death. For example, a mother who does not provide medical care when her child complains of chronic pain after a fall may be neglecting a medical need. Getting more information in situations like this is crucial, because the lack of medical care may be due to an inability to take off work, financial barriers, and so on.

Educational Neglect

Educational neglect involves the failure to provide adequate educational resources to a child of school age. If enrolling in private or public schools is not desired, participation in a home-schooling program is required. Additionally, not requiring school attendance of a child who is school age may be considered educational neglect. Because so many skills are developed and acquired at school, a lack of attendance can have serious social, emotional, psychological, and educational consequences. A father who allows his teenage daughter to skip school for weeks at a time may be neglecting an educational need of his daughter.

Emotional Neglect

Emotional neglect is more difficult to define and prove in a court of law. How can we prove that an action may hurt a child's psyche? How do some children experience emotional neglect and maltreatment and appear unscathed while others crumble and have significant issues? Some of these differences may be due to **protective factors**. Protective factors are characteristics that mitigate, or lessen, the impact of negative experiences. Access to support systems, access to resources, coping skills, and close, healthy relationships are some examples of protective factors. These, along with other individual characteristics may help explain the differences we see in the presentation of victims of emotional neglect and maltreatment.

Emotional, or psychological, neglect may include engaging in unstable interactions in front of the child (domestic violence), refusing access to mental health care, withholding affection, name-calling, ignoring, rejecting, isolating the child, threatening/terrorizing, or exploiting. Poor emotional development can lead to severe psychological consequences, including social skill concerns, substance abuse, poor self-esteem, and/or destructive decision making For example, a mother who calls her son names multiple times a day and withholds affection and praise may be neglecting his emotional needs.

Perpetrators of neglect may lack understanding of child development (which may lead to unnecessary frustration or a lack of necessary care), may be single parents, may be in financial distress, may report greater mental health concerns, may have a history of substance abuse, may have been previously victimized, and may be younger in age (Children's Bureau, 2011).

Treatment of Neglect

The primary goal in dealing with neglectful families is safety and prevention of additional harm. Fortunately, neglectful families are often able to remain united and can improve functioning with access to services and some mental health assistance. Parent Child Interaction Therapy, or PCIT, may be a useful treatment method for families in distress. It aims to improve the skills of parents, decrease negative interactions between children and parents, increase positive and prosocial communications, and decrease parental stress. According to the National Child Traumatic Stress Network (NCTSN), PCIT is an evidence-based treatment method that provides live coaching sessions to parents to improve the child/caregiver relationship (NCTSN, 2008). This treatment method might be particularly useful in cases of emotional neglect, whereas gaining access to resources might be a more useful intervention method for the other forms of neglect discussed. Individual therapy may be another option for parents or caregivers who are feeling overwhelmed, unmotivated, or stressed. Because of the dangers associated with child neglect, ensuring safety of the children involved is crucial, as well as improving future functioning.

 Consider This

Sometimes people believe, in a misguided fashion, that their neglect of their children is a part of their children's development and training. Try to imagine scenarios where this belief system may be active. How would a professional deal with these cases?

CHILD PHYSICAL ABUSE

Physical abuse is defined as "non-accidental trauma or physical injury caused by punching, beating, kicking, biting, burning or otherwise harming a child.... [P]hysical abuse is the most visible form of child maltreatment" (American Humane Society, p. 1). Like other forms of maltreatment, specific definitions and legal implications surrounding physical abuse vary state to state. Some states require physical injury to rise to the level of abuse while others do not (NCTSN, 2009). There is some debate associated with definitions of child physical abuse, particularly with corporal punishment. In many states, corporal punishment (spanking) is not illegal unless it crosses reasonable means. What is reasonable when considering spanking? If marks or bruises are left on the body? If an object is used? If the child is unable to sit or stand? These questions, and others, make this discussion difficult as people feel differently about what is reasonable or appropriate or not.

In 2011, there were more than 118,000 victims of child physical abuse (DHHS, 2011). The consequences of physical abuse can be significantly impairing to its victims, with death being the most severe result possible. These numbers pale in comparison with victims of neglect being more than 500,000, however, one victim of child abuse is one too many.

Risk Factors for Child Physical Abuse

When considering victims of child physical abuse, it is important to discuss potential risk factors associated with physical abuse. According to Rodriguez and Tucker (2011), poor attachment was considerably related to both dysfunctional child-rearing practices and increases the likelihood of child abuse victimization. These results emphasize the importance of the child/parent relationship and abuse potential. Additionally, these authors mention that in general, research supports that harsh or inappropriate discipline as a child may be related to harsh or inappropriate (and abusive) parenting styles (Coohey & Braun, 1997; Craig & Sprang, 2007).

As can be found in almost any introductory psychology textbook, Bandura's social learning theory supports these claims—what we see is often what we do. We can become desensitized to harsh parenting techniques over time, particularly if it becomes our "normal." Think about your own childhood for a moment. Are there things that were abnormal or strange that you did not realize were strange until you became an adult? Even in nonabusive households, we often find things that our parents did simply because their parents did, so on and so forth. When unhealthy parenting practices are carried from one generation to another, the cycle of abuse will be continued until someone or something breaks the cycle. What is the best predictor of *future* behavior? *Past* behavior. Knowing this, we can identify individuals who might be high risk for becoming perpetrators or victims of child abuse and provide services and interventions that might assist them in not crossing an inappropriate boundary.

Attachment and parenting style may also be related to child physical abuse. Rodriguez and Tucker (2011) studied at-risk mothers and found attachment to one's parents was significantly related to an increased child abuse potential and dysfunctional disciplinary style independent of individual maltreatment history. According to Cloitre, Stovall-McClough, Zorbas, and Charuvastra (2008) individuals with poor attachment histories may have characteristics such as difficulty regulating emotions, poor management of managing negative emotions, and distrustful of others. Thus, this suggests that an unhealthy attachment with one's parents may have personality characteristics that may make them more susceptible in engaging in poor parenting practices. Interestingly, poorest attachment was apparent in the mothers with reported personal histories of abuse and those women may be the most likely to maintain the cycle of violence, consistent with earlier research on attachment quality and predatory behavior (Zuravin et al., 1996, in Rodriguez & Tucker, 2011). What research like this does help us understand is how risk factors are related to child abuse; it is the hope that we can use this information in preventing abuse in the first place. If professionals can recognize the relationship between attachment, parenting style, and abuse history, interventions can take place that might offset some risk factors for future abuse.

Consequences of Child Physical Abuse

The consequences associated with child physical abuse go beyond what many people think of initially. Not only are there potential physical injuries like broken bones, head trauma, abdominal injuries, skin injuries, and so on, there can also be behavioral, emotional, and psychological effects from exposure to abuse of this kind.

Research has found links between physical abuse, depression, and aggressive behaviors but the relationship among these variables appears different when looking at men versus women (Scarpa, Haden, & Abercromby, 2010). It appears that males and females react differently to trauma, with males engaging in more antisocial behaviors and females becoming more withdrawn. Several studies have reported that child physical abuse is a noteworthy predictor of depressive symptoms (Gover & Mackenzie, 2003; Hill, 2003; Kilpatrick et al., 2003, in Scarpa, Haden, & Abercromby, 2010). Depression can be a difficult disorder to live with as it can impact us personally and professionally, so understanding the link between depression and childhood trauma is an important area of study. In agreement, Cichetti, Rogosch, Gunnar, and Toth (2010), there are physiological differences between children who were exposed to abuse/trauma at a young age, and those who were not. Specifically, the stress hormone, cortisol, can be suppressed or released in extreme quantities (very high or very low), which can be related to health and development.

Additionally, because crucial brain development occurs early in life, any negative exposure during a formative period could lead to developmental issues. If children's abilities to adequately handle and adapt to stress are negatively impacted early on, this can be a consequence that causes life-long difficulties.

In the literature, there appears to be a link between eating disorders and early experiences of childhood abuse and trauma (Johnson, Cohen, Kasen, & Brook, 2002; Rorty, Yager, & Rossotto, 1994). Because eating disorders are often related to the desire to be in control, some believe the relationship between eating disorders and trauma could be due to the lack of control the victim experienced during the abuse situation. In general, individuals with eating disorders are more likely to report a history of child maltreatment.

Messman-Moore and Garrigus (2007) reported that women who experienced multiple forms of childhood abuse, of any kind, experienced more difficulties associated with eating behaviors (bulimic tendencies, preoccupation with weight, etc.). This suggests that the chronicity of the abuse, rather than the type, may have a more significant impact than we once thought. Additionally, women who experienced physical abuse as a child reported excessive concerns with dieting and weight and extreme measures to pursue thinness.

Treatment of Child Physical Abuse

As has been mentioned previously, keeping a family intact, if possible, is a goal of Child Protective Services. Children often function best in their biological homes, if those homes are nurturing, loving, and appropriate.

With physical abuse, treatment methods vary, and like neglect, ensuring safety of the victim (and other children as appropriate) is a primary goal. For victims of physical abuse, the predictability of their world is often disrupted and they may live in fear.

Therapy, particularly focusing on trauma and trauma-related symptoms, may be an effective intervention for victims of physical abuse. Trauma-focused therapies can assist participants by providing education about trauma, normalization of symptoms, safety planning, dispelling myths and cognitive distortions, and allowing for free expression of emotions and concerns.

For the perpetrator of physical abuse, treatment is also an important consideration. For many, learning to implement effective parenting practices is a chief concern. Educating parents on appropriate and inappropriate discipline methods, providing alternative techniques of gaining cooperation from their children, and dealing with any mental health concerns (of the child[ren] or parent) are all important. As was mentioned in the Treatment of Neglect section, Parent Child Interaction Therapy (PCIT) can be an effective technique in increasing positive interactions between parents and their children. Parents who are susceptible to "losing their cool" or crossing boundaries of appropriate punishment techniques might be urged to avoid any methods that might cause them to revert back to inappropriate practices.

Do you respond better to negative or positive feedback? Most of us would rather hear good things we are doing rather than all of the things we are doing wrong. Children are no different; if we can find ways to compliment them, even on small things, they are likely to respond more favorably. This can be easier said than done; however, experience tells us reinforcement is more effective in the long-term than punishment.

Consider This

Chapter 2 detailed the principles of reinforcement and punishment. Try to imagine how parents who rely on "positive punishment" and little positive reinforcement may eventually face a downward spiral in which the punishments need to become more severe to maintain effectiveness.

CHILD SEXUAL ABUSE

Child sexual abuse is another unfortunate reality for many of our youth. It can be uncomfortable to talk or read about, but we cannot help protect children if we are not willing to acknowledge the problem. Defining child sexual abuse can be somewhat complicated as it can encompass a diversity of behaviors and actions.

According to the American Humane Society, *child sexual abuse* is defined as sexual abuse and can include: sexual intercourse or its deviations, sexually touching a child (such as fondling, making a child touch an adult's sexual organs, penetrating the child's sex organs in any way with any object), as well as nontouching offenses (exposing children to pornography, deliberately exposing a child to sexual acts, including masturbation) or sexual exploitation (soliciting a child for the purposes of commercial sexual exploitation/human trafficking). As you can see, there are many behaviors and acts that can occur that would fall under the category of child sexual abuse.

According to the Children's Bureau (2011), more than 65,000 children were reported victims of sexual abuse in 2011. One of the difficulties surrounding statistics of abuse, particularly sexual abuse, is the underreporting that professionals know occurs. Because sexual abuse is often done in a secretive manner and because we cannot look at people and tell if they have been sexually abused (as we may be able to do for a child who has been neglected or physically abused), children can avoid disclosing their abuse for many years after it occurs, if they disclose at all. It is possible that we are only skimming the surface with these statistics we report related to the number of children who experience abuse. According to Olafson and Lederman (2006), there is agreement among researchers that there are a significant number of children that delay disclosure of their abuse experience until adulthood. Can you think of a reason why this might occur? There is often a lot of shame, guilt, and blame associated with abuse, particularly sexual abuse, and because of this, victims may not ever tell someone about their abuse experience. Although actual numbers vary, several research studies report between 28% and 70% of adults, who were victimized as children, delayed their disclosure until adulthood and many never reported abuse to authorities (Olafson & Lederman, 2006). This tells us that when we calculate statistics based on cases formally reported to law enforcement or child protective services, we may be missing a significant number of cases in our calculations. Additionally, research tells us children delay disclosure within childhood—meaning they often wait to report abuse experiences for months or years after the abuse occurs, which can also influence statistics. So, use caution when reviewing statistics related to child abuse and understand the numbers are likely quite a bit higher than we can imagine.

Characteristics of Sexually Abused Children

Because child sexual abuse encompasses such a wide range of behaviors and actions, summarizing the characteristics of its victims can be somewhat complex. Children often fall victim to sexual abuse in their homes, by someone close to them, but there are occasions when children are abused by a stranger or by someone who has lured them to engage in particular behaviors. The relationship of the offender to the child can impact the child's experience with the abuse. Additionally, how the children view their responsibility in the abuse can also influence their experience.

Compliant Victims

If a child meets someone online on a social networking site and gets involved in commercial sexual exploitation as a result of the new relationship, will she feel responsibility for her experience? It is easy for professionals to say she should not, she was the child involved, but the reality is that many children experience guilt or self-blame because of actions they took (or did not take) that they believe would have changed their fate. Or, consider a 13-year-old who meets a 37-year-old online and forms a romantic relationship, which does include sexual contact. This 13-year-old views the 37-year-old as her boyfriend—do you think she views herself as a victim? Most likely not and because of this, this is an example where the victim may be viewed as a **compliant victim**, or people who cooperate and participate in their victimization. Sometimes, compliant victims reluctantly participate in their victimization because of benefits such as money, clothing, and attention, or they may not view the situation as abusive at all, like the example provided with the 13- and 37-year-old. In either situation, complicity can make investigations more difficult and may make participation in the legal process complicated. In my experience, compliant victims often do not see themselves as victims, but as willing participants. They will often refer to the offender as their "boyfriend" and may, at first, be uncooperative to provide information about the relationship in question. As this textbook mentions, building rapport is an important consideration when interacting with victims of child abuse, and I find it especially critical when working with compliant victims. Sometimes investigators may feel it is their job to educate the victims on how dangerous their behavior has been; however, this can cause investigative difficulties. When interviewing child victims, it is no concern when the children refer to the offender as their boyfriend or girlfriend because it is their perception of the situation—if time is spent lecturing about how a 37-year-old has no business "dating" a 13-year-old, an opportunity might be lost to gather crucial information to support the case. Although safety is an obvious concern, it may be more appropriate for a victim advocate or parent to discuss these matters with victims, rather than law enforcement officials who are trying to build a case for prosecution. If you remember being a teenager, your opinions were likely strong and important to you and when people tried to tell you something different than you thought or felt, it made you want to prove them wrong, right? We often look back and realize some of the choices we made as teenagers may not have been the smartest or safest, but it sometimes takes years for these realizations to occur. Thus, when talking with compliant victims, balance the need for gathering information with the need to educate the victim about the consequences of certain behaviors and actions. Sometimes, what is intended as educational may seem blaming, so it is important to keep this in mind when interacting with child victims. Consider this: "Susie, do you know what could have happened to you? You should never meet up with someone you met online because you could be killed! If you were my daughter, you would be grounded from your computer because there are some dangerous people out there!" Do you see how this could be interpreted as blaming the victim for her circumstance?

As you will learn in Chapter 7, a forensic interview is an appropriate investigative tool that can be used when interacting with child abuse victims and witnesses, including compliant victims. Some professionals believe is not necessary to forensically interview teenage victims; but, remember that children are not miniature adults and 13 is not a magic number where children can suddenly communicate at the same level as adults. Alternatively, teenagers can be egocentric in their communication and a forensic interview may be especially important to gather accurate details by asking developmentally sensitive and legally sound questions. Additionally, trained forensic interviewers have skills in dealing with various types of child victims and witnesses, including compliant victims and provide legally defensible testimony on behalf of those they interview.

The public may view compliant victims differently than those they view as "forced" into abuse because there is a lack of understanding on how or why children would cooperate or actively participate in victimization. There is often a lack of understanding about the manipulation and grooming techniques that will often initiate and maintain abuse. Education is critical to avoid blame being put on victims due to this complex phenomenon. The next section provides helpful information about how child sexual abuse begins and how it is secretly continued over time.

Dynamics of Child Sexual Abuse

As was mentioned, there can be a public lack of understanding about the dynamics of child sexual abuse. Some of this may be due to inaccurate information portrayed in the media, myths, and confusion about laws and statutes related to consent. There is often a misconception that children are more at risk for abuse by strangers (stranger danger). This is likely because it is easier to believe strangers could hurt our children, versus loved ones, and because of this, there can be confusion about the characteristics of abusive relationships.

Grooming

Child sexual abuse is often predatory in nature and techniques are often employed by offenders to groom the child victim and sometimes those close to the child victim (like parents). The term *groom* (or **grooming**) refers to techniques that initiate and/or maintain abuse. These techniques may include giving gifts, making threats, treating the victim like a significant other, and other behaviors and actions that may make the child maintain interest in the relationship for one reason or another.

According to Craven, Brown, and Gilchrist (2006), research suggests that there may also be "self-grooming" that occurs where the offender prepares himself (although we know women can be offenders, for the ease of discussion, we use a male offender for an example) for the abusive behavior and justifies his actions. This can take place in cognitive distortions where the offender reports that the child victim "came on" to him or that he was teaching the child victim about sex, for example.

Secondly, offenders often target children they view as vulnerable. This may include children who are isolated, have few friends, and have poor relationships with their family members. Offenders often become somewhat integrated into the victim child's life—which can make disclosure more difficult once abuse begins. This is why we see offenders becoming coaches, tutors, camp counselors, youth leaders, and so on, and placing themselves where they have regular access to the child victim (and other potential victims). As we know, all individuals who hold these positions are not sexual predators; however, the point is that sometimes, individuals seek these positions to increase their access to children. We have to consider that if an offender seeks a position of power and trust, the public may not view this person as a threat. It is difficult for us to think about the decorated football coach, the lead youth pastor at a beloved community church, or the director of a day care center being a sexual predator. I recall a case I worked a number of years ago where a child waited to disclose about her abuse because her mother had referred to the offender, a family friend, as a "really nice and upstanding gentleman," and she was worried her mother would not believe that he could have sexually abused her. Luckily, the child was wrong and her mom stood by her side and wholeheartedly believed her.

Grooming can also occur to individuals inside the child's frame of reference, such as parents, caregivers, and grandparents. Offenders may offer to babysit while the parents spend time outside the home or may provide gifts that the family couldn't afford. These actions may make it not only difficult for the child victim to disclose, but also difficult for the family to comprehend that someone who has been good to their family would betray them in this way.

Grooming is often gradual and can take place over a number of months or years. If children are *psychologically* groomed, this can lessen the likelihood they may disclose as they may be convinced the abuse is their fault, that no one will believe them, or that they will go to juvenile detention if they bring the concerns to light. With *physical* grooming, the contact will often begin as nonsexual touching and escalate to sexual touching as the relationship progresses. This will often desensitize the child victims and prepare them for increased sexual contact (Craven, Brown, & Gilchrist, 2006).

Grooming is a topic that is often neglected in discussion of child sexual abuse. Consider including information about this when working investigations of child sexual abuse to see if it helps paint a clearer picture of the child's experience. Imagine sharing with a jury that the reason a child didn't tell about the abuse is because she was provided free summer camp visits, given money and clothes, and promised a modeling career, and how much it would help them understand the dynamics of child sexual abuse and how abusive relationships are initiated and maintained. Participating in the relationship doesn't become the child victim's fault, but it does help us understand why it is complicated for the child to disclose or how the child may not realize the abusive relationship is inappropriate in nature.

Consequences Associated With Child Sexual Abuse

There is no checklist of characteristics that can be provided to you that all victims will exhibit or that are diagnostic of child abuse. Research and experience tells us that there are some commonalities among child abuse victims and some mental health concerns that can exist, particularly if trauma-related issues are not handled adequately.

According to research conducted by O'Leary, Coohey, and Easton (2010), mental health symptoms were related to a number of factors. Participants who were abused by more than one offender, who reported injuries due to their abuse, who were abused by a biological relative, and who did not disclose their abuse experience in-depth within 1 year of the abuse had a greater number of mental health symptoms.

Abuse victims and their parents often report varied symptoms following abuse experiences. Sometimes, children and their families report no significant difficulties or symptoms following abuse experiences and this may be due to protective factors (mentioned in an earlier portion of this chapter). Children who are victims of sexual abuse may experience internalizing (depression, anxiety, etc.) or externalizing (angry outbursts, bullying, etc.) symptoms. Some children may meet the criteria for various psychological disorders including posttraumatic stress disorder, major depressive disorder, oppositional defiant disorder, conduct disorder, and others. Some children may not meet the full criteria for disorders, but may have symptoms such as bedwetting, nightmares, crying spells, change in school performance, and irritability. Again, these disorders and symptoms can be present without a history of abuse, so these are not diagnostic and a psychosocial assessment can assist in developing a full clinical picture.

Consider This

Try to imagine the differing impact of gender on the way that children may feel about or even be willing to report the occurrence of child sexual abuse. What about males abused by females or males? What about females abused by males or females?

Treatment of Child Sexual Abuse

Treatment of the symptoms mentioned earlier will often include individual, family, and/or group psychotherapy and may involve the child victim, the nonoffender caregiver(s), and possibly siblings, if appropriate.

According to the National Child Traumatic Stress Network (2008), Trauma-Focused Cognitive Behavioral Therapy (TF-CBT) can be a highly effective treatment modality for children for not only abuse victims, but also for children who have experienced other forms of trauma. This treatment method follows the acronym PRACTICE and stands for **P**sychoeducation and Parenting Skills, **R**elaxation, **A**ffective Expression and Regulation, **C**ognitive Coping, **T**rauma Narrative, **I**n Vivo Exposure, **C**onjoint Child/Parent Sessions, and **E**nhancing Safety and Future Development. Each of these phases is flexible as to the time spent addressing each issue and based on the child and family's needs. This model seeks to provide therapeutic intervention to children who have experienced traumatic life events by providing new skills to help process and discuss thoughts and feelings surrounding the trauma. This method is the most well-supported and effective treatment for abused and traumatized children, so it is widely used in a therapeutic setting. It does require specific training, including participation in a learning collaborative, so clinicians who are adequately trained in TF-CBT can potentially do great work for children who are abuse victims. It is recommended that families are mindful of who they select as their therapist because some individuals may claim to be "trauma-focused" or "experts" in working with children who have experienced trauma, but they may have no specific training regarding these issues. Mental health is too important to risk seeing a clinician who is not adequately trained.

INTIMATE PARTNER VIOLENCE

Intimate partner violence (IPV) is an unfortunate phenomenon that many children witness on a regular basis. Professionals used to believe that the abuse had to actually happen to the children for it to impact them significantly; but, after years of research and experience, we now know that witnessing domestic violence can be as traumatic and damaging as actually experiencing abuse.

IPV, also known as domestic violence, is psychological, physical, or sexual harm by a significant other (current or former). Intimate partner violence, unfortunately, is also a common phenomenon, like other forms of child abuse and neglect. Children often witness these violent interactions and can be negatively impacted in many ways.

Unfortunately, those in violent relationships often stay much longer than is safe for them. There are various reasons for this, but a common reason is fear. In practice, we do see overlap among individuals who abuse children, their partners, and animals. Ascione (2000) examined 100 battered women and found that 50% of these women reported their partner had hurt or killed their pets and nearly 25% reported they delayed leaving because of concern for their animals. In these instances, animal abuse may have been used to gain control or silence from these women and likely kept them in harm's way longer.

Children who witness violence toward a parent may try to intervene and protect their parent and may get harmed because of this. Living in a constant state of fear can be detrimental to children in many ways and the unpredictability of their environment can be stressful and frightening. Wood and Sommers (2011) reported that children who witness intimate partner violence have short- and long-term consequences that impact their current and future relationships with same-sex peers and dating partners. Children may also exhibit symptoms of depression, anxiety, posttraumatic stress disorder, and externalizing and/or internalizing behaviors when they witness violent interactions in their home. Gender does appear to be a factor in symptomology as well, as Moretti, Obsuth, Odgers, and Reebye (2006) found. They reported that girls who witnessed their mothers engaging in aggressive behavior toward a partner exhibited more aggression in friendships. Additionally, boys who witnessed their fathers engaging in aggressive behavior toward a partner exhibited similar behavior in friendships. This suggests that modeling of the same-sex parent appears to predict hostility against friends. Witnessing chronic intimate partner violence or adding other forms of abuse directly to the child (neglect, physical abuse, sexual abuse, etc.) also may increase symptoms experienced.

Furthermore, witnesses to intimate partner violence may be at increased risk for intergenerational transmission of abuse; thus, intervening appropriately is crucial to stop the cycle of violence.

This information suggests that witnessing intimate partner violence may be as damaging as other forms of abuse, so professionals working in the field should consider how IPV impacts children and should inquire about other potential areas of concern (animal abuse) that may be occurring in the home to conduct thorough investigations.

Prevention of Child Abuse and Neglect

This chapter has included information about the widespread nature of child abuse and neglect, and the sad reality is that hundreds of thousands of children are impacted by child maltreatment on a regular basis. So, what can we do with this information? One thing that is important to talk about is prevention—we tend to be a "reactive" society where we wait for something to happen to care about or do something about it. We know that child abuse is an epidemic, so this next section discusses ways we can look forward and improve future generations' experiences in our community.

Because of the widespread nature of child abuse, prevention efforts emerged in the 1970s and increased in popularity in the 1980s. Prevention efforts varied, based on the type of abuse concerned. Efforts to prevent neglect or physical abuse often focus on adjusting caregiver behavior and increasing positive interactions between parents and their children. Efforts to prevent sexual abuse often focus on educating children about appropriate and inappropriate touches and cyber and personal safety. According to Wertele (2009), "most child-focused personal safety programs have these objectives in common: (a) helping children to *recognize* potentially abusive situations or potential abusers, (b) teaching children to try to *resist* by saying 'no' and removing themselves from the potential perpetrator, and (c) encouraging children to *report* previous or ongoing abuse to an authority figure" (p. 4). We need more than child-focused prevention efforts, however, because children cannot ultimately be the ones held responsible for their safety.

One of the difficulties surrounding prevention programs is the lack of evidence surrounding their efficacy at actually preventing abuse. Because of this, a comprehensive approach must be taken to reduce the number of children who experience abuse. Prevention programs; education for professionals, parents, caregivers, and those who interact with children; engaging the public in a "no tolerance" view of child abuse; and swift and strict punishment of offenders can be a start to reducing the number of child abuse victims. We must dispel myths about child abuse (i.e., stranger danger—although children can be abused by strangers, it is more likely someone they know) and provide useful information for our children about the facts of child abuse and ways to get help if they do fall victim. These conversations about child protection should occur early and often, so children feel empowered and comfortable with the knowledge they are given.

Child abuse is a reality that we should not have to discuss as an epidemic in 2014, but we have the ability to educate the public about child abuse, punish those who commit such crimes, and improve criminal and civil investigations when these crimes occur. As the next generation of professionals who work with children, remember how important your job is, even on the days when you are not sure why you decided to pursue a career in child protection. Frederick Douglass once said, "It is easier to build strong children than repair broken men." Remember this as you take on one of the most important tasks we can take on as a nation—protecting children. Child abuse will be discussed one day as a thing of the past and although many of us will not be around to see that time in our nation's history, to be a part of this movement will be one for the record books.

 Consider This

> Chapter 8 details what is known about true pedophiles and nonpedophilic abusers. Think through the problems that exist that make it difficult to provide complete protection for most of our children.

STUDY QUESTIONS

1. Define neglect and discuss the four types of neglect mentioned in the chapter.
2. Define physical abuse and discuss two risk factors that may lead to increased susceptibility to child physical abuse.
3. Discuss three consequences of physical abuse. How does age impact these consequences?
4. Why is emotional abuse so difficult to investigate in criminal proceedings?

5. How are body image issues/eating disorders related to a history of child abuse?

6. Define sexual abuse and discuss some of the statistical considerations mentioned related to child sexual abuse.

7. Discuss issues relevant to compliant victimization and child sexual abuse.

8. What is grooming and why is it important to understand as related to child sexual abuse?

9. Discuss how witnessing intimate partner violence impacts children.

10. Discuss prevention efforts and why these are important to child abuse and neglect.

GLOSSARY

abuse An act of commission; improper action toward other people that has the potential to hurt or injure them.

compliant victims People who cooperate and actively participate in their victimization but are legally unable to provide consent for these activities.

forensic interview A nonleading, objective, investigative interview with a child, typically ages 3 to 17, due to allegations of child abuse, child exploitation, or witnessing a crime.

grooming Techniques employed by offenders to initiate and/or maintain abusive interactions/relationships.

intimate partner violence Psychological, physical, or sexual harm by a significant other (current or former).

neglect An act of omission; failure to provide a necessary and adequate care to people who are unable to care for themselves.

physical abuse Nonaccidental trauma or physical injury caused by punching, beating, kicking, biting, burning, or otherwise harming a child; physical abuse is the most visible form of child maltreatment.

protective factors Characteristics that mitigate, or lessen, the impact of negative experiences.

sexual abuse Sexual intercourse or its deviations, sexually touching a child (such as fondling, making a child touch an adult's sexual organs, penetrating the child's sex organs in any way with any object), as well as nontouching offenses (exposing children to pornography, deliberately exposing a child to sexual acts, including masturbation) or sexual exploitation (soliciting a child for the purposes of commercial sexual exploitation/human trafficking).

REFERENCES

American Humane Society (n.d.). *Child neglect*, 1. Retrieved from http://www.americanhumane .org/children/stop-child-abuse/fact-sheets/child-neglect.html

Ascione, F. (2000). *Safe havens for pets: Guidelines for programs sheltering pets for women who are battered*. Logan, UT: Author.

Children's Bureau. (2011). *Child maltreatment 2011*, 1–251. Retrieved from http://www.acf.hhs .gov/sites/default/files/cb/cm11.pdf#page=28

Cichetti, P., Rogosch, F., Gunnar, M., & Toth, S. (2010). The differential impacts of early physical and sexual abuse and internalizing problems on daytime cortisol rhythm in school-aged children. *Child Development, 81*(1), 252–269.

Cloitre, M., Stovall-McClough, C., Zorbas, P., & Charuvastra, A. (2008). Attachment organization, emotion regulation, and expectations of support in a clinical sample of women with childhood abuse histories. *Journal of Traumatic Stress, 21*(3), 282–289.

Coohey, C., & Braun, N. (1997). Toward an integrated framework for understanding child physical abuse. *Child Abuse & Neglect, 21*(11), 1081–1094.

Craig, C. D., & Sprang, G. (2007). Trauma exposure and child abuse potential: Investigating the cycle of violence. *American Journal of Orthopsychiatry, 77*(2), 296–305.

Craven, S., Brown, S., & Gilchrist, E. (2006). Sexual grooming of children: Review of literature and theoretical considerations. *Journal of Sexual Aggression, 12*(3), 287–299.

Gaudin, J. (1993). U.S. Department of Health and Human Services. *Child neglect: A guide for intervention*, 1–103. Retrieved from https://www.childwelfare.gov/pubs/usermanuals/neglect_ 93/neglect_1993.pdf

Gover, A., & MacKenzie, D. (2003). Child maltreatment and adjustment to juvenile correctional institutions. *Criminal Justice and Behavior, 3*, 374–396.

Hill, A. (2003). Issues facing brothers of sexually abused children: Implications for professional practice. *Child & Family Social Work, 8*(4), 281–290.

Johnson, J. G., Cohen, P., Kasen, S., & Brook, J. S. (2002). Childhood adversities associated with risk for eating disorders or weight problems during adolescence or early adulthood. *American Journal of Psychiatry, 159*, 394–400.

Kilpatrick, D., Ruggiero, K., Acierno, R., Saunders, B., Resnick, H., & Best, C. (2003). Violence and risk of PTSD, major depression, substance abuse/dependence, and comorbidity: Results from the National Survey of Adolescents. *Journal of Consulting and Clinical Psychology, 71*(4), August, pp. 692–700.

Messman-Moore, T., & Garrigus, A. (2007). The association of child abuse and eating disorder symptomology: The importance of multiple forms of abuse and revictimization. *Journal of Aggression, Maltreatment and Trauma, 14*, 51–72.

Moretti, M., Obsuth, I., Odgers, C., & Reebye, P. (2006). Exposure to maternal vs. paternal partner violence, PTSD, and aggression in adolescent girls and boys. *Aggressive Behavior, 32*, 385–395.

National Child Traumatic Stress Network. (2008). *Trauma informed interventions*. Retrieved from http://www.nctsnet.org/nctsn_assets/pdfs/promising_practices/PCIT_General.pdf

National Child Traumatic Stress Network. (2009). *Child physical abuse fact sheet*. Retrieved from http://www.nctsnet.org/sites/default/files/assets/pdfs/ChildPhysicalAbuse_Factsheet.pdf

Olafson, E., & Lederman, J. C. (2006, Winter). The state of the debate about children's disclosure patterns in child sexual abuse cases. *Juvenile and Family Court Journal*, 27–40.

O'Leary, P., Coohey, C., & Easton, S. (2010). The effect of severe child sexual abuse and disclosure on mental health during adulthood. *Journal of Child Sexual Abuse, 19*, 275–289.

Rodriguez, C., & Tucker, M. (2011). Behind the cycle of violence, beyond abuse history: A brief report on the association of parental attachment to physical child abuse potential. *Violence and Victims, 261*, 246–256.

Rorty, M., Yager, J., & Rossotto, E. (1994). Childhood sexual, physical, and psychological abuse in bulimia nervosa. *American Journal of Psychiatry, 151*, 1122–1126.

Scarpa, A., Haden, S., & Abercromby, J. (2010). Pathways linking child physical abuse, depression, and aggressiveness across genders. *Journal of Aggression, Maltreatment & Trauma, 19*, 757–776.

Wertele, S. (2009). Preventing sexual abuse of children in the twenty-first century: Preparing for challenges and opportunities. *Journal of Child Sexual Abuse, 18*, 1–18.

Wood, S., & Sommers, M. (2011). Consequences of intimate partner violence on child witnesses: A systematic review of the literature. *Journal of Child and Adolescent Psychiatric Nursing, 24*, 223–236.

Zuravin, S. J., McMillen, C., DePanfilis, D., & Risley-Curtiss, C. (1996). The intergenerational cycle of child maltreatment: Continuity versus discontinuity. *Journal of Interpersonal Violence, 11*(3), 315–334.

6

Internet Exploitation of Children

GOALS OF THIS CHAPTER:

1. Readers will understand the history and evolution of technology and how it relates to Internet exploitation.
2. Readers will become familiar with the typical characteristics of Internet exploitation victims and perpetrators.
3. Readers will understand how to better protect children from online offenders.

> *CheerGurl98*: Lol, u know I can't do that . . . . . ☺*
>
> *GuitarMike14*: Come on, send a pic, I bet u r sexy with ur clothes off ;)*
>
> *CheerGurl98: **POTS, brb*
>
> *GuitarMike14: y don't u go to another rm?*
>
> *CheerGurl98: tbh, I'm scared to send a pic*
>
> *GuitarMike14: y would you b scared? U can trust me, I just want to c how sexy u r :->.*
>
> *CheerGurl98: what if some1 sees them*
>
> *GuitarMike14: u can make ur own decisions and if u don't want to b w/me, u can't keep leading me on like this*
>
> *CheerGurl98: ya, I've never been w/an older guy sry.*
>
> *GuitarMike14: age is just a number, I told u I'll never tell anyone—y don't u trust me!*
>
> *CheerGurl98: I do, pls don't b mad!*

---

*This is a fictional depiction of an online interaction between two individuals named Sarah and Joe for illustrative purposes. Any similarity to real individuals or cases is by chance and is not intended.

**POTS—Parents over the shoulder

BRB—Be right back

TBH—To be honest

SRY—Sorry

LOL—Laugh out loud

GuitarMike14: U aren't really gonna meet me tmrw, r u? R u not a sexual person? Do u not want to mess around like u said?

CheerGurl98: I do, I've just never had sex

GuitarMike14: we could have fun lots of other ways. do u want to?

CheerGurl98: I think I want to—u sure u r cool w/age thing?

GuitarMike14: ya, r u?

CheerGurl98: I just don't wanna get in trouble, ya know?

GuitarMike14: y would u get in trouble? i said i would never tell anyone—not their biz what we do.

CheerGurl98: so, u r gonna be at my school tmrw at 2? I am ditching art, so I shld b able to get out.

GuitarMike14: i got us a hotel rm so we can take some pics and then have some fun. Hope u can handle me, lol.

CheerGurl98: u promise not to show any1 the pics?

GuitarMike14: i sd i wouldn't and even if I do, its bc I want every1 to know how sexy u r.

CheerGurl98: ok ... i am just nervous.

GuitarMike14: don't b. i'll be gentle and u will like what u see. i can't wait to finally meet.

CheerGurl98: k, i am gonna go 2 bed. see ya tmrw.

GuitarMike14: can't wait, you won't be sry

CheerGurl98: k

The earlier list contains an example of an online chat conversation between Sarah, a 13-year-old female, and Joe, a 38-year-old male. Sarah and Joe had met a few weeks prior in a chat room for teenagers interested in meeting people. Before signing up to chat, participants are asked to check a box confirming they are less than 18 years of age. Joe told Sarah he was 21 and snuck into the chat room because he wanted to know if any teenagers might be interested in modeling for an agency he wanted to open. Sarah had always wanted to model and saw this as a perfect opportunity to get her foot in the door. Sarah's parents are not together anymore and her mom works constantly, trying to make ends meet. Sarah does not get much supervision and spends a lot of her time watching her younger siblings, Stephen and Sammy, ages 7 and 9. Sarah spends about 4 hours a day online and reports interacting with about 20 people over the last few months that she has never met in person.

Joe is the first person Sarah planned to meet in person and the first one to ask. Joe and Sarah started talking about modeling at first, but it quickly turned into discussions regarding sex, alcohol, and meeting up to get to know each other better. Sarah tried to avoid conversations of this nature on multiple occasions, but Joe would get upset; even threatening, from time to time. Sarah felt as if she was in way over her head, but when she considered discussing the situation with her parents, she was concerned that she would be found responsible.

Sarah decided to meet up with Joe the next day. Sarah was not entirely convinced she even wanted to meet Joe, but anytime she expressed concern or reservation, he would make comments that would make her feel guilty about doubting him. They had been talking for a while and she hoped she would not have anything to worry about, like Joe had said. Joe did not look 21, he looked older, but when Sarah questioned him about his age, he blew up. Things quickly escalated and before Sarah knew it, she found herself having sex in a local hotel room. Joe did not have a condom, but promised Sarah he would not "give her anything or get her pregnant." Sarah had never had sex before and felt like she had to trust Joe that he was telling her the truth.

A few weeks went by and there was virtually (pun intended) no sign of Joe. Sarah had tried messaging and texting him and he would never respond. Sarah was confused, particularly because she thought Joe truly cared about her, since he had said so many nice things about her.

Several weeks later, Sarah found out she was pregnant. As a result of meeting Joe in the chat room a few months ago, Sarah's life had changed forever. She had not listened to her gut instincts that something was not right with this situation and she was regretting that very much.

Sarah was not Joe's only victim. An investigation began shortly after Sarah discovered she was pregnant from her contact with Joe. Joe had lured other teenage girls through this website and had seven other victims, two of whom ended up pregnant by Joe. Only two of Joe's victims were cooperative with the investigation against him. Joe eventually pleaded guilty and was sentenced to 11 years in prison.

Were you able to completely understand the chat exchange between Sarah and Joe? If not, you are not alone. There are many acronyms used in chat rooms, email, web blogs, and text messages that can be difficult to understand and dangerous for children. Many people, even those who claim to be relatively Internet-savvy, are not aware of many of the popular acronyms and lingo available. How can we protect children from what we do not understand? This question continues to plague parents, child advocates, educators, and researchers.

This chapter is intended to provide you with information related to Internet child exploitation. This chapter just skims the surface with the information available, but it is my hope that you will enhance your own understanding of technology and how it relates to and perpetuates the abuse of children.

INTERNET EXPLOITATION AND EXPOSURE

It is no secret that children have been victims of abuse for many years. General research suggests that one in four girls and one in six boys will be a victim of sexual abuse before the age of 18 (Centers for Disease Control and Prevention, 2005). Prior to the widespread availability of the Internet, predators had to be in close proximity of children in order to gain access to victims. The instant communication available because of the Internet allows easy access to **child exploitation** networks; finding a victim may just be a mouse-click away. According to Harris Interactive-McAfee (2008), 63% of teens said they know how to hide what they do online from their parents. You remember being a teenager, right? Did you tell your parents everything that you did? Most people would say no and now it is much easier to hide interactions with others because we can now engage in relationships easily from the privacy of our own home. Children and teenagers are not just talking online with individuals; approximately 14% of students in 10th to 12th grades have accepted an invitation to meet an online stranger in person, which has the potential to be a dangerous situation.

In a survey conducted in 2008, Sabina, Wolack, and Finkelhor reported that 93% of boys and 62% of girls had been exposed to online **pornography** during adolescence. Additionally, these authors found that girls reported more involuntary exposure than boys, while boys reported being exposed to pornography at a younger age, seeing it more regularly, and seeing content such as rape and child pornography more frequently than their female counterparts (Sabina, Wolack, & Finkelhor, 2008). This is not to say that all exposure that children and teenagers have to exploitation materials is involuntary; however, the degree of exposure to abnormal and paraphilic sexual activity and materials is concerning and may have violated criminal laws, particularly the viewing of child pornography. Thus, even if children seek access to sexual materials, what they are exposed to may be more than they desired and may cause legal trouble as well.

With the increased use of smartphones, children and teenagers do not need access to a desktop computer or laptop to stay connected to the World Wide Web or send pictures to others. More than 14% of students, usually the same individuals who have accepted the invitations mentioned earlier, have invited an online stranger to meet them in person (Rochester Institute of Technology, 2008). If these strangers are child predators, inviting them to one's home or hometown puts the entire family and community at risk. We have to remember that children and teenagers are often **groomed** by child predators, so they often believe the person they are interacting with cares about them, may have promised them the world, and possibly have used threats or manipulation to get them to agree to do things they otherwise may not have. Additionally, predators will often groom parents, which can also maintain the abuse process. For example, a child predator might target a lower income family who is typically unable to afford much, aside from paying bills and making ends meet. A child predator might offer to buy the victim clothes, cell phones, computers, summer camp stays, or other enticing items to help alleviate the financial stress the family may be experiencing. The family may view the predator as generous, kind, and as an asset to the family, when the motive of the child offender is predatory. Material things can be quite important in the relationship, particularly to families that are unable to afford much on their own. The goods and services provided by the offender can become integral to the day-to-day functioning of the families and can be difficult to consider losing. In my experience, child predators have functioned as tutors, have bought multiple goods for victims and families, have paid for summer or church camp, have provided babysitting services, and so on. This phenomenon is one of many reasons that families also need to be educated about the manipulative and coercive behaviors that child predators will often engage in, so they can help keep their children safe. Families often report feeling blindsided and ashamed when they are taken advantage of by child predators; however, these predators are manipulative and good at what they do and can go undetected for significant periods of time.

Children are taught not to talk to strangers, but for many children and teenagers, those they interact with and "meet" online are not considered strangers and might mistakenly be identified as safe people for children and teenagers to be around. Additionally, people may be operating under a fake profile (also known as "catfish"), meaning they create a bogus profile and use false information (pictures, information, etc.) to lure children to develop relationships with them. The numbers of children and teenagers interacting with individuals they do not know online suggest that as technology becomes more advanced, so do the skills of children and teenagers using them.

Online child pornography/child sexual exploitation investigations accounted for 39% of all investigations worked under the FBI's Cyber Division in fiscal year 2007. Additionally, according to Internet Watch Foundation (2011), child pornography and exploitation is a growing crime and the content is becoming much more explicit. In 2011, it found 12,966 URLs on 1,595 individual child abuse domains (web addresses) and many were housed in the United States (Internet Watch Foundation, Annual Report, 2011). Additionally, like other forms of child abuse, child pornography is underreported. Technology is evolving so rapidly that policing these sites is nearly impossible; when one site is shut down, several more are being created simultaneously and law enforcement cannot keep up with the demand for these sites.

SEXUAL SOLICITATION

According to the National Center for Missing and Exploited Children (NCMEC, 2007), one in seven youth surveyed received unwanted sexual solicitations or approaches. Furthermore, approximately one-third of youth surveyed reported they had unwanted exposure to sexual material such as sexual pictures when Internet searches (unrelated to sexual material) were conducted. Similarly, 4% of all youth Internet users received aggressive sexual solicitations, which threatened to spill over into "real life" because the solicitor asked to meet the youth in person, called them on the telephone, or sent them offline mail, money, or gifts. More than 55% of children were solicited for photographs of themselves, with 27% of those requests being sexual in nature (NCMEC, 2007). Because many children and teens have regular access to cell phones, computers, and tablets, monitoring access can be a daunting task.

Children and teenagers are not just subject to what they would view as positive interactions when they interact with others online. One study that discusses youth experiences on the Internet is the Youth Internet Safety Study.

The Youth Internet Safety Study (YISS) found 31% of children and teenagers were targets of aggressive solicitation. Because this research was done several years ago, we can assume these numbers are somewhat higher at this point. In this instance, aggressive solicitation is defined as an aggressor attempting to make offline contact with youth. In these cases:

- Seventy-five percent of solicitors asked to meet youth in person.
- Thirty-four percent called youth on the telephone.
- Eighteen percent came to youths' homes.
- Twelve percent gave youth money, gifts, or other items.
- Nine percent sent offline mail (letters, etc.) to youth.
- Three percent bought travel tickets for youth (NCMEC, 2005).

What do all of these statistics mean to you? They mean Internet exploitation and crimes against children is a growing problem, and with child pornography becoming one of the fastest growing businesses online, protecting children has become a more difficult job than ever before. If you are considering a career in forensic psychology, social services, or criminal justice, it is important to know what you are up against. The next portion of the chapter discusses the evolution of technology and how it applies to Internet exploitation.

SEXTING

Because the Internet is readily available via computers, cell phones, tablets, and so on, ways to interact with others are almost endless. Sexting, or texting sexually explicit messages, photographs, or videos among individuals, has become an increasingly popular activity among children and teenagers. Some might argue that a 14-year-old girl sending a provocative picture to her 16-year-old boyfriend is not pornography, but this is inaccurate and in some states possession of child pornography is charged for offenses like these. The ease of sending pictures and videos is what makes sexting an even bigger concern; phone sex and sexually explicit letters and conversations have been around for generations, so as technology advances, so do the means of communication. Because of the digital footprint that is left once an image has been sent to someone else (or posted online), the image is there for good and cannot be "taken back." Some sexters may be required to register as sex offenders and appear on the sex offender registry at a young age, which has extremely negative consequences. Ostrager (2010) discusses restructuring of laws to include categories of sexting for juveniles to avoid prosecuting these individuals as adults when sexting crimes have been committed. Because of the cost involved with incarceration, some literature supports diversion or rehabilitative/educational programs in lieu of jail time when sexting has occurred. Consider this example: Jennie and Brandon, both 16, have been dating for a year. Jennie regularly sends Brandon sexually explicit pictures and messages, assuming they are for his eyes only. After a huge fight, Jennie breaks up with Brandon. Brandon is angry and decides to send the provocative pictures to 16 people, including Jennie's parents. Jennie's parents want to press charges against Brandon for possession and distribution of child pornography. If convicted, Brandon will have to register as a sex offender and will be prohibited to live in certain areas or work with children, among other things. What do you think? Does the punishment fit the crime in this instance? Should juveniles be tried as adults and should they be lumped into the same category as pedophiles? Some would argue that Jennie is also guilty in this instance; others would argue the actions were meaningless until Brandon purposely distributed these pictures in a malicious manner. This is another debate in the field of forensic psychology.

We want to share this information with children and teenagers and educate them about the penalties associated with these behaviors because we cannot always predict the legal ramifications of our actions. Any time someone sends or receives a picture that is sexual in nature of someone who is a minor, it could be considered child pornography. This is something we need to be enlightening children, teens, parents, and professionals about because many children feel immune to these considerations and do not consider the potential long-term consequences of their actions.

EVOLUTION OF INTERNET EXPLOITATION AND TECHNOLOGY

Technology has evolved rapidly over the past few decades and advancements make it more and more difficult to catch online offenders. Online resources such as peer-to-peer networks and file servers allow the transmission of illegal material to move faster, in significantly greater quantities, than ever before. Policing these sites is nearly impossible as these images can be hidden among what seem like harmless files. Additionally, software is available to erase electronic footprints and other proof of inappropriate behavior. Unprotected wireless networks are like a playground for offenders as they may secretly gain access to wireless networks to download pornographic material. This is one reason it is so important for individuals and businesses to password protect their wireless networks. Would you want child pornography downloaded to someone else's computer and linked to the IP address associated with your apartment or home? Certainly not.

And where is the downloaded material stored? If it were in obvious locations, the job of investigators would be much easier; however, surreptitious locations for data storage exist such as video game consoles, watches, and MP3 players.

Although it is convenient to have the Internet available 24/7, this can be as harmful as well; it makes access to children and teenagers much easier for child predators. According to Nurenberg (2002), Stevenson, who poses as an underage chat room visitor, reports that he has received as many as 30 hits within a couple of minutes, while in the chat rooms. Stevenson also reports that there is not necessarily a good or bad time when it comes to online predators because they are online all of the time. This is a frightening thought considering how easily accessible the Internet is for children and teenagers. The Internet is second nature to many individuals, who often use it as a significant means of communication and interaction with others; very few use it to only check email.

The World Wide Web has been available since 1989 and since that time, technology has evolved rapidly (Ferraro & Casey, 2005). Some of the more popular Internet applications include email, e-groups/mailing lists, discussion/bulletin boards, social media sites, chat rooms, instant messaging, web camera applications, and peer-to-peer file sharing networks. With so many options, online predators can "pick their poison," and easily gain access to thousands of children who may be using these applications for school research, to talk with friends, and so on. If you are not familiar with the applications mentioned earlier and more specifically, ways they can be utilized to lure children to predators, this is an important area to research when working in the field of child abuse. Policing these applications has become increasingly difficult as they are evolving so rapidly.

Consider This

Think through the changes in technology that have happened in the past 20 years, or even the past 10. Now imagine the technology that might be available in the next 10 or 20 years. Try to imagine how people (who are trying to protect children) will both create safety in current technology, and prevent ever newer ways for technology to bypass those attempts.

VICTIMS OF INTERNET EXPLOITATION CRIMES

Victimization in Internet exploitation crimes has been on the rise over the past decade and has become a multibillion-dollar revenue stream over the past decade (Federal

Bureau of Investigation, 2012; Gallagher, 2007; Internet Watch Foundation, 2011; NCMEC, 2007). Although no child is immune to victimization by Internet crimes, there are characteristics that many victims share. According to Gallagher (2007) victims (of cases examined) were most often females living in economically disadvantaged single parent or reconstituted family homes, ranging in age from below age 5 to adolescence. For many victims, Internet exploitation was not the first maltreatment they had experienced; there were some histories of sexual abuse. Victims and offenders were often related in some way; offenders were generally parents, extended family members, acquaintances, or individuals responsible for the care of the child. Therefore, the stranger danger we often talk about is providing a disservice to children in many ways; it is more likely the danger of child abuse occurs at the hands of someone they know.

Of the offenders arrested between 2000 and 2001, 83% had images involving children between ages 6 and 12; 39% had images of children between ages 3 and 5; and 19% had images of infants and toddlers under age 3 (NCMEC, 2005). The majority of victims were female and Caucasian in race. This would suggest that school-aged/prepubescent children are the most common victims associated with child pornography and exploitation crimes.

Research suggests that female victims tend to exhibit more internalizing behaviors, such as depression, anxiety, posttraumatic stress, and suicidal ideation (Feiring, Taska, & Lewis, 1999). Conversely, male sexual victims are more likely to have externalizing problems such as oppositional behavior, aggression, substance abuse, and impulsivity (Beitchman, Zucker, Hood, DaCosta, & Akman, 1991 in Wells & Mitchell, 2007; Kendall-Tackett, Williams, & Finkelhor, 1993). In support, Wells and Mitchell (2007) reported that a survey of mental health practitioners found differences among symptom presentation in child exploitation victims. Mental health practitioners reported that female clients concerns included depression, anxiety or phobias, a specific life stressor, suicidal ideation or attempt, parent-child conflict, disciplinary problems at home, social withdrawal, trouble making friends, failing grades at school, disciplinary problems at school, sexual victimization, and sexual acting out. Male youth clients experienced depression, anxiety or phobias, a specific life stressor, parent-child conflict, disciplinary problems at home, social withdrawal, trouble making friends, failing grades at school, disciplinary problems at school, aggressive acting out or conduct problems, and sexual acting out. For both genders, parent-child conflict was reported more than 70% of the time, so this suggests that when clinicians, teachers, and so on, see children with parent-child conflict, they may want to consider the possibility of child abuse or Internet exploitation as a reason for the conflict. Nonetheless, these symptom presentations are not diagnostic and may be indicative of other experiences, other than child abuse.

Taken together, these are imperative considerations when exploring treatment options for victims of child exploitation. The clinical presentation of male versus female victims is different and is important to consider in designing treatment plans and interventions and to avoid misdiagnosis—all children and teenagers who are abuse victims will not respond or behave the same way and this is important to identification and treatment of victims of child abuse and Internet exploitation.

PERPETRATORS OF INTERNET EXPLOITATION CRIMES

Let us start with a story about someone who was not only an online predator, but also a pedophile who offended many young boys in his community. Again, the names and nature of the situation have been changed to avoid identification to any actual cases, but this will help further illustrate the characteristics of online sexual offenders. A 13-year-old boy (we call him John) comes from a lower income family and begins a relationship with a tutor at his middle school and youth pastor at a local church who he met online a few months before he started tutoring at John's school. The tutor (we call him Steve) is a 24-year-old male who is very involved in his community and at face value, appears to be doing great things for young boys in the area. Steve reports he works for a local party planning company and having access to cell phones, gaming systems, iPods, and other materials left at parties he has worked. John thinks it is pretty cool this tutor also likes to party and that he is so nice to him. He offers to buy him some new clothes because of a bonus he got at work and even offers to let him borrow one of the extra cell phones the tutor has lying around his apartment. John comes from a hardworking family, but also a lower-income one, and he hardly sees his mom, who works two jobs as a single parent to three boys. Mom starts to wonder where her son is getting new clothes and a cell phone from, but feels thankful someone is willing to help her family out.

Once the relationship progresses, Steve asks John if he would like to stay the night at his apartment so they can hang out. Again, he thinks this is pretty cool that this tutor is being so nice to him; people his own age are too immature for him, the young boy believes. Once he starts hanging out at the tutor's apartment, Steve lets the boy drink alcohol, smoke cigarettes, and even watch pornography, which is something he is never able to do at home! One night, when John is preparing to go to sleep on the couch, Steve offers him his bed. The couch is pretty uncomfortable, so John jumps at this opportunity, assuming Steve will take the couch for a night. Once John gets situated in Steve's bed and is almost asleep, Steve comes into the room and is not wearing any clothes. He crawls into bed and starts touching John in his genital area and John is frozen; he does not know what to say or what to do, so he does nothing. Steve tells John to do some sexual things he is not comfortable with and when John tries to say no, Steve threatens to take his clothes back, take his cell phone back, and tell John's mom about his drinking, smoking, and other behaviors at his house. John feels stuck. He continues spending time with Steve to avoid getting into trouble and the sexual contact between them becomes more involved and John has no idea how he has gotten to this point.

Eventually, someone tells on Steve, because John is not his only victim. Steve has lured more than 40 young boys into relationships with him from a fake social networking profile where he portrayed a young female and he continued to exploit young boys by obtaining employment in agencies where he could have easy access to them. No one ever suspected the tutor, party planner, and youth leader to be a sexual predator, and the community was devastated by the news. When the boys were asked why they did not tell sooner, they reported videos being made of them of sexual contact and continued threats of exploiting these materials—these boys had fear of being labeled as homosexual and/or being held culpable for their actions. Fortunately, Steve was convicted of his crimes against many of the boys he offended and those boys and the community are on their way to healing from the devastation Steve caused.

The Internet can be used by offenders to establish contact with potential victims and can be a means to remain somewhat anonymous while doing so. How do we really know who we are talking online to is really who she says she is? Additionally, the Internet can be a tool aiding offenders in contacting other offenders or providing them with ways to research techniques and methods associated with maltreatment.

Gallagher (2007) suggests that offenders of Internet exploitation crimes may be males with low socioeconomic status and unemployed. In agreement, Reijnen, Bulten, and Nijman (2009) reported Internet offenders lived alone more often, were more frequently single, and rarely had children. Many may be divorced or separated and their ages typically range from late teens/early 20s to 60 or more years. Also, although most offenders identified as heterosexual, some identified as bisexual or homosexual (Gallagher, 2007). These offenders may also be married, with children, and with prominent positions in the community, so it is impossible to predict everyone who might be at risk for being an offender and we cannot rule someone out as an offender because they do not fit a profile of a "typical offender." I recall a case I worked years ago where an online child predator was married for years with two children who he had not offended. His wife was shocked and had no idea he was living a double life; this is why child predators can be so difficult to catch because they are often manipulative and secretive about their behaviors and actions and can go undetected for many years. The hypothesis that social isolation might lead to these behaviors does not fit the mold for someone who is married with a family. Some research suggests that social isolation and social skill deficits could lead to child pornography viewing and/or downloading, while others believe these individuals purposely isolate themselves to engage in these socially unacceptable behaviors (Reinjen et al., 2009).

Burgess, Mahoney, Visk, and Morgenbesser (2008) suggest the largest category of occupations associated with Internet offenders are people in positions of authority to the child like physicians, clergy members, or law enforcement officers, which aligns with other research that reports that sexual predators are often known to the child victim. When the child knows the offender, it can impede the disclosure process, due to complexities in the relationship. If the child is receiving benefits from the relationship such as money and gifts, or being threatened in some way, the reasons to keep the relationship a secret may outweigh the reasons to tell someone.

Reijnen et al. (2009) studied 22 child pornography offenders and compared them to more than 100 perpetrators of other types of crimes and found no distinct profile on the Minnesota Multiphasic Personality Inventory-2 (MMPI-2) for child pornography offenders as compared to other types of offenders. This means that with symptoms like "typical" associated with child victimization, we do not have a distinct profile of online offenders, which can make them harder to identify. Treatment of online offenders can be complicated due to the differences among offenders and their behaviors, preferences, and actions. Reijnen et al. (2009) did note that child pornography downloaders were younger than other sexual offenders but did not differ in average age from their nonsexual offending counterparts.

According to Malesky (2007), when examining behaviors of 31 individuals who had contacted or attempted to contact minors for the sexual purposes, "three-fourths of the participants monitored chat room dialogue and almost one-half reviewed online profiles of minors in an attempt to identify potential victims" (p. 1). The participants examined in Malesky's study (2007) reported being drawn to posts by children who mentioned wanting to engage in sexual contact with older men, demonstrated knowledge about sex or interest in sex, a user ID associated with their age (Susie, 13, for example), and/or a willingness to chat openly. Once the actual contact was established, many reported sending pornographic pictures to and engaging in explicit, sexual conversations with these minors. More than 80% of the offenders examined purposely entered chat rooms where they anticipated minor participation (Malesky, 2007). Child offenders scour the Internet looking for vulnerable children and once the children are engaged in conversation, these offenders have varying techniques to accomplish their goals. These are important points as children should be aware that the things they post online may entice child predators to contact them. A good rule of thumb is to avoid contact with individuals you do not know and if a conversation turns sexual in nature to immediately alert an adult. In my experience, children and teenagers frequently report "friending" someone they do not know on social networking sites and talking with strangers in chat rooms/messaging programs, so this task is easier said than done.

Reoffending or **recidivism** rate is a concern for offenders of all types, but particularly those who commit crimes against children. Offenders are often not caught until they have offended against multiple children and because some report a sexual preference toward children (versus adults) treatment can be difficult. According to Eke, Seto, and Williams (2011), predictors of new aggressive contact in offenders included prior offenses, younger age at first offense, and violent criminal history. For some of the offenders examined, about half of those on conditional release accessed the Internet and were in contact with children again upon their release.

✍ Consider This

Even adults can be lured into believing things others say about themselves on the Internet. How many Internet dates turned real have not been as imagined? Now think about reasons that children may be even more vulnerable to the Internet presentations of others. What makes adults more likely to be suspicious?

CHILD PORNOGRAPHY DEBATE

Some argue that child pornography is less harmful than actual abuse (Diamond, Jozifkova, & Weiss, 2011). The difficulty with this assumption is that there is research to suggest the overlap is quite high among actual offenders and possessors and viewers of child pornography. In a study of arrested child pornography possessors, 40% had both sexually victimized children and were in possession of child pornography. Between 2000 and 2001, of those arrested for child pornography possession, 83% had images involving children between the ages 6 and 12; 39% had images of children between ages 3 and 5; and 19% had images of infants and toddlers under age 3 (NCMEC, 2005). Although some argue that viewing child pornography might satiate the desire to actually engage in abusive behavior toward children, research suggests the overlap is extensive between viewers, possessors, and offenders. Supporting this, Seto, Cantor, and Blanchard (2006) found that child pornography offending is a better diagnostic indicator of pedophilia than is sexually offending against child victims. Additionally, Bourke and Hernandez (2009) found that Internet offenders of child pornography were significantly more likely than not to have sexually abused a child in a hands-on act and were more likely have more than one victim as well, with an average of 13.56 victims reported.

It appears that those who claim to be merely "collectors" of child pornography or those who believe child pornography is not as harmful as actually offending on a child, might consider the research in the studies mentioned above. Just as cocaine can be a gateway drug to other drugs, viewing, possessing, or manufacturing child pornography may be a gateway into committing other offenses against children.

APPLICATIONS FOR SMARTPHONES AND TABLETS

It is important to be familiar with applications (apps) available for smartphones and tablets that might replace or enhance features related to cell phones. In a quick search done this morning, more than 500 apps are available for the iPhone to send and/or receive picture messaging (more than 2,100 are available when searching for applications with just text messaging features). One particular app, SnapChat, allows for real-time picture chatting and control over how long a picture is viewable. For example, you can send a picture to a friend and the app will only make the picture viewable for 10 seconds; after 10 seconds, the picture will be deleted from your phone and the recipient's phone. At face value, this may seem like a great idea that might protect children and teenagers from sexual pictures being distributed over the World Wide Web. Although this is a potential benefit, it may be more of a temptation for a child or teenager to feel more comfortable in sending a picture to someone they do not know and tracking what is being done on cell phones and tablets becomes more challenging as well.

Parents may feel like they are protecting their children by turning text or picture messaging off on their children's cell phones, but with more than 2,500 apps available that can replicate this feature, children are still able to send and receive text messages and pictures freely.

GEOTAGGING

Geotagging (or geolocating) is a relatively new and unfamiliar phenomenon that has the potential for locating victims even more easily, by recording longitude and latitude of locations where pictures are taken and uploaded. According to Kuzma (2012), geotagging is the "process of storing longitude and latitude data within an image" (p. 55), and has become a common occurrence, with many websites (Photobucket, Flickr, Instagram, etc.) offering the tools to create and access such images. Author Rachel Fondren Happel argues that although this practice poses a danger to anyone, leaving them at risk for robbery or general privacy violations, children (either the subjects of the photo or in the background) are especially vulnerable due to their lack of consent or even knowledge about such pictures and technology. Consider an upcoming family vacation and how excited everyone would be for the trip—if every family member posts "two days until we head out to Mexico" with a picture of their new luggage, it can alert predators to the exact location of the family's home and when the home will be vacant.

Kuzma (2012) reports there are no direct laws that address geolocation privacy, and those that have been applied predate social networking sites and are therefore inadequate. It takes action on the part of the person taking the picture to remove geotagging, as it is often a default setting with many websites (how many of you knew about this?). Children likely do not know what geotagging is or the harms associated with it, which puts them at additional risk for online predators to locate them. Many smartphones, tablets, and applications associated with them come with the "location services" feature automatically enabled, so many children, teenagers, and adults are communicating their location to everyone around them without a second thought. Did you know that if you use a hashtag (#), a person on Instagram can pull up anything associated with that particular hashtag, even if they are not someone you know? For example, if I posted a picture with the hashtag #birthdaychick, anyone on Instagram searching for hashtags associated with chicks could see my photo and the exact location where I took the picture. This means that children and teenagers do not even have to say where the picture was taken; it is communicated for them.

This study identified the 50 highest-income zip codes in the United States and analyzed photographs of children uploaded to Flickr from these areas. Researchers found that each of the areas had an average of 116 photos of children that had been geotagged, leaving them susceptible to privacy violations and security risks. Thus, this is not a problem reserved for a particular socioeconomic status group and can impact anyone with a camera or a camera phone.

Kuzma (2012) concludes changes should be implemented by the Internet sites like Flickr that host such photos, legislation should be updated to address the needs of younger individuals, and users of these sites should be made more aware of the geolocation data so more informed decisions regarding their photos can be made. Until a legislative change can occur, education is key in this underresearched area to help better protect children. How many pictures have you taken that have been geotagged? How many of your followers on Instagram now know where your pictures have been taken? Most individuals have never heard of this concept, let alone are familiar with the dangers of this occurrence.

LEGAL ISSUES WITH INTERNET EXPLOITATION CRIMES

Legal issues exist when discussing Internet exploitation crimes, their victims, and their offenders. An important point raised by Lam and Seto (2010) suggests there is a disconnect between perceptions of offenders of crimes against children (in general and Internet-related) and what empirical evidence supports. This disconnect has implications for public policy and laws regarding management and punishment associated with sex offenders.

According to Rogers (2008), some view possession of child pornography as a victimless crime. Until we can come to an agreement regarding the harm of child pornography in general, prosecuting these crimes may be difficult. The author states that there is immense evidence supporting the theory that the U.S. criminal justice system believes child pornography possession is a victimless crime; we may not verbalize this, but by providing acquittals, lenient sentencing, and/or not prosecuting these crimes, we communicate this message. Researchers found an example of this when examining cases where child pornography possession had occurred. An elementary school teacher was found with 360 child pornography images in his possession, yet only received 4 months' imprisonment. Another individual possessed 68 images, some depicting infants being raped, but was only given 5 years of probation. Similarly, a case involving images of the rape of 2- and 3-year-olds, a defendant received a single-day sentence. Although these specific examples were eventually reversed, other cases were granted similarly lenient sentences. Educating juries about the dangers of possessing child pornography as well as the statistics associated with this leading to other crimes, is an extremely important duty.

According to a judge in New York, "a person can view hundreds of these images, or watch hours of real-time videos of children subjected to sexual encounters, and as long as those images are not downloaded, printed or further distributed, such conduct is not proscribed" (Ribeiro, 2012). What do you make of this thought? When much of the research supports the danger of child pornography, to have legislation that decriminalizes it may be a step in the wrong direction.

EVIDENCE COLLECTION

Preserving and collecting evidence properly is vital to investigations of this type. Ensuring evidence-collection materials (chat logging collection mechanisms, for example) are working properly is an important consideration. Additionally, educating yourself about suspected offenders to be able to more appropriately interact and/or interrogate them is a central concern as well. Slang terminologies are often used in the online environment, and becoming familiar with the terminology will help individuals conducting investigations.

Documentation must be done quickly, appropriately, and accurately. Any document created during an investigation can become part of a court record and this should be kept in mind when creating these documents. According to Ferraro and Casey (2005), documentation is particularly important when conducting thorough Internet searches, as some information obtained may be irrelevant and not pertinent to the case. A summary of helpful information can be useful to highlight important items found during investigative online searches. Collecting evidence often requires search warrants and these warrants require advance preparation to ensure successful evidence acquisition—and proper documentation is one step in the right direction.

WHERE DO WE GO FROM HERE?

What can be done to protect children from Internet crimes? As was previously mentioned, education is extremely important for children and those responsible for the care of children. We cannot fix what we do not understand and we must take time to educate ourselves about the continued threats associated with evolving technology.

Talk with local legislators to make changes to the things that are not working in your community. Megan's Law (sex offender registration), Jessica's Law (sentencing law in Florida), and other laws and acts have been created because individuals spoke up against an injustice to children.

Talk to children about the dangers of the online environment. Provide them with supervision, skills, and information that can help protect them from online predators. Let children know they cannot always trust the person sitting on the other end of the online conversation and that meeting someone in person is extremely dangerous.

Consider regular monitoring of Internet usage. Regular perusal of social networking contacts might be a useful tool. Ask children to list three things they know about their Facebook, Twitter, and MySpace friends and how they met their friends. If people request to be "friends" with children and they are strangers, encourage them to say no. The number of friends one possesses on these sites may provide bragging rights, but may also increase exposure to child predators and other unsafe individuals.

Teach children to limit personal information available online. Any personally identifying information can be ammunition for an online predator. Things such as full name, pictures, phone number, address, and school attended can provide offenders with information needed to locate a child. Remind children that information they post online or send from a cell phone may *always* be there. A decision they make at 13 years old may be something that haunts them for the remainder of their lives.

Additionally, educating children to be responsible when they use the Internet can be very helpful. Children who have been provided with safety tips are more likely to approach parents, guardians, teachers, counselors, and so on, with concerns or situations that have made them uncomfortable.

Once society becomes more comfortable discussing the topic of child abuse and, more specifically, Internet exploitation, we can present a united front against child predators. It is our responsibility to protect those who cannot protect themselves.

STUDY QUESTIONS

1. Discuss the history and evolution of technology and how it relates to child exploitation.

2. How prevalent is child exploitation? Why will we not ever know the true numbers associated with this form of abuse (like other forms of abuse)?

3. Describe the characteristics of a child exploitation victim. If they present in therapy, what will they "look" like?

4. Describe the characteristics of online sexual predators. How has the Internet perpetuated these types of crimes?

5. What is geotagging and why is it important in the discussion of child exploitation?

6. What are some considerations related to evidence collection for online crimes?

7. Discuss some of the legal issues related to child exploitation crimes.

8. Discuss the child pornography debate. Is looking at child pornography less harmful than hands-on offending? Why or why not.

9. How can we protect children from the dangers of the Internet?

10. Discuss sexting and the legal implications of this behavior.

GLOSSARY

child exploitation Possession, distribution, manufacturing, viewing, and so on, of child pornography; enticement of a child for sexual purposes, child trafficking, or tourism.

geotagging (geolocating) Identification of geographic location, including latitude and longitude, of an object, such as a home or picture.

groom (groomed, grooming) Process by which perpetrators manipulate and maintain the abuse process with the victims themselves and potentially, their parent(s). May come in the form of coercion, gifts, threats, and so on, and can engage and sustain the abuse with children.

pornography Visual recording of sexual abuse or sexual exploitation of a child or adult, often performing a sexual act or engaging in sexually explicit poses or actions.

recidivism Act of reoffending an undesirable act; tendency to relapse into a previous, undesired behavior or action.

sexting Sending sexually explicit messages, photographs or videos between individuals.

REFERENCES

Bourke, M., & Hernandez, A. (2009). The "Butner Study" redux: A report of the incidence of hands-on victimization by child pornography offenders. *Journal of Family Violence, 24*, 183–191.

Burgess, A., Mahoney, M., Visk, J., & Morgenbesser, L. (2008). Cyber child sexual exploitation. *Journal of Psychosocial Nursing, 46*(9), 38–45.

Centers for Disease Control and Prevention. (2005). *Adverse childhood experiences study: Data and statistics.* Atlanta, GA: Centers for Disease Control and Prevention, National Center for Injury Prevention and Control. Retrieved from http://www.cdc.gov/nccdphp/ace/prevalence.htm

Diamond, M., Jozifkova, E., & Weiss, P. (2011). Pornography and sex crimes in the Czech Republic. *Archives of Sexual Behavior, 40*, 1037–1043.

Eke, A., Seto, M., & Williams, J. (2011). Examining the criminal history and future offending of child pornography offenders: An extended prospective follow-up study. *Law and Human Behavior, 35*, 466–478.

Federal Bureau of Investigation. (2012). *Innocent images national initiative.* Available from http://www.fbi.gov/about-us/priorities/innocent-images

Feiring, C., Taska, L. S., & Lewis, M. (1999). Age and gender differences in children's and adolescents' adaptation to sexual abuse. *Child Abuse and Neglect, 23*, 115–128.

Ferraro, M., & Casey, E. (2005). *Investigating child exploitation and pornography: The Internet, law and forensic science.* Boston, MA: Elsevier Academic Press.

Gallagher, B. (2007). Internet-initiated incitement and conspiracy to commit child sexual abuse (CSA): The typology, extent and nature of known cases. *Journal of Sexual Aggression, 13*, 101–119.

Harris Interactive-McAfee. (2008). *The secret lives of online teens.* Retrieved from http://promos.mcafee.com/en-US/PDF/lives_of_teens.pdf

Internet Watch Foundation. (2011). *Annual report.* Retrieved from http://www.iwf.org.uk/accountability/annual-reports/2011-annual-report.

Kendall-Tackett, K., Williams, L., & Finkelhor, D. (1993). The impact of sexual abuse on children: A review and synthesis of recent empirical studies. *Psychological Bulletin, 113*, 164–180.

Kuzma, J. (2012). Children and geotagged images: Quantitative analysis for security risk assessment. *International Journal of Electronic Security and Digital Forensics, 4*(1), 54–64.

Lam, A., Mitchell, J., & Seto, M. C. (2010). Lay perceptions of child pornography offenders. *Canadian Journal of Criminology and Criminal Justice, 52*(2), 173–201. doi:10.3138/cjccj.52.2.173

Malesky, L. (2007). Predatory online behavior: Modus operandi of convicted sex offenders in identifying potential victims and contacting minors over the Internet. *Journal of Child Sexual Abuse, 16*(2), 23–32.

Ostrager, B. (2010). OMG! LOL! TTYL: Translating the law to accommodate today's teens and the evolution from texting to sexting. *Family Court Review, 48*(4), 712–726.

National Center for Missing and Exploited Children. (2005, 2007). *Child pornography statistics.* Retrieved from http://www.missingkids.com/missingkids/servlet/NewsEventServlet?Language Country=en_US&PageId=2064

Nurenberg, G. (2002). *Cracking down on online predators.* Retrieved from http://www.techtv.com/news/print/0,23102,3397013,0.html

Reijnen, L., Bulten, E., & Nijman, H. (2009). Demographic and personality characteristics of Internet child pornography downloaders in comparison to other offenders. *Journal of Child Sexual Abuse, 18*(6), 611–622.

Ribeiro, J. (2012). Viewing child porn on web not a crime in New York, court rules. *IT World.* Retrieved from http://www.itworld.com/internet/276358/viewing-child-porn-web-not-crime-new-york-court-rules

Rochester Institute of Technology. (2008). *Online abuse and crime by youth: Results from the Rochester Institute of Technology (RIT) survey of Internet and at-risk behaviors.* Retreived from http://www.enough.org/inside.php?tag=statistics

Rogers, A. (2008). Child pornography's forgotten victims. *Pace Law Faculty Publications, 28,* 847–863. Retrieved from http://digitalcommons.pace.edu/lawfaculty/541

Sabina, C., Wolack, J., & Finkelhor, D. (2008). The nature and dynamics of Internet pornography exposure for youth. *Cyber Psychology & Behavior, 11*(6), 691–693.

Seto, M., Cantor, J., & Blanchard, R. (2006). Child pornography offenses are a valid diagnostic indicator of pedophilia. *Journal of Abnormal Psychology, 115*(3), 600–615.

Wells, M., & Mitchell, K. J. (2007). Youth sexual exploitation on the Internet: DSM-IV diagnoses and gender differences in co-occurring mental health issues. *Child & Adolescent Social Work Journal, 24*(3), 235–260.

7

Process of Forensic Interviewing

GOALS OF THIS CHAPTER:

1. Readers will understand the purpose of child advocacy centers related to forensic interviews.
2. Readers will become familiar with some of the available protocols for conducting forensic interviews.
3. Readers will understand the mechanics associated with forensic interviews including controversies surrounding media for interviewing children.

Below, there is an excerpt of a portion of a forensic interview with an 8-year-old child. This interview is following the CornerHouse Forensic Interview Process (as of 2012), also known as RATAC. CornerHouse has recently updated their protocol to include more free narrative. Although the dialogue below is fictional, it is created using several years of forensic interviewing experience and is based on actual events.

Child:	Then, he touched it.
Interviewer:	Tell me about that.
Child:	About what?
Interviewer:	Tell me about when he touched it.
Child:	He put his hand on it.
Interviewer:	And then what happened?
Child:	He rubbed it and said, "Do you like that?"
Interviewer:	And then what happened?
Child:	I said I didn't like it and told him to stop.
Interviewer:	Where were your clothes?
Child:	They were off.

Interviewer: How did your clothes get off?

Child:　　　Daddy took them off.

Interviewer: And then what happened?

Child:　　　Then he started touching my pee pee.

Interviewer: (using the anatomical drawings). Earlier, when we talked about parts on the body, you called this (pointing to female genital area) a pee pee. Are you talking about that part or something else?

Child:　　　That part (pointing to female genital area).

Interviewer: What did he touch your pee pee with?

Child:　　　His hand.

Interviewer: Then what happened?

Child:　　　He rubbed my pee pee hard.

Interviewer: Did he say anything when this was happening?

Child:　　　He said that all daddies do this with their little girls.

Interviewer: Did he say anything else?

Child:　　　He said if I told Mommy about what he was doing that he would go to jail.

Interviewer: And then what happened?

Child:　　　He told me to touch it to make it bigger.

Interviewer: What did he want you to touch?

Child:　　　His thingy.

Interviewer: (using the anatomical drawings). Earlier, when we talked about parts on the body, you called this (pointing to male genital area) a thingy. Are you talking about that part or something else?

Child:　　　That part (pointing to male genital area).

Interviewer: Did you have to touch that part?

Child:　　　Yes, he made me.

Interviewer: Tell me about that.

Child:　　　He took my hand and put it on his thingy and made me rub it.

Interviewer: Was that on top of clothes or under clothes or something else?

Child:　　　Under clothes.

Interviewer: Did you see his thingy?

Child:　　　Yes.

Interviewer: Tell me about that.

Child:　　　It got bigger when I touched it and it was hairy.

Interviewer: What was daddy doing when you touched it?

Child:　　　He was moving my hand faster.

Interviewer: Then what happened?

Child:　　　Mommy got home, so Daddy rushed around and told me to go in the other room.

Interviewer: Is this something that happened one time or more than one time?
Child: More than one time.
Interviewer: Tell me about another time when something happened.

The **abuse** of children is a continuing problem in most communities. Few societies find sexual contact between children and adults to be morally appropriate and because of this, many states make such contact punishable with significant consequences, including lengthy prison terms and/or continuous identification as a sexual perpetrator against children. Accurately identifying the occurrence of child abuse is an extremely important duty. False negatives and false positives of alleged abuse can be equally problematic. According to Babiker and Herbert (1998), the cost of a false accusation is determined by decisions about the tradeoff between the two potential types of error: misclassifying children who are being abused and putting them at risk for future abuse versus misclassifying children who are not being abused and possibly subjecting them, their families, and others to unnecessary stress. It is important, when investigating allegations of child abuse, that procedural fairness is provided to the alleged perpetrator to reduce concerns of false accusations and convictions.

An important consideration of the criminal justice system is that the child victims are often the only witnesses to child abuse events and their testimony can be the key evidence in criminal proceedings. In an ideal situation, when children are asked to be witnesses and report on events, the experienced events would be recalled and reported in the most accurate manner possible (Fanetti & Boles, 2003). However, this is not always the case and there are many theories related to the inaccuracy of children's reports (see Chapter 4 for information about child memory). Obtaining accurate information from children about their experiences is important in enhancing safety in our communities as well as providing impartiality to those accused of child abuse crimes. It is important, for this reason and others, that child victims are interviewed by individuals who are adequately trained in **forensics**, child memory, **linguistics**, and so on. Children are not miniature adults and it is important to understand communication style, abilities, developmental considerations, legal implications, and suggestibility when engaging in investigative practices with children.

☞ Consider This

Try to imagine, using real people that you know, the various possible consequences for both false positives (people found to be guilty but did not abuse a child) and false negatives (people who did abuse a child but were acquitted of the charges). Either result can be very problematic for a child and the adults in their lives.

MULTIDISCIPLINARY TEAMS

Have you ever heard the saying, "There is no 'I' in team"? There is an "I" in multidisciplinary team (actually several), but the saying does ring true, even related to child abuse investigations. One person cannot do a child abuse investigation alone as effectively as a team could perform the same duties. The use of a multidisciplinary team allows for individuals to share investigative responsibilities and play on their strengths and rely on others for their weaknesses. **Multidisciplinary teams** (or MDTs as they are commonly called) are teams composed of law enforcement officials, child protective services (CPS or children's division [CD] in some states) personnel, child advocacy center staff, juvenile office investigators, attorneys, and others as appropriate. According to Pence and Wilson (1994), the use of multidisciplinary teams to conduct joint investigations is not a new concept and can be used to share case information, discuss information, and share investigative responsibilities. The use of multidisciplinary teams during child abuse investigations can increase efficiency, help lessen duplication of efforts, and may reduce **trauma** to children and families by promoting interagency cooperation and communication. Multidisciplinary teams can build on the skills and abilities of its members and can provide support to both its members and the children and families they work with. Using a team approach to conduct investigations can allow for team members to share duties and responsibilities and can provide opportunities for improvement by reviewing cases after completion for strengths and weaknesses to improve future efforts. Multidisciplinary teams often participate in the investigative process from beginning to end and can be present during forensic interviews. A nice benefit of multidisciplinary team members' attendance at forensic interviews is that it may reduce the number of times children are asked to report their story and can allow for cooperation and communication between the forensic interviewer and the remainder of the MDT members. The remainder of this chapter discusses forensic interviews and some of the research associated with this investigative interaction.

FORENSIC INTERVIEW CONSIDERATIONS

Forensic interviews are one method of gathering information from children who are alleged victims of abuse. A **forensic interview** is an interview with a child, typically between 3 and 17 years of age, who is an alleged victim of abuse or witness to such a crime. Forensic interviews vary in location, length, and protocol, but are often conducted in child advocacy centers. Child advocacy centers (or CACs) were introduced in the 1990s as a way to offer child-friendly options for forensic child-abuse investigations. Currently, more than 800 child advocacy centers are in operation in the United States (National Children's Advocacy Center, 2012). Child advocacy centers vary on the specific services they provide, but two of the most common services provided by these agencies are forensic interviews and medical examinations.

A mission of child advocacy centers is to reduce further trauma by limiting the number of interviews and investigative exposures child victims experience while providing a child-friendly and comfortable environment. If, during an investigation, a child's trauma can be reduced or eliminated because of good investigative practices, this is a success for the multidisciplinary team and the criminal justice system as a whole.

Although there are several popular, research-based protocols available for questioning children, these protocols have more similarities than differences. Before learning about the individual protocols available, it is important to set the stage by discussing some general considerations related to questioning children to assist in your understanding of why these protocols were developed and how they are executed.

SUGGESTIBILITY

Suggestibility is the degree to which someone responds to and is influenced by suggestions made by someone or something. Research suggests that younger children are typically more susceptible to suggestive questioning techniques than older children and adults (Bruck & Ceci, 1999; Garven, Wood, Malpass, & Shaw, 1998). However, some research suggests that suggestive questioning can also influence older children. In fact, even children older than 6 years of age may be susceptible to suggestion about a wide range of topics (Bruck & Ceci, 1997). Have you ever fallen victim to a suggestive selling technique? Many of us have purchased an item that would provide us with longer, stronger hair, or a more desired physique, or have joined a pyramid scheme in hopes of becoming a millionaire. We know these items are not likely to work as painlessly and easily as they suggest, but despite our better judgment, we often succumb to suggestive selling techniques. This supports research that even adults can be influenced by suggestive techniques. Even the accuracy of adults' recollections of events may be compromised by suggestive questioning techniques (Loftus & Pickrell, 1995).

According to Lyon (2002), "children with stronger memories are less susceptible to repeated questions" (p. 25). Repeated questions can decrease accuracy of reports and can be related to suggestibility concerns. Additionally, Lyon suggests that children will be less likely to change responses (when asked repeated questions) when the detail is related to a major event or detail as compared to a trivial event or marginal detail (Lyon, 2002). It is important that professionals remember suggestibility research and avoid questioning techniques that may be more susceptible to suggestibility, such as repeated or developmentally inappropriate questions, which may lead children to changing their responses or guessing to provide an answer.

TRAUMA AND MEMORY

Some research has been conducted to examine whether a traumatic experience or a series of traumatic experiences impact the memory of children. We cannot remember or report what we do not encode, so research has been interested in how trauma relates to memory in children. Does trauma damage or strengthen memories?

According to Berliner, Hyman, Thomas, and Fitzgerald (2007), memories for traumatic events may be shallowly encoded, which may lead to hazier or less salient memories. Additionally, cognitive avoidance strategies may be used by someone experiencing a traumatic experience (i.e., dissociation), which may decrease encoding of certain details associated with the experience. For example, if during a rape a child cognitively goes to her "happy place" during the incident and starts picturing she is at the circus, she may not encode all of the stimuli available during the event itself. Have you ever tried to think about something else when something bad was about to happen to you? For many, considering a visit to the doctor and a subsequent shot might elicit a memory where you did something to try to keep your mind off of something that is unpleasant. We do not like to experience pain or suffering and may do things to try to protect ourselves from negative experiences. If we do this while the negative event is occurring, it may change our perception and memory of the experience. Additionally, as time passes, our memories often become less detailed, with some small details being difficult to recall at all.

This is not to suggest that reports made by children who have experienced trauma are inaccurate—it is important to note that there may be errors in sequencing, time frame, and lack of certain details, but this does not mean the report as a whole is necessarily inaccurate. Children who have experienced trauma may report less sensory or coherent detail in reports of their experiences (Berliner et al., 2007).

Some research suggests that trauma may not significantly impact memory or reports of abuse incidents. According to a study conducted by Valentino, Cicchetti, Rogosch, and Toth (2008), abused and maltreated children did not differ in the occurrence and frequency of false recall, when compared to their nonabused counterparts. This would suggest that trauma may not significantly impact memory or reports of experiences. These authors found, consistent with other research, that maltreatment does not appear to obstruct or negatively impact development of basic cognitive skills (Valentino et al., 2008). The findings from their research suggest that the experience of maltreatment does not increase or decrease susceptibility to false recall.

In agreement, Chae, Goodman, Bederian-Gardner, and Lindsay (2011) found that abuse status (abuse versus neglect histories, etc.) had less to do with noted memory differences than did self-reported trauma symptoms, age, and psychopathology.

Taken together, research is mixed when examining trauma and memory relationships in children. Overall, research appears to agree that abused children are not more susceptible to providing false information regarding their experiences, but may have less detail and coherence to their reports due to varying factors.

TECHNIQUES AND OTHER CONSIDERATIONS

The form of a question may also influence a child's responses in an interview. Dale, Loftus, and Rathbun (1978) attempted to determine whether preschoolers' responses to yes/no questions are influenced by very subtle differences in the form of questions. Their results suggest that if a question was asked about a thing that was present in the experimental film, the manner in which the question was asked did not have a significant effect. However, if a question was asked about a thing which was *not* present in the film, the form of the question significantly affected the probability of a yes response. It is believed that children in this study were able to infer the interviewer's belief about the existence of objects (which did not really exist) by using specific identifiers in the questions (e.g., "the" object) rather than nonspecific identifiers ("an" object).

Using more coercive questioning styles, Thompson, Clarke-Stewart, and Lepore (1997) examined the influence of suggestive interviews on young children's reports of an adult's [janitor] behavior. The results of their research demonstrate that suggestive interviews can dramatically alter children's reports and recollections of a personal experience with an adult. Children who were interviewed in a neutral manner interpreted the janitor's actions correctly and children who were interviewed in a suggestive manner interpreted the janitor's actions correctly only when it was consistent with what the interviewer had suggested. The suggestion in this case is revealing to the child the "beliefs" of the interviewer about what had happened. In both cases, interviewers were able to increase the probability of memory errors in children by allowing the children to infer what the interviewer believed had happened.

Next, the use of open-ended versus closed-ended questions also appears to affect event recall, especially in forensic settings such as child sexual abuse assessments, like forensic interviews. Children make more detailed disclosures when asked open-ended (i.e., narrative) questions, especially in the beginning stages of a forensic interview (Dale, Loftus, & Rathbun, 1978; Lamb, Orbach, Hershkowitz, Esplin, & Horowitz, 2007; Sternberg, Lamb, & Hershkowitz, 1997; Wood & Garven, 2000). Some researchers have found that open-ended questions may yield responses up to 3 times longer and more detailed than other forensic interviewing techniques without negatively impacting accuracy (Wood & Garven, 2000). Interviewers sometimes may not ask open-ended questions because they may be trained to look for evidence to support their opinions about a situation or they may get into habits of asking more direct questions than open-ended. Try this: Ask your parent, spouse, roommate, boy/girlfriend, friend, and so on about their day. Ask questions that are only open-ended—start with "Tell me everything about your day from beginning to end." How much information did you get by asking that question? Now, ask people about their day, but use only yes/no or forced-choice questions, start with—"Did you sleep well? Did you eat breakfast? Did you have cereal for breakfast?" The amount of information you get is likely smaller and less specific and you had to do a lot more work! People are more inclined to tell us more when we ask open-ended questions, versus forced-choice. We should keep this in mind when asking questions of children in the forensic setting, as they often respond well to open-ended question types. This does not mean that there is no place for directed questioning, just that questioning styles more likely to yield accurate and complete data should be utilized first. Once those question types are exhausted, being more specific can be beneficial and elicit additional details. A good analogy when considering question types and forensic interviews is an *accordion*—start with an open-ended question, move into a more specific question as necessary, and then open the discussion back up with an open-ended question, and so on.

Now that you have a better understanding about questioning types, research related to suggestibility, and areas of caution, this next section discusses specific protocols available as well as tools utilized to conduct forensic interviews. This list is not comprehensive, but discusses frequently utilized interviewing protocols, as well as popular media used to communicate with children during forensic interviews.

 Consider This

Using what you know of memory and suggestibility (from this and earlier chapters), try to explain how children might come to believe in a version of events that does not reflect what actually happened. How is this even possible?

FORENSIC INTERVIEWING PROTOCOLS

The next section describes some of the protocols available to conduct forensic interviewing, but is not an exhaustive list. These protocols have many similarities and some differences and are often used based on jurisdictional preference. It is important for individuals conducting forensic interviews to be trained in a research-based protocol like the following.

National Children's Advocacy Center Forensic Interviewing Protocol

The National Children's Advocacy Center (NCAC) opened in 1985 in Huntsville, Alabama and had a goal of developing a more effective way to interact with child victims.

Prior to the development of the first child advocacy center, children would be interviewed multiple times, by individuals who were not always properly trained, and in environments that were not appropriate for children. With the development of the child advocacy center, came the development of the *NCAC Forensic Interviewing Protocol*, a semi-structured process of interviewing child victims. Additionally, the National Children's Advocacy Center also trains professionals using a multidisciplinary team approach to investigating alleged crimes against children.

Leading questions are discouraged in NCAC's protocol, like all others that are discussed in this chapter (and likely any protocol utilized in the United States). Operationally defining what a leading question is and how to avoid using them within interactions with children is an important consideration for those training professionals to question children. A leading question is a question that suggests an answer to the interviewee. For example, "Mommy hit your arm in the bedroom, didn't she?" would be deemed a leading question as it suggests an answer to the interviewee. A forensic interviewer should always avoid leading questions to avoid contamination of the interviewee's report. Interviewers are even encouraged to avoid leading questions in rapport building phases as this can set the stage for children feeling as if they must agree with the forensic interviewer. Something that may seem harmless like, "Well, these are comfortable chairs, aren't they?" can ask for agreement and can set up a dynamic where the children feel like they must agree with the person conducting the interview. It is important to be careful with all questions and responses, start to finish in a forensic interview, to avoid issues. As was mentioned previously in this chapter, open-ended questions should be attempted first, if the child is developmentally able to respond to those types of questions.

The phases in the NCAC protocol include introductions, rapport building, developmental screening, question formation guidelines, transition questions, abuse-specific inquiry guidelines, obtaining details regarding any disclosure(s) made (using open-ended narrative or narrative inquiries), and interview closure (Steele, 2003). Due to the semi-structured nature of this protocol, all phases may not be used in each forensic interview and the order of the phases may change based on individual needs (age, development, etc.) of the child being interviewed. Some children know why they are participating in a forensic interview and may be prepared to discuss allegations at the beginning, while others may need additional time building rapport to feel comfortable and interviewers have the liberty of adapting the protocol accordingly.

CornerHouse Forensic Interview Protocol

In 1989, CornerHouse, a private, nonprofit child advocacy center opened in Minneapolis, Minnesota and soon after came the development of the *CornerHouse Forensic Interview Protocol*. Professionals trained between 2005 and 2012 who were trained in this protocol referred to its phases as **RATAC**, which stands for **R**apport, **A**natomy Identification, **T**ouch Inquiry, **A**buse Scenario, and **C**losure, each representing a phase in the interview process (CornerHouse Interagency Child Abuse Evaluation and Training Center, 2013). It has recently been amended based on research related to best practice in the forensic interviewing field. The protocol increased their use of open invitations/free narrative early in the interview and redefined their closure phase. Their phases now are referred to as Build Rapport, Seek Information, Explore Statements, and End Respectfully (Anderson et al., 2013).

It is also a semi-structured protocol that allows for the cognitive, behavioral, developmental, and social abilities of each child who is interviewed using this method. During this interview process, use of anatomical drawings or anatomical dolls may be appropriate. These tools are discussed later in this chapter.

According to Anderson et al. (2013), CornerHouse partnered with the National Child Protection Training Center (NCPTC) and has reportedly trained more than 23,000 professionals from 48 states and 9 foreign countries. The training related to this protocol is referred to as Child First, formerly Finding Words. Similar to the National Children's Advocacy Center, providing training and continuing education opportunities to multidisciplinary team members is a goal of their agency.

CornerHouse suggests there are various question types available for use in forensic interviews. By using the "Process of Inquiry" as a means of understanding the different types of questions available in forensic interviews, we can gather a better understanding of these question types (Anderson et al., 2010). Free recall, focused recall, multiple-choice, yes/no, and leading (or misleading) are the question types Process of Inquiry discusses. Ultimately, the discretion of question type is the choice of the forensic interviewer, but like NCAC, CornerHouse cautions against the use of leading questions. Additionally, CornerHouse suggests age, ability, and developmental or cognitive concerns can influence the appropriateness of a question type. They recommend a "balanced" use of open-ended and "focused" questions to minimize suggestibility.

One difference between CornerHouse and other available protocols is the introduction of rules during a forensic interview. CornerHouse does not provide an introduction of interview rules at the onset of the interaction; rather, it provides an explanation of the rules at a more natural part in the interview. Said another way, rather than telling children at the beginning of the interview that saying "I don't know" is okay if they do not know the answer to a question asked, the CornerHouse method waits for the child to say "I don't know," and then encourages the child to say "I don't know" from that point further. Something like, "It's okay if you don't know. I just want to know what you do know. If there is anything else I ask you that you don't know, you can tell me that," might be a way to have this discussion.

State of Michigan Forensic Interviewing Protocol

Poole and Lamb (1998) created a forensic interview protocol that has been adapted by the state of Michigan with permission from the American Psychological Association. This phased interview protocol has similar beliefs as other protocols that have been discussed in this chapter related to audio/video recording, number of interviews, avoiding use of leading questions, and so on (State of Michigan, 2008).

According to the State of Michigan protocol (2008), interviewers should be hypothesis-testing rather than hypothesis-confirming, be child-centered, avoid making promises, avoid suggesting feelings to the child, and stay relaxed throughout the interview to avoid adding additional stress on the child. There are eight phases of this protocol, which allows for a semi-structured, but organized interaction with the child.

Interviewers do have the ability to make the interview more personalized based on the child's age and needs, as is the case in the other protocols discussed in this chapter. This phased protocol does not recommend use of anatomical drawings or dolls to elicit disclosures due to the controversy surrounding these tools. Authors report these tools can be suggestive and lack diagnostic ability (State of Michigan, 2008). This is discussed more fully in the Media for Interviewing Children section of this chapter.

National Institute of Child Health and Human Development Protocol

Another available protocol for forensic interviewing was developed by the **National Institute of Child Health and Human Development (NICHD)**. According to Lamb et al. (2007), this protocol contains all phases of an investigative interview. This protocol is structured, as compared to the previous protocols discussed, meaning there are specific questions and interactions that are intended to take place during each stage of the forensic interview. Some argue that a structured protocol may reduce the likelihood of the use of leading questions (since specific question wording is provided to the interviewer), which may be true; however, one pitfall to structured protocols may be a lack of flexibility. Essentially, this protocol acts similar to a decision tree in that the interviewer determines which question to ask next dependent on the response the child gives. Only after free-recall prompting has been exhausted, will interviewers move to more directive questioning.

This, like other interviewing protocols, requires significant training to utilize most effectively in the forensic interview setting. It is extremely important that directions are followed closely to implement this protocol appropriately.

Extended Forensic Interview Model (NCAC and RATAC)

Because many children experience chronic or multiple abuse events, there is some concern about allowing one opportunity to share their story (referring to a one forensic interview model) is sufficient. There is growing popularity in the use of the extended forensic interview model (formerly known as the forensic evaluation model) when allegations of abuse arise, but these extended interviews are not available in all states and jurisdictions. This is a "multiple-interview" model that allows children more than one opportunity to disclose abuse and may be in various ways in a criminal investigation. An extended interview model might be beneficial or appropriate if children are unable, unprepared, or unwilling to disclose about their abuse experience in a single forensic interview; if children present with positive medical findings indicating sexual contact, but have not disclosed; or if children simply need more time to disclose their experience fully and accurately.

As was mentioned previously in this chapter, there can be dangers associated with multiple interviews and/or repeated questioning of children. On the other hand, research is available that supports the notion that children who have been abused may not be willing to disclose this given the short-term nature of the relationship presented in a one-interview model (Olafson & Lederman, 2006; Sorenson & Snow, 1991). The intention of extended interviews is not to repeat a forensic interview, but to spread the interview process over a greater amount of time and reduce rapport-barriers such as lack of trust. Extended forensic interview protocols keep similar considerations in mind as single forensic interviews and, in fact, the stages in the extended forensic interview model are designed to be similar to those that take place during single forensic interviews. Multiple interviews are not fundamentally more suggestive, but it is imperative to consider the increased possibilities of contaminating or suggestive interviewing techniques that could take place during multiple contacts with children (Rooy, Lamb, & Pipe, 2009, in Kuehnle & Connell, 2009).

To be a forensic interviewer in many states, it is not required that the person be a mental health professional. Forensic interviews are significantly different from therapy; so many CACs do not require advanced training in psychology as a job requirement. According to Carnes (2001), professionals who conduct extended interviews are intended to be mental health professionals with training similar to those who conduct single forensic interviews in subjects related to forensics, linguistics, suggestibility, and so on.

TRUTH/LIE DISCUSSION

Another topic of concern in forensic interviewing research is related to the promise to tell the truth during the forensic interview. Research suggests that asking a child to promise to tell the truth does not always increase the veracity of their statements. Due to the brevity of the truth-lie discussion that occurs in forensic interviews, some researchers suggest that a discussion like that does little to increase truth-telling behaviors within the forensic interview (Huffman, Warren, & Larson, 1999). Researchers found that study participants who were given an extended truth-lie discussion did provide more accurate details, thus suggesting that forensic interviews may benefit more from prolonged explanations of truth versus lies (Huffman et al., 1999). Poole and Lamb (1998) suggest that inappropriate truth-lie discussions may make children appear less credible and should be used with caution.

Other research suggests that even brief truth-lie discussions may be beneficial (London, 2001). In agreement with Huffman, Warren, and Larson (1999), London (2001) found that whether children could articulate an understanding of truth versus lie did not predict their veracity or measure competency to participate in court proceedings. If a truth-lie discussion occurs, one that demonstrates the competence of the interviewee and takes age, development, linguistic, and cognitive abilities into account should be utilized. This may help demonstrate children's competencies to enhance acceptance of interviews as evidence in court proceedings.

Wandrey, Quas, and Lyon (2012) conducted a study and found that children are better at identifying truthfulness or dishonesty when the acts they are questioned about are good/positive. Essentially, these authors report that including bad behavior in truth-lie scenarios may underestimate children's abilities related to their understanding of the meaning of lying. It is suggested, in the literature, that children's understanding of lying may be so broad that it also includes bad words, mistakes, immorality, and so on (Peterson, Peterson, & Seeto, 1983; Piaget, 1932/1965 in Wandrey, Quas, & Lyon, 2012).

In summary, valence can impact children's understanding of truth versus lie and particularly when considering this from the legal standpoint, we should keep this in mind when performing forensic interviews, doing competency assessments, and interacting with children in general.

MEDIA FOR INTERVIEWING CHILDREN

Due to the sensitive nature of child abuse topics, helping children discuss abuse allegations can be a difficult thing. Imagine talking to a stranger about one of the worst experiences of your life? This is what children face when they participate in a forensic interview.

One way children can communicate is through the use of media in a forensic interview setting. The use of tools, when used properly and with appropriate training, may assist in recall, comfort, and communication. There is some controversy surrounding the various tools available for use in the forensic setting and some of those concerns are also discussed later.

DRAWINGS

Because children lack vast communicative abilities, they may be more comfortable and/or competent using art, drawings, or other media to assist them during the forensic interview. According to Anderson et al. (2010), reporting from clinical experience and research, drawings can provide an additional communication tool for children, may reduce the intensity of the forensic interview at various stages, and may also assist in clarification. The CornerHouse Forensic Interview method uses Face Pictures with younger children to check for abilities associated with making a representational shift, an ability necessary to utilize anatomical dolls (which are discussed shortly). A representational shift is a person's ability to see an object as a representation of him or herself (Anderson et al., 2010). Additionally, Family Circles, where children are asked to discuss their living situation, can invite communication and clarification, as well as build rapport. Drawings may be used throughout forensic interviews as a tool for children who cannot or are not willing to verbally articulate an experience. If a child is having difficulty describing the setup of a room, for example, it may be a useful communication tool to ask the child to draw a picture of the room to allow for clarification.

Poole and Bruck (2012) found no evidence that interviewing props made children more comfortable than verbal questions alone, so it contradicts the thought that drawings and other media might put children at greater ease and elicit more detail during a forensic interview. There is certainly much more debate surrounding body diagrams and anatomical drawings than other types of drawings, and those controversies are discussed in the next section of this chapter.

ANATOMICAL/HUMAN FIGURE DRAWINGS

One tool available for use during forensic interviews is **anatomically detailed (or human figure) drawings**. Typically, when anatomically detailed drawings are utilized in forensic interviews, it can be used to determine the child's ability to differentiate between genders, arrive at a common language for names of body parts, and as a clarification tool. Anatomical drawings might "break the ice" in a sense, too; if names for body parts are discussed and no one gets in trouble or overly embarrassed, children may be more comfortable discussing these body parts, if necessary, at a later point in the forensic interview. According to Anderson et al. (2010), anatomical drawings have been identified as a popular tool for use in the forensic interview, so they are widely used. For example, if a child discloses his private part was touched, an anatomical drawing could be used to clarify what private part he is talking about. For many children, "private part" might represent multiple parts on their bodies and criminal charges can vary based on where touching took place, so making assumptions is not a good idea in the forensic interview setting.

Prior to 2000, research on anatomical dolls and diagrams supported their use, but following 2000, much research that has occurred is fairly critical and cautionary regarding their use (Lyon, 2012). In some research, anatomical drawings have been reported as unhelpful, have elicited false reports of touching, and therefore, may be leading. Poole and Dickinson (2011) suggest use of open-ended questions regarding touch prior to using a body diagram and caution against body diagram use in early phases of forensic interviews. This supports research that suggests using anatomical drawings as a last resort with older children and avoiding them with younger children, if possible. Aldridge et al. (2004) reported that following an exhaustive verbal interview, the use of anatomical drawings elicited additional information from the children in the study, but it was unclear if the information was reliable or not. Brown, Pipe, Lewis, Lamb, and Orbach (2007) caution against the use of dolls after an exhaustive verbal interview because in their research, body diagrams did not elicit more information than verbal questions alone and did not appear useful when introduced at later points in the interview. As you can tell, research is mixed in this arena.

In the end, there is research to support both schools of thought and both sides make valid points. This research often comes into question when discussing reluctant, embarrassed, tentative children because they may benefit most from an additional tool to aid in communication. Again, familiarizing yourself with all relevant literature can help you educate yourself, other professionals, and jurors, as needed.

ANATOMICAL DOLLS

When you hear the phrase "anatomical doll," what do you think of? Would you be comfortable holding a doll that had genitals and using it in an interaction with a child? For many, it is difficult to wrap our minds around a doll that has anatomically detailed body parts. But, they do exist and can be utilized in various ways in the forensic interview setting. I (Rachel Fondren Happel) was shaking and very anxious the first time I used an anatomical doll in a forensic interview; I was certainly more nervous than the child was and I was concerned the child would pick up on my discomfort. This was when I made a commitment to gain comfort with the tool or stop using it because I was concerned it would be counterproductive if I used the tool ineffectively.

Research is mixed on the use of anatomical dolls and drawings during forensic interviews (Koocher et al., 1995). Anatomical dolls are typically used in forensic interview settings as a clarification aid and communication tool, to arrive at a common language for the names of body parts, and to assess the child's ability to differentiate between genders and/or make a representational shift. There are risks associated with the use of anatomical drawings and dolls, especially if the person using them is not adequately trained or introduces the media at an inappropriate time. According to Boat and Everson (1994), anatomical dolls can serve distinct functions in the interview process—for this reason, it is important not to endorse or condemn anatomical dolls without understanding the function for which the doll is serving in the forensic interview.

Faller (2005) reviewed some of the relevant literature associated with the use of anatomical dolls. She found that these dolls are rarely suggestive to children with no history of abuse (and that those who were likely to have been abused were significantly more likely to engage in sexualized behavior with the dolls), and dolls are valuable in facilitating responses about abuse compared to not using props, but not necessarily *better* than another prop such as a body map (Faller, 2005). Additionally, Faller reported that dolls can be useful for children to communicate through demonstration and may increase a child's willingness to discuss details about abuse because it may be less embarrassing to demonstrate on an anatomical doll. In support, Hlavka, Olinger, and Lashley (2010) found that in a survey of 500 interviews, the dolls "enhanced children's verbal disclosures through demonstration" (p. 540) and facilitated the disclosure of sexual abuse despite the child's embarrassment or verbal/cognitive limitations. Additionally, Thierry, Lamb, Orbach, and Pipe (2005) found that younger children used them more often as a language-substitution and older children used them mostly as a memory-retrieval mechanism.

Research suggests when anatomical dolls are used improperly they can be leading and suggestive, and may negatively interfere in the disclosure process (Faller, 2007). Additionally, because children often lack cognitive sophistication to make a representational shift or use as a "map," dolls may be ineffective (Dickinson, Poole, & Bruck, 2005). Research suggests that by the age of 4, many children have that ability (Anderson et al., 2010).

Anatomical dolls must only be used after a child has made a disclosure in the forensic interview. If the dolls are used in another way, they may be leading or suggestive. Dickinson, Poole, and Bruck (2005) report that concerns about the use of anatomical dolls include eliciting play behavior in children that could be mistaken as a sign of abuse and note the potential for reporting errors, concerns about cognitive abilities, and concerns about training and education of interviewers using anatomical dolls. These authors also conclude, upon a review of literature, that there is insufficient evidence suggesting the benefits of using the dolls outweigh the risks. In support, Bruck, Ceci, Francoeur, and Renick (1995; Bruck, Ceci, & Francoeur, 2000) found that the novelty of the dolls may prompt children to play, rather than use the doll as a demonstration aid.

When considering use of a controversial tool in a forensic interview, the interviewer should weigh the pros and cons of using the tool and be familiar with the research supporting and cautioning against its use. This will inform the forensic interviewer with relevant literature and help them make a determination of best practices. The interviewer has to weigh the pros and cons and consider the consequences particularly if a child or other children might be at risk for future abuse. Being familiar with all sides of the anatomical doll and drawing arguments can better prepare forensic interviewers for court testimony as well, which can be an important part of their job. With anatomical dolls and drawings, it is important that the interviewer is adequately trained in the research and delivery associated with these tools.

Forensic interviewing should be a child-centered, successful way to gather information from children who are alleged victims of abuse or witnesses to such crimes. Despite the controversies involved regarding the most effective protocol, discussion of truth and lie, the use of anatomical dolls and drawings, and others, forensic interviews can be a very useful instrument in child abuse investigations. Understanding the research and jurisdictional preferences of the area where you work is an important task. With sensitive interactions, like forensic interviews, it is important that you do not just know *what* to do, but *why* you are doing it. This will help when testifying in court and in avoiding burnout by empowering professionals to fully understand the importance of everything we do to advocate for child victims.

 Consider This

> Spend some time to consider the similarities and differences between the various interviewing models discussed in this chapter. Do you think this reflects a gradual convergence of "best practices" or agreement about how these interviews should be done? Why or why not?

STUDY QUESTIONS

1. Discuss some of the types of questions available to use in forensic interviews. Are any question types more or less effective? Why or why not?

2. What is suggestibility? Why is it important in the forensic interview setting?

3. What is a multidisciplinary team? What are some of the benefits of the "team approach" in child abuse investigations?

4. Discuss two of the forensic interview protocols available. What are the similarities? Differences?

5. Discuss the forensic evaluation model. How does it differ from traditional forensic interviewing?

6. How can drawings be utilized as a communication aid in forensic interviews?

7. What are the controversies associated with anatomical dolls?

8. What are the controversies associated with anatomical drawings?

9. Discuss the literature on the truth-lie discussion in forensic interviews.

10. How does trauma impact the memory of children?

GLOSSARY

abuse An act of commission; improper action toward other people that has the potential to hurt or injure them.

anatomical doll Anatomically detailed doll used in forensic interviews to provide clarification following a disclosure.

anatomical drawing Anatomically detailed drawing, or body diagram, used as a communication aid during a forensic interview.

forensics (also known as forensic science) Techniques or scientific approaches used in investigations of crimes.

forensic interview A nonleading, objective, investigative interview with a child, typically ages 3 to 17, due to allegations of child abuse, child exploitation, or witnessing a crime.

linguistics The scientific study of language.

multidisciplinary team (MDT) A team of individuals (typically composed of law enforcement officials, child protection workers, mental health professionals, child advocacy center personnel, juvenile officers, and medical personnel) who work together to provide investigative services to a child and his/her family when allegations of abuse arise.

representational shift A person's ability to see an object as a representation of him or herself.

suggestibility The degree to which someone responds to and is influenced by suggestions made by someone or something.

trauma An emotional response to an experience, typically negative, such as abuse, natural disaster, or accident.

REFERENCES

Aldridge, J., Lamb, M., Sternberg, K., Orbach, Y., Esplin, P., & Bowler, L. (2004). Using a human figure drawing to elicit information from alleged victims of sexual abuse. *Journal of Consulting and Clinical Psychology, 72*, 304–316.

Anderson, J., Ellefson, J., Lashley, J., Lukas-Miller, A., Olinger, S., Russell, A., ... Weigman, J. (2010). The CornerHouse forensic interview protocol: RATAC. *T.M. Cooley Journal of Practical & Clinical Law, 12,* 194–331.

Babiker, G., & Herbert, M. (1998). Critical issues in the assessment of child sexual abuse. *Clinical Child and Family Psychology Review, 1*(4), 231–252.

Berliner, L., Hyman, I., Thomas, A., & Fitzgerald, M. (2003). Children's memories for traumatic and positive experiences: Relationship to psychological symptoms. *Journal of Traumatic Stress, 16,* 229–236.

Boat, B., & Everson, M. (1994). Exploration of anatomical dolls by nonreferred preschool-aged children: Comparisons by age, gender, race, and socioeconomic status. *Child Abuse and Neglect, 18*(2), 139–153.

Brown, D., Pipe, M., Lewis, C., Lamb, M., & Orbach, Y. (2007). Supportive or suggestive: Do human figure drawings help 5- to 7-year-old children to report touch? *Journal of Consulting and Clinical Psychology, 75,* 33–42.

Bruck, M., & Ceci, S. J. (1997). The suggestibility of young children. *Current Directions in Psychological Science,* 75–79.

Bruck, M., & Ceci, S. J. (1999). The suggestibility of children's memory. *Annual Review of Psychology, 50,* 419–439.

Bruck, M., Ceci, S. J., & Francoeur, E. (2000). A comparison of three and four year old children's use of anatomically detailed dolls to report genital touching in a medical examination. *Journal of Experimental Psychology: Applied, 6,* 74–83.

Bruck, M., Ceci, S. J., Francoeur, E., & Renick, A. (1995). Anatomically detailed dolls do not facilitate preschoolers' reports of a pediatric examination involving genital touch. *Journal of Experimental Psychology: Applied, 1,* 95–109.

Carnes, C., Nelson-Gardell, D., Wilson, C., & Orgassa, U. (2001). Extended forensic evaluation when sexual abuse is suspected: A multisite field study. *Child Maltreatment, 6,* 230–242.

Chae, Y., Goodman, G., Bederian-Gardner, D., & Lindsay, A. (2011). Methodological issues and practical strategies in research on child maltreatment victims' abilities and experiences as witnesses. *Child Abuse & Neglect, 35,* 240–248.

CornerHouse Interagency Child Abuse Evaluation and Training Center. (2013). *Basic forensic interview training at CornerHouse.* Retrieved from http://www.cornerhousemn.org/basicinterview.html

Dale, P. S., Loftus, E. F., & Rathbun, L. (1978). The influence of the form of the question on the eyewitness testimony of preschool children. *Journal of Psycholinguistic Research, 7*(4), 269–277.

Dickinson, J., Poole, D., & Bruck, M. (2005). Back to the future: A comment on the use of anatomical dolls in forensic interviews. *Journal of Forensic Psychology Practice, 5*(1), 63–74.

Faller, K. (2007). *Interviewing children about sexual abuse: Controversies and best practice.* New York, NY: Oxford University Press.

Fanetti, M., & Boles, R. (2003). Forensic interviewing and assessment issues with children. In W. T. O'Donohue (Ed.), *Handbook of forensic psychology* (pp. 245–265). New York, NY: Academic Press.

Fanetti, M., & Boles, R. (2004). In W. O'Donohue & E. Levensky (Eds.), *Handbook of forensic psychology* (pp. 249–262). San Diego, CA: Elsevier Academic Press.

Faller, K. C. (2005). Anatomical dolls: Their use in assessment of children who may have been sexually abused. *Journal of Child Sexual Abuse, 14*(3). doi:10.1300/J070v14n03_01

Garven, S., Wood, J. M., Malpass, R. S., & Shaw, J. S. (1998). More than suggestion: The effect of interviewing techniques from the McMartin preschool case. *Journal of Applied Psychology, 83*(3), 347–359.

Huffman, M., Warren, A., & Larson, S. (1999). Discussing truth and lies in interviews with children where why and how. *Applied Developmental Science, 3*(1), 6–15.

Hlavka, H. R., Olinger, S. D., & Lashley, J. L. (2010). The use of anatomical dolls as a demonstration aid in child sexual abuse interviews: A study of forensic interviewers' perceptions. *Journal of Child Sexual Abuse, 19*, 519–553.

Koocher, G., Goodman, G., White, C., Friedrich, W., Sivan, A., & Reynolds, C. (1995). Psychological science and the use of anatomically detailed dolls in child sexual abuse assessments. *Psychological Bulletin, 118*, 199–122.

Kuehnle, K., & Connell, M. (2009). *The evaluation of child sexual abuse allegations: A comprehensive guide to assessment and testimony.* Hoboken, NJ: Wiley.

Lamb, M., Orbach, Y., Hershkowitz, I., Esplin, P., & Horowitz, D. (2007). Structured forensic interview protocols improve the quality and informativeness of investigative interviews with children: A review of research using the NICHD Investigative Interview Protocol. *Child Abuse and Neglect, 31*(11–12), 1201–1231.

Loftus, E., & Pickrell, J. (1995). The formation of false memories. *Psychiatric Annals, 25*, 720–725.

London, K. (2001). Investigative and courtroom interviews of children: Examining the efficacy of truth/lie discussions in increasing the veracity of children's reports. *Dissertation Abstracts International, 62*(3-B), 1618.

Lyon, T. D. (2002). Applying suggestibility research to the real world: The case of repeated questions. *Law and Contemporary Problems, 65*, 97–126.

The National Children's Advocacy Center. (2012). *History.* Retrieved from http://www.nationalcac.org/history/history.html

Olafson, E., & Lederman, J. C. (2006). The state of the debate about children's disclosure patterns in child sexual abuse cases. *Journal and Family Court Journal, 57*(1), 27–40.

Pence, D., & Wilson, C. (1994). *Team Investigation of child sexual abuse: The uneasy alliance* (pp. 9–29, 30–42). Thousand Oaks, CA: Sage.

Peterson, C., Peterson, J., & Seeto, D. (1983). Developmental changes in ideas about lying. *Child Development, 54*, 1529–1535.

Piaget, J. (1965). *The moral judgment of the child.* New York, NY: Macmillan. Original work published 1932.

Poole, D., & Bruck, M. (2012). Divining testimony: The impact of interviewing props on children's reports of touching. *Developmental Review, 32*, 165–180.

Poole, D., & Dickinson, J. (2011). Evidence supporting restrictions on uses of body diagrams in forensic interviews. *Child Abuse and Neglect, 35*, 659–669.

Poole, D., & Lamb, M. (1998). *Investigative interviews of children: A guide for helping professionals*. Washington, DC: American Psychological Association.

Rooy, D., Lamb, M., & Pipe, M. (2009). Repeated interviewing: A critical evaluation of the risks and potential benefits. In K. Kuehnle & M. Connell (Eds.), *The evaluation of child sexual abuse allegations*. Hoboken, NJ: Wiley.

Sorenson, T., & Snow, B. (1991). How children tell: The process of disclosure in child sexual abuse. *Child Welfare, 70*(1), 3–15.

State of Michigan. (2008). *Forensic interviewing protocol*. State of Michigan Governor's Task Force on Children's Justice and Department of Human Services. Retrieved from http://www.michigan.gov/documents/dhs/DHS-PUB-0779_211637_7.pdf.

Steele, L. (2003). Child Forensic Interview structure, National Children's Advocacy Center. *APSAC Advisor, 15*(4).

Sternberg, K. J., Lamb, M. E., & Hershkowitz, I. (1997). Effects of introductory style on children's abilities to describe experiences of sexual abuse. *Child Abuse & Neglect, 21*(11), 1133–1146.

Thierry, K., Lamb, M., Orbach, Y., & Pipe, M. (2005). Developmental differences in the function and use of anatomical dolls during interviews with alleged sexual abuse victims. *Journal of Consulting and Clinical Psychology, 73*(6), 1125–1134.

Thompson, W. C., Clarke-Stewart, A., & Lepore, S. J. (1997). What did the janitor do? Suggestive interviewing and the accuracy of children's accounts. *Law and Human Behavior, 21*(4), 405–426.

Valentino, K., Cicchetti, D., Rogosch, F., & Toth, S. (2008). True and false recall and dissociation among maltreated children: The role of self-schema. *Development and Psychopathology, 20*, 213–222.

Wandrey, L., Quas, J., & Lyon, T. (2012). Does valence matter? Effects of negativity on children's early understanding of truths and lies. *Journal of Experimental Child Psychology, 113*, 295–303.

Wood, J. M., & Garven, S. (2000). How sexual abuse interviews go astray: Implications for prosecutors, police and child protection services. *Child Maltreatment, 5*(2), 109–118.

CHAPTER

8

———✦———

Understanding Pedophilia

GOALS OF THIS CHAPTER:

1. To become familiar with the concepts of pedophilia and child molestation.
2. To understand how pedophilia is diagnosed and treated.
3. To understand the legal and social impact of pedophilia and child molestation.

"Pedophilia" is a combination of two Greek words meaning children (*pedo*) and love or attraction (*philia*). The love or attraction involved in this word refers to an *adult's sexual or erotic attraction* as opposed to an adult's normal attraction or love of children in which the adult regards children are "cute" and perhaps wants to be around them based on this feeling, nurture them, and make sure they are safe and healthy. Pedophilia belongs to a larger class of mental disorders in the *Diagnostic and Statistical Manual of the American Psychiatric Association* (American Psychiatric Association [APA], 2013) called paraphilic disorders. *Para* means outside and again *philia* means love or attraction. The basic idea is that individuals suffering from this group of disorders have a sexual attraction or orientation that is **outside the norm**.

In pedophilia the adult finds children sexually arousing and usually has sexual fantasies about children and, in the typical case, desires to have some sort of sexual contact with the child. **Pedophilia**, unsurprisingly, is considered a mental disorder in the *DSM-5* (APA, 2013). (It is also important to note that there is another technical term, *hebephilia*, which indicates an attraction to individuals—early adolescents— that are still regarded as too young for an adult to be attracted to them—say 14- or 15-year-olds. Hebephilia is an attraction to postpubescent adolescents who are still below the legal age of consent in the state, which admittedly varies tremendously across states. Despite the efforts of some, hebephilia currently is not considered a mental disorder in the *DSM-5* and thus hebephiles are regarded as pedophiles.)

It is useful to actually examine the *DSM-5* diagnostic criteria for pedophilia (APA, 2013, pp. 697–698). Basically, the diagnosis of pedophilia involves four specific criteria:

A. The person has had to experience recurrent and intensive sexually arousing urges, fantasies, or behaviors involving sex with a prepubescent child (13 or younger) for at least 6 months.

B. This individual was disturbed by the events described in A or acted on them.

C. The individual is at least 16 years old and at least 5 years older than the child that they are aroused by.

D. And then there are subtypes, specifically:
    a. Only attracted to children vs. also attracted to adults.
    b. Which genders they are attracted to (just girls, just boys, or both).
    c. And then whether it is limited to incest.

It is important to note that the *DSM-5* also makes a distinction between a *pedophilic sexual orientation* and a *pedophilic disorder*. Basically, if the adult is sexually attracted to children but is not distressed by these feelings, is not functionally impaired by these feelings, and has never acted on these urges then, according to the *DSM-5*, the adult simply has a pedophilic sexual orientation. This is not regarded as a mental disorder or a pathology in the *DSM*. (This may be a weakness of the current *DSM*.) However, if the adult is sexually attracted to children and is distressed, or functionally impaired, or has acted on these urges then the adult, according to the *DSM-5*, suffers from a pedophilic disorder. O'Donohue (2010) has argued that this distinction between a pedophilic *orientation* and a pedophilic *disorder* is not useful and not valid. He argued that a sexual orientation toward children in itself is disordered and the additional criteria needed to be met in the *DSM-5* are superfluous—for example, if someone is not distressed by being attracted to children, this in fact is just a further abnormality rather than something that somehow overrides the pathological orientation. According to O'Donohue (2010), the notion of a "contented pedophile"—an adult who is happy with their sexual attraction to children—is still to be regarded as disordered.

Five Interesting Facts About Pedophilia According to DSM-5

1. **By far, most pedophiles are male.** The *DSM* suggests that the "highest possible" prevalence of pedophilia in the male population is 3% to 5% and that the prevalence of pedophilia in the female population is unknown but believed to be a small fraction of what it is in the male population.

2. **Pedophilia is a lifelong condition.** There is no cure for this mental disorder; it is not an acute problem that waxes and wanes like the flu where one "gets it" for a period but overcomes it a little bit later. Later we discuss how the best research

evidence indicates that sexual orientations are relatively fixed; for most people these tend not to change much if at all.

3. **There is a relationship between pedophilia and antisociality.** Antisociality is another psychological problem in which individuals do not have a normal sense of morality and many important rules without guilt or remorse. These individuals are usually also deceitful and impulsive. Thus, we find that many individuals with pedophilia also have these kind of antisocial traits. This makes them much more difficult to treat.

4. **Many adult males who suffer from pedophilia also report being sexually abused as children (this may be partly related to their antisociality).** The *DSM* is careful to indicate that this correlation should not be interpreted as causation. For example, it is also important to recognize that most victims of childhood sexual abuse are females, but because it is very rare that females suffer from pedophilia, it cannot be said that childhood sexual abuse causes pedophilia. If it did, then we would expect to see many more females who suffer from pedophilia.

5. **Some individuals admit to their pedophilic disorder but many other individuals deny or minimize this orientation or abusive behaviors associated with it.** Thus, diagnosis can be difficult. The client is often stating that either they simply did nothing that the victim or victims have said that they did or that the (alleged) victim is misconstruing his behavior (e.g., the touch was accidental or nonsexual). Even after a trial and a conviction, the individual may still claim they suffered an injustice, due to their poor lawyer, scheming ex-wife, and so on. This denial and minimization makes both assessment and treatment very difficult. In most cases when clients come to see a therapist they are giving accurate information (e.g., "I have panic attacks" or "My marriage is on the rocks") but in this is not the case with pedophilia.

Other Information Known About Pedophiles

- **When they victimize a child, in most cases the child is known to them**—for example, the child is a relative or acquaintance. However, this is a trend and not a universal rule: Sometimes, although more rarely, the victim is a stranger to the pedophile.

- **Pedophiles display a fairly high relapse rate.** Reoffense rates for untreated sex offenders, who primarily target children, range from 10% to 40%. Reoffense rates for treated pedophiles may be slightly less than this but are still unacceptably high.

- **There is no "profile" of a pedophile.** That is, beyond being male one cannot see other markers or "signs" of a pedophile. They do not have a certain look. They may be extraverted or introverted, rich or poor, tall or short.

Consider This

Think about the children in your own life, be they siblings, offspring, nieces or nephews, and so on. At what point would they be "able" to consent to sexual behavior? At what point do you think they would be able to consider all of the variables associated with sexuality? At what point would they be able to effectively say no to unwanted advances? These are precisely the problems with which most societies must deal.

THE OTHER PARAPHILIAS

It also may be useful to take a look at what other kinds of problems the *DSM-5* classifies as a **paraphilia**. This can be important as there is some evidence that in some cases substantial comorbidity exists between the paraphilias (Abel, Becker, Cunningham, Mittelman, & Rouleau, 1988). That is, many individuals suffer from more than one paraphilia:

Voyeuristic disorder. Sexual gratification that requires viewing others, especially those who do not know, essentially "peeping."

Exhibitionistic disorder. Sexual gratification that requires exposing one's genitals in front of other people, especially those who have not consented.

Frotteuristic disorder. Sexual gratification that requires touching or rubbing against others, especially those who have not consented.

Sexual masochism disorder. Sexual gratification that requires being beaten, bound, or pain and suffering.

Sexual sadism disorder. Sexual gratification that requires causing pain and suffering to others.

Fetishistic disorder. Sexual gratification that requires being aroused by a nonsexual object such as by feet or shoes.

Transvestic disorder. Cross-dressing, or wearing clothing that typically is indicative of the opposite gender.

Paraphilia not otherwise specified (NOS). This category is a catchall for less frequent paraphilias such as obscene phone calling.

It should be apparent that these are *para* (outside) *philias* (attractions). More commonly these are often called *perversions*. Although many people may "play" with some of these behaviors, the important differences are related to consent and severity.

Now that there has been a bit of an overview of pedophilia, we examine some diagnostic issues in a bit more detail.

ARE THE *DSM-5* DIAGNOSTIC CRITERIA FOR PEDOPHILIA CLEAR?

O'Donohue (2010) has argued that the diagnostic criteria in the *DSM* have at least two problems. For example:

1. There are no data to show that two clinicians will apply these diagnostic criteria in the same way and make the same diagnoses. That is, if the same patient were to see two different clinicians, we would want the clinicians to arrive at the same conclusions (to either agree that pedophilia should be ruled in or ruled out). However, for many decades the field has been missing data that this consistency would occur. This is known by a technical term in psychometrics, *interrater reliability*. Historically, this has been a problem for many *DSM* diagnoses. Some diagnoses in earlier versions such as *DSM-I* and *DSM-II* were shown to have very low interrater reliability for problems such as schizophrenia, bipolar disorder, and even depression. (There is a psychometric principle that problems in reliability show up as problems in validity.) The *DSM-III* tried to use clearer behavioral criteria to overcome this problem and was at least partially successful for some of the diagnoses. However, we still do not know if clinicians will agree on the *DSM-5* diagnoses of pedophilia—the problem being that diagnoses become not what the client presents with, but the clinician introduces problematic variability and heterogeneity. When patients receive a health care diagnosis, they do not want to think that if they just go to another clinician, then the diagnosis might disappear. Studies need to be conducted to see the extent to which disagreements regarding diagnoses exist.

2. Some of the terms in the *DSM-5* diagnostic criteria are unclear and require significant judgment on part of the clinician, which can lead to diagnostic unreliability. For example, the terms,

   a. "Recurrent"—How many times do these have to occur—2, more than 2, 30 … ?

   b. "Intense"—How does one measure the intensity of a sexual fantasy or sexual urge—can the client be counted on to report this accurately? If not, what are other measurement options?

   c. "Acted on the urges or fantasies"—Certainly, abusing a child would count as acting on these, but what about choosing a career to have more contact with a child such as becoming an elementary school teacher? What about gazing at a child a few seconds longer—is this not acting on an urge? Do clinicians agree on this? Even if they do, can clients be trusted to report this accurately?

   d. "Marked distress"—What exactly is marked distress? Does one need a full-blown *DSM* diagnosis such as major depressive episode? Does being somewhat perturbed by this fall short of being "markedly distressed"? If the person is not bothered but say his wife is, and he is bothered by his wife's reaction, does this count?

As one can see, there are a number of terms that are not perfectly clear and may result in diagnostic unreliability.

AGE AND PHYSIOLOGICAL DEVELOPMENT

The *DSM* diagnostic criteria refer rather vaguely to age—remember these state "generally age 13 years or younger" and there is also reference to a developmental stage "prepubescent." Basically the idea is that normal sexual attraction meets one of two conditions:

1. If a person is a mature adult then the person will be attracted to other mature adults (although the age range may be quite large—a 40-year-old may find 18-year-olds attractive as well as 50-year-olds).
2. However, if these people are children or adolescents, it is normal for these people to be attracted to those around their age or maybe even a little older (for example, it is normal for a 12-year-old boy to be attracted to roughly 10- to 16-year-olds—it should be clear that it is a difficult and tricky task to set these ranges—nothing is set in stone). Thus, it is not diagnosable pathology for a person who is 12 to be attracted to someone who is 10, 11, 12, 13, 14, and so on.

Sometimes scholars have tried to add a bit more precision by using a developmental scale called the **Tanner scale**. There are five Tanner stages of physical development for both males and females, with Tanner Stage 1 indicating prepuberty and Tanner Stage 5 indicating full maturation (Tanner, 1978). Tanner stages focus on breast development and pubic hair growth in females, and on genital development and pubic hair growth in males. The first three stages (Stages 1 to 3), representing physical immaturity and thus relevant to the diagnosis of pedophilia, are:

Tanner Stage 1: Girls, no palpable breast tissue; boys, genitals similar to early childhood; both sexes, no pubic hair at all.

Tanner Stage 2: Girls, breast bud stage; boys, enlargement of scrotum and testes, with change in both the color and texture of scrotal skin; and in both sexes, sparse growth of long, slightly pigmented downy hair, appearing mainly along the labia or base of the penis.

Tanner Stage 3: Girls, further enlargement of breast and areola with no separation of their contours; boys, growth of the penis and testes to half adult size or less;

both sexes, pubic hair is darker and coarser, but lesser in quantity and different in quality from adult type.

Again, basically the idea is that these boys and girls have not developed physically into adult bodies and it is abnormal for an adult to be sexually attracted to them.

It is also important to note that we do not know all that the individual suffering from pedophilia is attracted to—certainly it seems that the attraction is to the physically immature body, but others have hypothesized that individual suffering from pedophila may also be attracted to the powerlessness of the child, the obedience of a typical child, and even their immature voices, and simplicity.

✍ Consider This

Using the idea of the Tanner scale and differences in development for different growing children, what difficulties might arise for those who progress more quickly than average through the Tanner scales? How might this put them at more, or less, risk for sexual contact by predators who are either pedophilic or not?

WHAT MAKES PEDOPHILIA ABNORMAL?

This can be an important question, partly because there are some that have argued that viewing adult-child (or what they often call *intergenerational*) sexual attraction wrong is simply a prejudice or sexual hang-up. There are actually a few organizations that are trying to instigate social movements to correct what they see as this societal wrong or prejudice. Two of the most prominent of these are the Rene Guyon Society and the North American Man-Boy Love Association (NAMBLA). Their view is that sexuality throughout history has often been harshly and inappropriately judged and that there has been a series of successful sexual revolutions in the past century. For example, in their literature they claim the first sexual revolution was realizing that women's sexuality was often inappropriately judged—women were not supposed to enjoy sex; to be sexual was to be unladylike, it was worse for a woman to engage in premarital sex (they were labeled a "slut") than for a man to do the same thing (men would be "studs"), and so on. Individuals in these organizations then state that there was a sexual revolution for women around the turn of the 20th century in which women's sexuality was viewed as more equal to males and as acceptable and healthy. The second sexual revolution for them occurred when gay rights were recognized and homosexuality was taken out of the *Diagnostic and Statistic Manual* in the latter half of the 20th century. They argue that now a further revolution is needed in which societal prejudices against "man-boy love" (NAMBLA is oriented toward only this) and intergenerational sex are overcome.

They argue that an older person can sexually "mentor" a younger person and this is a good, healthy way to learn about sex. One of their mottos is something along the lines "Sex before 8 or else it is too late."

O'Donohue (1987) and others (de Young, 1987) have argued against this line of reasoning. De Young has astutely analyzed the rhetoric (basically attempts at persuasion) of this movement and has suggested that they use a number of *tropes* (rhetorical strategies) in which members of these organizations illegitimately take on the role of victim (they are being discriminated against); they ally themselves with past positive social movements (women's rights and suffrage movements); and speak in philanthropic and amelioristic terms (they are about helping children). Thus, their rhetoric may be shrewd but this does not mean the substance of their argument or their goals are sound.

O'Donohue (2010) has argued that the core reason that adult-child sexual contact is wrong (morally and legally) is that children, by virtue of their being children, are not capable of consenting to sexual interactions with an adult because they are developmentally incapable of the relatively complex cognitive tasks associated with this. Basically, the idea is that when two adults decide to have sex, they are both more or less capable of making an informed decision and thus giving consent to the sexual contact. Two adults can consider factors like: Do they actually like this person; what is the risk of venereal disease or pregnancy; what impact might this have on them socially; is this consistent with their morals; will the person treat them well. The key problem is that children are immature not only physically but also cognitively and intellectually and thus cannot appraise these factors because they do not have all the information or the abilities to process this information rationally. Thus, it would be a very unequal negotiation between the adult and the child. For the same reasons, all states have laws that prohibit children entering into contracts: Due to their cognitive unsophistication they might think incorrectly that a fair trade may be to sell a house for three Barbie dolls. Thus, because sex can be very consequential (on self-image, health, and social variables) and because informed consent is critical and because children are cognitively incapable of the information and processing needed to consent to sex, then sex with children is properly considered to be both morally and legally wrong. Thus, the idea is that an attraction to do this is a mental disorder because it inclines one toward this immoral and illegal act.

AN IMPORTANT DISTINCTION: THE DIFFERENCE BETWEEN A "CHILD SEXUAL ABUSER" AND A "PEDOPHILE"

This is an important distinction. Remember that a pedophile is someone who has an abnormal attraction to a child. A child sexual abuser is someone who has actually sexually abused a child. These are not identical terms because their extensions are not the same:

- Some pedophiles have not acted on their abnormal attraction and thus have not sexually abused a child. Thus, these individuals suffer from pedophilia but are not child molesters.
- Some individuals sexually abuse children for other reasons than a pedophilic attraction. The field does not know all these pathways but examples include:
  a. Some individuals suffering from antisocial personality disorder abuse children.
  b. Some individuals due to their substance abuse problems and intoxication sexually abuse children.
  c. Some individuals due to their cognitive problems (e.g., dementia, mental retardations) sexually abuse children.
  d. Thus, because of these other pathways to abuse, not all child abusers suffer from pedophilia

HOW WILL A PEDOPHILE BEHAVE?

Sometimes an individual suffering from pedophilia will act just like everyone else. Again, there is not a *typical* profile of a pedophile. However, compared to individuals who do not suffer from pedophilia they will tend to:

- Seek out and use child pornography (which is itself a crime).
- Seek out contact with children (for sexual reasons). They might volunteer for babysitting or become a coach or a school bus driver. They may even marry to get access to their spouse's children. Just as you as an adult will seek out people you are sexually attracted to, individuals suffering from pedophilia will do the same—but with children.
- May *groom* children. **Grooming** is a technical term with historically a wide range of meanings. Basically it means the "seduction" of children. Thus, pedophiles may give expensive or inappropriate gifts to children they are sexually interested in (maybe bikinis or bras). They may talk to them about sex, even under the guise of "sex education." They may show them inappropriate films—for example, they may show a 5-year-old an R-rated romance.

WHAT CAUSES PEDOPHILIA?

A simple and true answer is that we do not know what causes pedophilia. This is an important question but a difficult one. Special research methodologies must be used in order that a *causal inference* can be made (i.e., "This caused that"). Remember the old saying, "correlation is not causation." Thus, it is not enough to show that some higher than expected percentage of child abusers (again, remember this is not the same construct as "pedophile") have been abused as children. This shows a correlation—perhaps a very interesting one—but it does not show causation. It does not *prove* that undergoing abuse as a child will cause a person to become an abuser.

In general, behavioral science looks to both nature (genetics) and nurture (environment) in order to understand causes of behavioral conditions (e.g., schizophrenia, extraversion). In general, we find that both kinds of causal factors are important. That is, conditions have a heritable, genetic component (we are physiologically predisposed toward a specific behavior by our genes) but that the environment also plays a role (we are more likely to engage the behavior in some contexts). That is, our life experiences impact this inborn potentiality. Take a simple example. Genetics clearly play a role in determining your adult height. If both your parents are unusually tall, you will generally have the genes to also be tall (generally less *unusually* tall than your parents—this is called *regression toward the mean*). However, say that during your gestation (when you were in the womb) and even during your childhood you were very poor and did not consume much protein. This lack of proper diet is an environmental factor. In general, severe protein deprivation will reduce your adult height—even though you had the genetic potential to be a few inches taller, because you did not get the right nourishment from your environment, this genetic potential was not fully actualized. This general phenomenon is called a *genetic-by-environment interaction*—it shows the important role of both kinds of factors.

What do we know about sexual orientation in general? J. Michael Bailey of Northwestern University has done some important studies. In 1993, along with Richard Pillard, he published some twin studies investigating the role of genetics and environment in determining sexual orientation. Studying twins is generally thought of as the "gold standard" method for understanding the roles of nature versus nurture. The logic of these twin studies is as follows. Both monozygotic (identical) and dizygotic (fraternal) twins are studied. We know by definition that identical twins have 100% of the same genetic makeup. We know also by definition that dizygotic twins have exactly half of this—that is, their genetic makeup is only 50% the same. Thus, if we find that the same ratio is found in some trait (this is called by a technical term *concordance*) we can infer that there is a genetic component to the trait. In addition, if we find that the concordance rate is less than 100% in identical twins, this generally means that the trait is not completely due to genetics—that the environment also plays a role. (The astute reader might also notice that another factor plays a role here—how the environment may treat identical twins more similarly [after all they are identical] than fraternal twins. The best twin studies also examine adopted identical and fraternal twins as this adoption can control for environment—if they are adopted to different families then they no longer share the same environments.)

Bailey has not studied pedophilia with the twin study methodology—unfortunately, no one has. Instead, he studied sexual orientation and more specifically homosexual orientation. However, their conclusions can possibly shed some light onto this question. In their first study they found the concordance rate of monozygotic gay twins at 52% and with dizygotic twins at 22% (i.e., roughly one half the rate). That is, if one identical twin was gay there was a 52% likelihood that the other identical twin was gay; but if a fraternal twin was gay there was only a 22% likelihood that the other fraternal twin was gay. Also, for the adoptive siblings of the same sex who are not twins the concordance rate was 11%. However, subsequent research by Bailey and his colleagues did not replicate these high concordance rates. In monozygotic twins he found a concordance rate of 20% for males and 24% for women, suggesting a much smaller role for genetics. Bailey suggests that the first study might have had a biased sample as he advertised for gay twins, and he thinks twins might have considered the sexual orientation of their twin before deciding to participate.

These data suggest that sexual orientation is at least partially genetically determined. These data also show an important role of the environment (the concordance rates for identical twins were not 100%). Also, fraternal twins and brothers are similar genetically yet fraternal twins have nearly twice the concordance rate of brothers who were adopted—this points to the role of environmental factors. To be sure, we would have to extrapolate these findings to pedophilia and this must be done with caution. We need to return to our previous statement: We as a field do not know what causes pedophilia, but there are some data to show that sexual orientation has a moderate genetic component. However, there are still environmental factors that have a role and we do not know what these are.

Consider This

Try to imagine situational contexts in which a person with a pedophilic sexual orientation would not become a child abuser. Furthermore, try to imagine situational contexts in which a person with a normal sexual orientation would become a child abuser.

HOW IS PEDOPHILIA DIAGNOSED?

Typically, the clinician uses several assessment procedures to arrive at this diagnosis. These include a record review, clinical interview, paper and pencil testing, collateral contacts, and sometimes even physiological testing called the *penile plethysmograph*. The clinician then takes all this information and determines the extent to which reasonable conclusions can be made regarding whether the diagnostic criteria set forth in the *DSM-5* (APA, 2013) are met. Typically, though, the clinician is also assessing a few other important issues:

- Whether the client suffers from other problems (sometimes called comorbid problems) such as antisocial personality disorder, depression, substance abuse, another paraphilia.
- The extent to which the client is admitting to his problems versus the extent to which he is minimizing or in denial. Typically, treatment requires that the client admit that he has these kinds of problems. If the client is in complete denial he may first be required to enter into an intervention targeting his denial so that treatment may begin.
- As we see later, the most common treatment for child molesters suffering from pedophilia is called *relapse prevention* (RP). In order to administer this treatment, the clinician needs to have a fairly good understanding of each episode of abuse. Each episode is viewed as a self-control failure, which was a result of a chain of behaviors that had several links: for example, a fight with the wife resulted in feeling angry, which resulted in drinking, which resulted in feelings of sexual arousal and entitlement, which resulted in isolating the child, which resulted in abuse of the child. Each link of the chain represents to the clinician an important point of intervention. Thus, assessment needs to be what is called *treatment relevant* and uncover the kinds of information that may be targeted in treatment. This includes:
  a. The person's lifestyle balance.
  b. The person's victim empathy.
  c. The person's willingness to accept responsibility for any crimes or past abuse.
  d. The person's cognitive distortions regarding sex or children.
  e. The person's risk factors.
  f. The person's problem of immediate gratification (lack of self-control).
  g. Areas in which the person is immature.
  h. The person's ability to regulate emotions such as anger.

Thus, assessment is often complex and may take several sessions. Again, assessment is complicated if the person is not maximally cooperative or if they are lying, denying, or minimizing.

A BIT MORE ABOUT THE MAJOR ASSESSMENT TECHNIQUES

Clinical Interview

This is a formal name for asking questions to find out more about the person and their past. The clinician may get a history from the clients finding out about their childhood, past sexual experiences, previous contacts with mental health professionals or law enforcement, work history, marital history, and so on. The interview may cover the extent to which the person is motivated for treatment and what past abuse they will admit to. The interview may also question the clients about their willingness to participate in therapy, which may take years. Finally, the clinician may ask questions about topics covered earlier—that is, comorbid problems—and topics such as victim empathy, emotional regulation, and lifestyle balance.

Record Review

Because individuals with these problems are often reluctant to be perfectly honest, it is important to examine records. Of particular importance are the statements of past victims (these are usually gathered by police as part of routine evidence gathering). The clinician typically sees the extent to which the client's self-report in the assessment session matches the victim's statements. For example, if the victim says the abuse happened 10 times over 1 year and the client says it happened only twice, the victim statement is viewed as more accurate and the client then is viewed as minimizing. The client may be confronted with this discrepancy to see how he reacts. Records are also reviewed for past arrests, past statements from spouses or partners, and past mental health treatment.

Collateral Contacts

"Collateral" literally means "on the side." Given consent the clinician may deem it useful to speak with certain key individuals to gain more information on the client. They may interview current or past spouses, current or past employers, current or past therapists, and even past victims. Clinicians want to both check up on what the client tells them about these situations and to get impressions of these individuals who know the person well. The clinician may ask questions such as: How well did they control their emotions? What did you observe about their substance use? Did they ever behave in ways that you thought were strange or inappropriate? How well did they function as a spouse, parent, or employee?

Paper and Pencil Testing

There are a variety of tests that can be given. The clinician may routinely give common tests such as the Minnesota Multiphasic Personality Inventory-2. This test is commonly used as a broad screen for psychopathology and it has scales both for antisocial tendencies as well as lying or faking validity scales, which can be of interest to the clinician. Some clinicians then will give other tests depending on the view of the client (depression scales such as the Beck Depression Inventory; or Empathy Scales; or Cognitive Distortion Scales).

Penile Plethysmograph

Most clinicians do not have the equipment or the skills to administer this test, and thus if they think it critical they will refer the client to someone to administer this. This is fairly specialized testing and a referral can be difficult. This test is also controversial. In this test a client places what is called a *strain gauge* on his penis—this gauge is used to measure the physical circumference of his penis. Obviously when the circumference changes, this means that the person is becoming physiologically aroused. The client is then shown a variety of stimuli (e.g., slides of nudes of various ages). The basic idea is that if a person shows a physiological response (penile engorgement—an erection) to a certain kind of stimuli, then they are attracted sexually to this kind of stimuli. Typically the data are recorded by a computer and then a printout of circumference changes by type of stimuli is then available to the clinician. Certainly, this measure is not perfect and there are ways around it (not viewing the stimuli, masturbating before the test so that they are not aroused by anything, pinching themselves) but in general the reliability and validity of this procedure has been well studied and is quite good (O'Donohue & Letourneau, 1992).

The clinicians look at all the data—from their review of records, from their clinical interview, from their paper and pencil testing, and from the specialized testing—and arrive at some diagnostic conclusions as well as some treatment recommendations.

REPORTING REQUIREMENT

All mental health professionals are what is called *mandated reporters*. That is, if they have reason to suspect that a child has been abused they must report these suspicions to either the police or to the department of child welfare. It is important to note that clinicians do not have to do an investigation to become absolutely convinced that a child has been abused, they just have to form a reasonable suspicion. This is relevant because sometimes during this assessment phase, an offender will disclose new victims or new incidents of abuse. These trigger mandated reporting requirements and the clinician must inform either the police or the department of child welfare. The basic rationale for this rule is that society was to be maximally vigilant and to discover and help all children who have been abused, particularly when their abuser has not been identified and thus may abuse them or others again. Chapter 12 in this book is specifically dedicated to mandated reporting laws.

HOW IS PEDOPHILIA TREATED?

In some important sense pedophilia is *not* treated—it is viewed as a sexual orientation that has not been shown to be *able to be changed*. Perhaps much like your sexual orientation, you cannot imagine that going into therapy could suddenly cause you to switch these—from say being straight to being gay. Instead, more research in this area has focused on taking child abusers and attempting to help them learn how to not abuse any additional children in the future. The idea has been that their attraction to children may remain, but can we as therapists give them enough tools so they will never act on this deviant attraction? You might think that this is not an easy task. You would be right. The outcome data from these sorts of interventions are often disappointing—there are too many relapses despite years of therapy. However, we review the most common model used—called *relapse prevention*—and also briefly review some of the best designed outcome research investigating this model's effectiveness.

CAN SEX OFFENDERS BE TREATED THROUGH MEDICATIONS?

An important professional association related to the assessment and treatment of pedophilia is called the Association for the Treatment of Sexual Abuse (ATSA; www.atsa.com). This organization has made a statement regarding what is commonly called *chemical castration*, that is, treating individuals with sexual offending problems by essentially giving them chemicals to wipe out their sex drive. These chemicals are also called **antiandrogens**. Androgens are the male sex hormones such as testosterone. Both males and females manufacture testosterone (although males have more of it) and these androgens are most responsible for a sex drive in both genders. Here are some of the most important of ATSA's conclusions:

> Findings from a meta-analysis examining the effectiveness of various treatment interventions for adult sex offenders indicated that, when used in combination with other treatment approaches, biological interventions like testosterone-lowering hormonal treatments may be linked to greater reductions in recidivism for some offenders than the use of psychosocial treatments alone. (Losel & Schmucker, 2005)

Other data, described later, suggest that nonhormonal psychotropic medications can also be effective supplements to standard therapeutic interventions for sex offenders.

A number of hormonal agents have been introduced as pharmacological treatments for reducing testosterone and sexual drive in individuals with paraphilias and/or who have engaged in sexually abusive behaviors. Primary examples include medroxyprogesterone acetate (MPA—Depo-Provera), leuprolide acetate, cyproterone acetate, and gonadotropin-releasing hormone analog. These chemical agents, referred to as *antiandrogens*, act by breaking down and eliminating testosterone and inhibiting the production of luteinizing hormone through the pituitary gland, which in turn inhibits or prevents the production of testosterone. Because testosterone is associated with sexual arousal, the use of these agents generally results in a reduction of sexual arousal. This reduction in sexual arousal is assumed to also reduce the motivation for sexually offending in individuals predisposed to such behaviors.

- Some research suggests that offenders treated with antiandrogens, when compared to those who have not received such treatment, have lower rates of detected sexual recidivism as well as decreased sexual arousal in response to offense-specific stimuli by self-report and physiological evidence (e.g., Maletzky, Tolan, & McFarland, 2006; see also Briken & Kafka, 2007). However, there is also evidence that offenders treated with hormonal agents alone show similar rates of sexual recidivism following a standard course of pharmacotherapy and follow up than their nonhormonally treated counterparts (e.g., Maletzky, 1991; McConaghy, Blaszczynski, & Kidson, 1988). In all, well-designed control studies are lacking, and more empirically rigorous research is needed in this area.
- The use of antiandrogens carries negative and punitive connotations (i.e., linked with the idea of "castration"), and testosterone-lowering agents have significant medical side effects (e.g., breast enlargement or swelling, weight gain, blood clots, depression, gallstones, diabetes mellitus, osteoporosis, hot flushes). As a result, individuals may be prone to decline such treatments, or to demonstrate later noncompliance after initially agreeing to a treatment regimen.
- The limited outcome data on all testosterone-lowering agents make definitive treatment recommendations premature. Because of significant side effects, the prescription of such medications should be restricted to paraphilic patients and sexual offenders with an at least moderate or high risk for hands-on sexual offenses. Additionally, because other etiologies and risk factors are present, the use of hormonal agents should be combined with empirically supported psychotherapy practices (Briken, Hill, & Berner, 2003).
- Studies of sexual offenders, men with paraphilias, and those with nonparaphilic expressions of hypersexuality suggest that mood disorders (dysthymic disorder, major depression, and bipolar spectrum disorders), certain anxiety disorders (especially social anxiety disorder and childhood-onset posttraumatic stress disorder), psychoactive substance abuse disorders (especially alcohol abuse), attention-deficit/hyperactivity disorder (ADHD), and neuropsychological conditions (e.g., schizophrenia, Asperger's syndrome, and head injury) may occur more frequently than expected in sexually impulsive men, including sexual offenders (for example, Kafka & Hennen, 2002; Kafka & Prentky, 1994, 1998).

- Empirically established effective pharmacological treatments for mood disorders, ADHD, and impulsivity are well documented. These conditions affect prefrontal/orbital frontal executive functioning and are associated with impulsivity; therefore, amelioration of such conditions could certainly affect, if not markedly ameliorate, the propensity to be sexually impulsive.
- Though much evidence exists demonstrating the efficacy of these treatments for other Axis I disorders, few empirical studies have examined the role of these interventions in the reduction of sexual arousal or sexual aggression. One retrospective study reported significant reduction in paraphilic activity among participants (Kraus et al., 2007), all of whom had received selective serotonin reuptake inhibitor (SSRI) medications and psychotherapy.
- Literature supporting the prescriptive use of the mood stabilizers such as limbic anticonvulsants and atypical neuroleptics for sexual offenders is lacking. There have also been sporadic case reports of the prescriptive use of naltrexone for adults with "compulsive sexual behavior" (Raymond, Grant, Kim, & Coleman, 2002).
- Research support for the effectiveness of pharmacological treatments such as testosterone-reducing agents is mixed. Without clear data regarding the efficacy of such treatments, providers should be sure to balance the risks of such interventions with the potential benefits of treatment.
- When pharmacological intervention is utilized, physicians should be included as a part of the treatment team.
- Pharmacological treatments should not be used as "stand-alone" interventions, and are ideally combined with other therapeutic treatment modalities, most commonly cognitive-behavior–based treatments, along with community-based interventions and supervised probation or parole. These treatments show promise as one significant aspect of sexual offender management.

OTHER IMPORTANT ISSUES

Civil Commitment

As of 2010 approximately 20 states (Arizona, California, Florida, Illinois, Iowa, Kansas, Massachusetts, Minnesota, Missouri, Nebraska, New Hampshire, New Jersey, New York, North Dakota, Pennsylvania, South Carolina, Texas, Virginia, Washington, and Wisconsin) and the District of Columbia have passed laws permitting the **civil commitment** of sexual offenders. In addition, the federal government passed legislation allowing civil commitment for federal sex offenders. The term "civil commitment" means that even after a convicted sex offender (this term applies to both rapists and child molesters) has fully served their prison term, they can, after certain legal proceedings showing their continued high risk of reoffending, be confined to a secure treatment facility for future treatment and in order to further protect the public. This civil commitment (civil because no additional crime has been committed) can last for many years—until treatment providers believe that the risk of reoffending has been reduced to a level in which it is safe to release the person. This law was passed partly based on past incidences in which offenders served their complete terms and treatment providers had good evidence that they would hurt other children if released, and these predictions turned out to be true. For example, in California a child molester who sexually violated and physically harmed children served his full prison term. While in treatment he stated that if released he would harm another child. He was released once he served his full term and immediately kidnapped a child and even bit off his penis. Officials wanted a legal mechanism to prevent this sort of occurrence so fairly predictable future incidences of abuse could be prevented.

This kind of law has been controversial. There have been criticisms along three major lines: (1) the field is not all that accurate at predicting future risk and thus due to this error rate, some individuals will be incorrectly committed; (2) relatedly, the field is not all that effective at reducing risk, that is, our treatments are somewhat weak and thus is it only to require someone to receive a relatively weak treatment until they are substantially changed by this; and (3) is it constitutional to confine someone based on the (flawed) prediction of a future crime. In general our system confines based on past crimes after due process. There are, however, exceptions to this—for instance, a person may be confined against their will because they are dangerous to themselves (e.g., they are suicidal).

Sex Offender Registration Laws

A final forensic issue is that the federal government passed a sex offender registration law (this often applies to a wide range of sexual offenders—child abusers, rapists, and even exhibitionists and voyeurs). This was spurred by a 1989 abduction of an 11-year-old boy in Minnesota. In 1994 a federal law was passed mandating all sexual offenders to register with their local law enforcement agencies so that their location could be known. In 1996 President Clinton signed what is commonly known as "**Megan's Law**," which required all states to disseminate this registry information to the public. In 2006 the law as also modified by the so-called Adam Walsh Sex Offender Registration and Notification Act, which also created a national registry for classifying sex offenders based on their type of offense for which they were convicted. All 50 states are also mandated to have websites so that the public can become informed about who is a sex offender and where they are living. The overall goals of this law is to both (1) enable law enforcement to track past offenders, and (2) help the public protect itself by allowing potential victims to understand where a past offender lives or works. Currently it is estimated that there are more than 600,000 registered sex offenders in the United States (ATSA, 2010). These laws are controversial and have been criticized for the following three reasons: (1) There is little research showing that these laws actually produce the intended outcomes, for example, they actually reduce future victimization; (2) they may violate the privacy of these convicted individuals, which may be a constitutional violation of rights; and (3) there are some data to suggest that these offenders and even their families receive problematic consequences due to these laws, such as job loss, threats, or property damage.

STUDY QUESTIONS

1. Explain the concept of paraphilia and how pedophilia is one of them.
2. Explain how a penile plethysmograph is used to assess sexual orientation.
3. What are the different ways that pedophilia is assessed and diagnosed?
4. What are some treatment options for those with pedophilic disorder?
5. What are the long-term legal consequences for those who are convicted of child sexual abuse charges?
6. Although there is no profile of pedophilic child abusers, what are some ways that they are different than others?
7. What is the Tanner scale and how is it used?

GLOSSARY

antiandrogen treatment A treatment choice in which those with pedophilic sexual attraction are given chemicals that are designed to reduce the sexual urge by decreasing the concentrations of testosterone. Sometimes referred to as *chemical castration.*

civil commitment (of sexual offenders) The right of many states to commit sexual child abusers to indefinite commitment in a mental health institution after criminal incarceration has concluded, presumptively to prevent future reoffending.

grooming Adult behavior that serves to ingratiate, train, or bring closer children for the purposes of increasing the chances of sexual contact or behaviors.

hebephilia Sexual attraction to children who are typically older than puberty, but usually considered too young to be viable or acceptable sexual consenters.

Megan's Law Laws requiring the registration of convicted child sexual abusers, as well as databases of convicted offenders that can be shared state to state.

paraphilia A sexual disorder that involves the necessary inclusion of (normally) non-sexual objects, behaviors, or situations as part of the sexual act.

pedophilia A sexual disorder that involves a sexual attraction to children.

penile plethysmograph A physiological assessment that involves using technology to measure changes in the circumference of the penis while viewing sexually explicit material. A version, the vaginal plethysmograph, also exists for women.

Tanner scale A scale of physiological development of primary and secondary sexual characteristics. The scale ranges from 1 to 5 (full sexual maturity).

REFERENCES

Abel, G. G., Becker, J. V., Cunningham, J., Mittelman, M. S., & Rouleau, J. L. (1988). Multiple paraphilic diagnoses among sex offenders. *Bulletin of the American Academy of Psychiatry and the Law, 16*, 153–168.

American Psychiatric Association. (2013). *Diagnostic and statistical manual of mental disorders* (5th ed.). Washington, DC: American Psychiatric Publishing.

Association for the Treatment of Sexual Abusers. (2010). *Sexual offender residence restrictions.* Retrieved from www.atsa.com/sexual-offender-residence-restrictions

Bailey, J. M., Pillard, R., Neale, M., & Agyei, Y. (1993). Heritable factors influence sexual orientation in women. *Archives of General Psychiatry, 50*(3), 217–223.

Briken, P., Hill, A., & Berner, W. (2003). Pharmacotherapy of paraphilias with long-acting agonists of luteinizing hormone-releasing hormone: a systematic review. *Journal of Clinical Psychiatry, 64*, 890–897.

Briken, P., & Kafka, M. P. (2007). Pharmacological treatments for paraphilic patients and sex offenders. *Current Opinions in Psychiatry, 20*, 609–613.

Hanson, R. K., & Harris, A. J. R. (2000). Where should we intervene? Dynamic predictors of sexual offense recidivism. *Criminal Justice and Behavior, 27*, 6–35.

Kafka, M. P., & Hennen, J. (2002). A DSM IV axis I comorbidity study of males (n = 120) with paraphilias and paraphilia-related disorders. *Sexual Abuse: A Journal of Research and Treatment, 14*, 349–366.

Kafka, M. P., & Prentky, R. A. (1994). Preliminary observations of DSM III-R axis I comorbidity in men with paraphilias and paraphilia-related disorders. *Journal of Clinical Psychiatry, 55*, 481–487.

Kafka, M. P., & Prentky, R. A. (1998). Attention deficit hyperactivity disorder in males with paraphilias and paraphilia-related disorders: A comorbidity study. *Journal of Clinical Psychiatry, 59*, 388–396.

Kraus, C., Strohm, K., Hill, A., Habermann, N., Berner, W., & Briken, P. (2007). Selective serotonin reuptake inhibitors (SSRI) in the treatment of paraphilia: A retrospective study [in German]. *Fortschritte der Neurologie Psychiatrie, 75*, 351–356.

Losel, F., & Schmucker, M. (2005). The effectiveness of treatment for sexual offenders: A comprehensive meta-analysis. *Journal of Experimental Criminology, 1,* 117–146.

Maletzky, B. M. (1991). The use of medroxyprogesterone acetate to assist in the treatment of sexual offenders. *Annals of Sex Research, 4,* 117–129.

Maletzky, B. M., Tolan, A., & McFarland, B. (2006). The Oregon Depo-Provera program: A five-year follow-up. *Sexual Abuse: A Journal of Research and Treatment, 18,* 303–316.

McConaghy, N., Blaszczynski, A., & Kidson, W. (1988). Treatment of sex offenders with imaginal desensitization and/or medroxyprogesterone. *Acta Psychiatrica Scandinavica, 77,* 199–206.

O'Donohue, W. T. (2010). Critique of the proposed DSM-V diagnosis of pedophilia. *Archives of Sexual Behavior, 39,* 587–590.

O'Donohue, W. T., & Letourneau, E. (1992). The psychometric properties of the penile tumescence assessment of child molesters. *Journal of Psychopathology and Behavioral Assessment, 14*(2), 123–174.

Raymond, N., Grant, J. E., Kim, S. W., & Coleman, E. (2002). Treatment of compulsive sexual behavior with naltrexone and serotonin reuptake inhibitors: Two case studies. *International Journal of Psychopharmacology, 17,* 201–205.

Sandyk, R. (1988). Naltrexone suppresses abnormal sexual behavior in Tourette's syndrome. *International Journal of Neuroscience, 43,* 107–110.

Tanner, J. M. (1978). *Foetus into man: Physical growth from conception to maturity.* Cambridge, MA: Harvard University Press.

CHAPTER

9

The Treatment of the Sexually Abused Child

GOALS OF THIS CHAPTER:

1. To understand the diversity of problems that may or may not occur for the sexually abused child.
2. To understand the complexity of assessments for problems associated with having been sexually abused.
3. To be a better prepared advocate in the search for intervention for children who have been sexually abused.

In order to really understand how a skilled clinician addresses the needs of a child who is sexually abused, we must first cover some basic information and issues involved in contemporary psychotherapy. The main five issues we cover are:

1. Is "sexual abuse" the right conceptual category regarding treatment? (We argue that it is not.)
2. What is known regarding victims' reactions? (Spoiler alert: There is some commonality, but their reactions are quite variable and we explain the reasons for this heterogeneity.)
3. Relatedly, what is known about clinical assessment and diagnoses related to these problems? (Assessment is complex and needs to be evidence-based.)
4. What is known about evidence-based treatment of these? (Short answer: Cognitive behavior therapy is the evidence-based therapy showing most effectiveness for a variety of problems experienced by sexually abused children.)

5. What are problems in contemporary health care delivery? (There are many problems: lack of access; high cost; problematic quality particularly in that many clinicians do not use evidence-based assessments and treatments.)

THE CATEGORY OF "SEXUALLY ABUSED CHILD"

A prominent philosopher, Gilbert Ryle (1949), came up with an interesting analysis of an intellectual mistake that he called "a category mistake." A category mistake, according to Ryle, occurs when a person misuses a term by making statements about a kind of thing that are simply inappropriate semantically for that kind of being. For example, it is perfectly meaningful (whether it is true or false is another matter) to say, "Most children are happy," because "happiness" is a kind of thing (conceptual category) "children" can experience. However, it would be a category mistake to say, "Most apples are happy." Apples simply are not the proper *kind* of entity that can be ascribed emotions such as happiness. The statement that "Most apples are happy" really then is not false but rather it is meaningless. The sentence seems syntactically well formed (it has a subject, a verb, and a predicate) but despite this outward appearance, semantically it is nonsense. Here is another sentence that is syntactically well formed but meaningless: "Green ideas sleep furiously." There are many category mistakes in this sentence—ideas are not the kind of thing that can be green—they are not the kind of thing that can sleep—and sleep is not the kind of thing that can be done furiously. Again, this sentence is not so much true or false as meaningless.

Some therapists claim that they treat "the sexually abused child." This phrase, though, might also be a category mistake. Let us explain first by using an example. It can be said with some meaning (but, also, as it turns out, problematically) that physicians treat "car accident victims." But really this, too, is a category mistake. There are no definitive medical protocols for treating "a car accident victim." There are, however, treatment protocols for treating a fractured tibia, or hemorrhaging, or cranial damage—medical problems and diagnoses, any of which may (or may not) result from a car accident. The point is that "car accident victim" may be an accurate descriptor of an historical event—the person while in a car was in a crash—and may even be the cause of the problem to be treated, but the wide variety of what can happen—the effects of this cause—to the person medically, makes the phrase "the treatment of a car accident victim" fairly useless for treatment planning. Most car accidents (fender benders), thankfully, result in no physical injury—and thus there needs to be no medical treatment for the "car accident victim." On the other hand, unfortunately, some accidents cause multiple life threatening injuries—perhaps to the brain, or perhaps to the heart—and these result in their own unique medical treatments.

👉 **Consider This**

If a physician were asked how to treat a "car accident victim," what kind of questions might they ask before venturing a treatment opinion?

The same ideas are true about the phrase "the treatment of the sexually abused child." There is too much heterogeneity in this phrase for it to be meaningful. Let us explore why there is this heterogeneity in the effects of abuse. This heterogeneity comes from five factors:

1. There is a lot of variance contributed by the term *sexual abuse*—sexual abuse can mean touching the child's chest while they were sleeping (and thus they might not even sense that it was occurring), or rubbing lotion inappropriately on a baby's genitals (they might not have the cognitive development to understand that they were being abused), or having repeated forced sexual intercourse with a 14-year-old stepdaughter. The abuse can have occurred one time or hundreds of times. Note that your intuitions would suggest that the child's reactions to these acts would probably vary a lot. And you would be right.

2. There is also a lot of variance in the term *child*. This is essentially a legal term and states vary on the age of majority (meaning when a person becomes an adult). But a child may be anything from a young baby, to, in some states, a 17-year-old. The reactions to abuse vary considerably by age.

3. Who abuses the child also can make a difference. Most abuse is what is called *intrafamilial*—a family member is the perpetrator. Whether the abuse is perpetrated by a father or by a stranger can have an impact on the child's reactions. The child's relationship to the abuser matters in the effects of the abuse on the child.

4. Finally, there are a host of other factors that mediate the effects of child sexual abuse (CSA) including whether the child is believed, social support during and after the child's outcry, the child's preabuse mental health status (whether they were already suffering from certain problems), whether they received good-quality therapy after the abuse if needed, how long the abuse occurred, whether the mother was complicit in the abuse, and so on. Other variables that may lessen or increase reactions to CSA include gender, age when first abused, age when abuse finished, and age at disclosure.

5. Finally, the effects of abuse can be thought to have various time courses. There can be *immediate effects* (minutes after the abuse—such as physical pain, fear,

shame); *midterm effects*—weeks or a few months after the abuse (e.g., PTSD, social problems); and *longer-term effects*—those that happen years afterward (e.g., substance abuse, sexual functioning problems, marital problems).

Thus, our view is that the better phrase is, for example, "the treatment of depression in a sexually abused child" or "the treatment of posttraumatic stress disorder in a sexually abused child"—because depression and PTSD are *the kinds of categories* mental health professionals treat. Or even "the treatment of academic difficulties of the sexually abused child"—because again academic difficulties may be the *kind of category* mental health professionals treat. So the bottom line on all of this is that really we have three issues:

1. There is no unique definite set of symptoms all sexually abused children experience. There are some trends (e.g., posttraumatic stress disorder is the most common *DSM-5* diagnosis; Foa, Keane, Friedman, & Cohen, 2008), but even with this, many children do not get this diagnosis.
2. Thus, each sexually abused child needs to be assessed individually to find out his or her unique set of symptoms, if any. (A point that is made is that thankfully some children seem to display no symptoms that merit treatment, just like some car accident victims—although they experienced a bad thing—do not display medical symptoms that they need medical treatment for.)
3. Thus, it is more meaningful and proper to talk about the treatment of PTSD and or depression, and so on, of the sexually abused child.

WHAT KINDS OF REACTIONS DO CHILDREN HAVE TO SEXUAL ABUSE?

Again, we have to recall the points we just made: There is no one symptom, no one set of symptoms, or no "pattern"—it depends too much on a host of mediating variables that were mentioned earlier (how long did the abuse occur, how many times was the child abused, at what age, by whom, what abusive acts occurred, how was the child doing before the abuse, how healthy was the child's support system, etc.). Having said this, however, certain problems are much more common than others. For example, sexual abuse causing someone to be psychotic (i.e., having delusions or hallucinations) is very rare; where abuse causing posttraumatic stress disorder is much more common (Foa et al., 2008).

Let us examine one study that illustrates many of these points. There was a recent study in New Zealand that examined 900 sexually abused children and followed them up for a number of years (Fergusson, McLeod, & Horwood, 2013). This longitudinal study allows an examination of different symptoms occurring over the course of time. Here's what the study found:

- Some of the children had no significant mental health problems (good news).
- There was a higher incidence of these disorders in children who were sexually abused:
  a. Depression
  b. Anxiety disorders, particularly PTSD
  c. Suicide ideation
  d. Suicide attempts
  e. Alcohol dependence
  f. Drug dependence
  g. Lower self-esteem
  h. Lower life satisfaction
  i. Decreased age of initiation of sex
  j. Increased numbers of partners
  k. Increased numbers of medical complaints

This pattern of results is fairly typical regarding sexually abused children. A good clinician will attempt to screen for these kinds of problems when seeing a sexually abused child or an adult who was sexually abused when they were younger. You can see that the assessment task is fairly complex as there are a number of problems to rule in or rule out. And again, individuals' reactions may be unique—they may have an eating disorder that either was premorbid to the abuse, exacerbated by the abuse, or caused by the abuse.

Clinicians sometimes classify the disorders of children into two broad categories: externalizing disorders and internalizing disorders (Achenbach, 1966). Roughly, externalizing disorders are behavioral excesses—hitting others, swearing, masturbating in public, disobeying rules, and so on. Internalizing behaviors are problems that are behavioral deficits or that are not as overt. For example, depression and anxiety are internalizing disorders. Someone who is depressed may do less due to their low energy. Someone who is anxious may have a lot of thoughts (internal states) that are related to worry and fear. In general, researchers have found that children can have either kind of problem after they have been sexually abused, but boys most often have externalizing problems while girls more often have internalizing problems (Ackerman, Newton, McPherson, Jones, & Dykman, 1998; Friedrich, Urquiza, & Beilke, 1986).

Finally, we would like to reemphasize the point that some children do not experience any mental health problems after they have been abused. This does not mean that the abuse was okay; it simply means that the child was not severely negatively impacted by the act. This could be due to a variety of reasons: The abuse was not particularly severe;

the child had a good support network; the child had good coping skills; and so on. It is wrong to think that every sexually abused child *must enter therapy. Many need therapy but some do not.* The second author (O'Donohue) has been directing a free clinic that treats sexually abused children for 20 years: A certain percentage of the children we assess (not the majority but around one in five) do not have any significant pathology that we need to treat. Again, this is good news: Children can be resilient.

WHAT IS NOT KNOWN

One has to read the preceding section very carefully. A useful and very important question is, "What is the probability that a child who has been abused will develop problem *x*?" where *x* can be anything like PTSD, depression, and so on. However, from the above, we can see that a number of variables mediate this relationship. This question becomes much more complex as each mediating variable needs to be properly accounted for in the question. Thus, the question becomes more like, "What is the probability that a 4-year-old girl, whose only premorbid problem was that she suffered from mild Asperger's disorder, who was abused by her stepfather, by his touching her chest one time, and immediately disclosed to a supportive mother, will develop problem *x* in the next year?" You hopefully can see how this question is appropriately nuanced. Unfortunately, these nuances make data collection more difficult. To answer this, we would need a representative sample of clients who have these characteristics (and, ideally, subjects who have all these characteristics who were not abused) to be in a control condition to see the base rates of these problems in the general population. Thus, if we had a sample of, say, 1,000 of these children and found that in a year 10% develop depression, while in the control group of identical children who were not abused the incidence of depression in a year was 5%, then we could infer that sexual abuse doubles the risk of depression, but still the majority of children with these characteristics do not develop depression (90% were not depressed). Note we need these control groups because children may develop problems for other reasons—their parents are not getting along, and so on ... we are actually interested in the difference between the base rate of problem development between children who have not been abused and children who have been abused. This is a reason why science and research is so important—if we hone our questions appropriately we see there is simply a need to conduct data in a controlled study.

Unfortunately our field does not have these kinds of studies. These are very difficult to conduct. Gathering a sample of these children with all the permutations of mediating variables is very, very difficult and expensive. So often we are left with the Socratic conclusion, that we do not know. We may have some relevant information—that it seems that sexually abused children often have a higher rate of depression—but often the exact frequency or a comparison to a similar group of children is not available

(Sbraga & O'Donohue, 2003). But to repeat one of the bottom-line points is just because there is research that shows that children who are sexually abused experience more problems does not mean *that the majority* of children who have been sexually abused experience this problem.

How can a child who has been sexually abused—which is a terrible event—not have problems?

This is an important question. Basically, it can be answered in two ways:

1. Remember some abuse (although always very wrong) is minor—just like some car accidents are minor and cause no medical problems. (Note also that just because the abuse does not result in a serious psychological problem for the child does *not* mean that the abuse was not wrong. Abuse is always wrong—because it mistreats a child—whether it results in diagnosable harm to the child).

2. Some children have very favorable mediating variables that cause them to be resilient and are able to cope with the negative events in their lives. They may have very loving supportive families, are blessed with no premorbid problems, or have a lot of strengths that they can bring to bear (intelligence, good problem solving, emotional stability, good support network) that allow them to cope with the negative event and not end up having a lot of psychological problems.

CLINICAL ASSESSMENT AND DIAGNOSIS

Assessment and diagnosis is about measurement. Measurement means the attempt to accurately detect whether something is present and perhaps to detect the magnitude of this kind of entity. For example, clinicians may want to measure whether you are depressed; and if they find out you are, whether your depression is mild (some minor crying and some minor decrease in energy levels) or whether it is severe (suicidal ideation, not functioning at all). In mental health the constructs one is attempting to measure has something to do with psychological constructs—perhaps diagnoses such as depression or PTSD, perhaps behaviors (amount of alcohol consumed per day), perhaps thoughts (frequency and intensity of suicidal ideation), perhaps what has happened in the past (exactly what did the abuse consist of), and so on.

Assessment is difficult. It is hard for a variety of reasons. Among these are:

- Clients sometimes just do not know the information we are seeking. We can ask about how many hours they slept last night and they can have difficulties providing us with this bit of information.
- Clients sometimes lie or distort. They can be embarrassed or want to "fake good" or "fake bad" for a variety of reasons.

- Therapists can make mistakes. At first we are often meeting a relative stranger (although we may have some phone intake information)—we face the classic problem of "we don't know what we don't know." What domains should we query? The child is young—say 10—should we ask about alcohol or drug use? It is not unprecedented at this age, but somewhat rare. We can make the mistake of not assessing a domain that actually needs to be queried.

- With children, we not only ask questions to them and about them, but we also ask questions to and about their caregivers. We do this because as adults they should be able to supply important information that their child may just be too young to know. But we also do this as the mental health of the caregiver impacts the well-being and the treatment of the child. A caregiver who suffers from depression and alcoholism will likely limit the success of treatment and create additional problems for the sexually abused child.

- It is a psychometric principle that all assessment methods contain error (this is discussed more later). The issue becomes, how much error? You might see this when you weigh yourself in the morning on your bathroom scale. Your scales are not perfect measurement devices—how you stand on them, whether your floor is perfectly even, and so on, can affect their reading. Take three measurements of your weight tomorrow morning. Chances are they are not all exactly the same. Your weight (the underlying construct to be measured) is not changing in these few seconds; it is simply your measurement device is showing its error. The same thing applies to measurement procedures in mental health—none are perfect. They all contain error. We have several important terms to describe the amount of error in measurement devices.
  - Reliability. **Reliability** simply refers to the consistency or repeatability of a measurement. The idea is that if the measurement reading is changing when we know the underlying thing to be measured is not changing, then we know we have error in our measurement. We saw this in the bathroom scale example above. If you get on the scale and it says 150, get off and get on again and it says 155, and get on and off again and it says 152, we know your scale is not reliable—there is no way you are gaining 5 pounds and then losing 2 pounds in a few seconds. The key saying in psychometrics is that if we know we have reliability problems then we know we have validity problems. Note a very interesting special case. If the bathroom scale consistently says 2 pounds; 2 pounds; 2 pounds, then the scale is reliable—the measurement is consistent—but unless you weigh 2 pounds—completely invalid. There are different types of reliability. Here are some of the major ones:
    - **Test-retest reliability**. The strategy here is to give the test two times, in a time frame where the underlying construct should not change, and to see

if one gets the same reading. The repeated use of the bathroom scales was a test-retest reliability.

- **Split-half reliability**. The strategy here is to see the consistency between, say, the first half of the test and the second half of the test. Thus, if I have a 100-item test I can see how the score of the first 50 items relate to the score of the second 50 items.

- **Interrater reliability**. This can be an important issue with respect to diagnosis. The question becomes, do two raters (e.g., clinicians) come to the same conclusions regarding a particular client. For example, do they both diagnosis her as depressed? Or do they both rule out panic disorder?

○ Validity. There are actually many kinds of validity. **Validity** refers to the accuracy of inferences made from a measurement.

- **Content validity** refers to whether the measure contains the right sort of items and the extent to which it comprehensively covers the domain. For example, solely having addition items on a test purportedly measuring mathematical knowledge would be an example of poor content validity—it does not have items on subtraction or multiplication, or geometry.

- **Construct validity** refers to the accuracy of inferences regarding the construct. If one is attempting to measure the construct of depression by using a bathroom scale, the issue is: How much do your weight measures correlate with the actual construct of depression? The higher the correlation (which is the preservation of rank order) the more the measure has construct validity. In this example, we would expect the bathroom scale measure of depression to have a low (although not zero correlation). Better correlations might be found with paper and pencil measures that ask the respondent actual questions about depressive symptoms (lower appetite, crying, feelings of hopelessness, etc.).

- **Predictive validity** refers to the extent that the measure can be used to make inferences about other points of time. Measures of suicide potential often seek high predictive validity. If we measure your suicide potential now, we are most interested whether in the future you will actually attempt suicide.

- **Discriminant validity** refers to the ability to make accurate inferences about the construct without noise being added by other constructs. Thus, if I want to measure intelligence I might worry my test results also are influenced by other constructs—for example, the motivation to do well on a test. Discriminant validity shows that I am measuring my construct of interest purely—and that I am not inadvertently also measuring other constructs.

- **Sensitivity** is the probability of a positive test among clients with the problem. That is, if a person actually has the disorder, will my test detect it? The sensitivity of a test tells me this.
- **Specificity** is the probability of a negative result in clients without the problem. That is, if the person actually does *not* have the problem, will my test tell me this—give me a negative reading—or will it falsely classify the person as positive?

Evidence-based assessment is a movement that suggests that clinicians should only administer measures that have known and good reliability, validity, sensitivity, and specificity. Certain well-known tests such as the Rorschach Inkblot tests generally fail regarding this (Wood & Lilienfeld, 1999), while other tests such as the MMPI or the Beck Depression Inventory generally have known and acceptable psychometrics—although again, not perfect. It is also important to recognize that these psychometrics are really not universal—one needs to ask what are the psychometrics of a test for a specific population and for a specific inference. For example, what is the predictive validity of the BDI for Hispanic women for predicting suicide? This, again, shows the need and the complexity of research into the psychometrics of clinical instruments.

Consider This

What would it mean to have an assessment of depression that was reliable but not valid. What about one that has no reliability? How would we know anything about validity in that case?

WHAT AN ASSESSMENT OF A SEXUALLY ABUSED CHILD MIGHT LOOK LIKE

There is usually a variety of assessment methods used. Here we describe the major ones.

Record review. It is important to review a variety of records in order to understand the child's history as well as current status. Each case will vary on what records are available. Typically the clinician will want to review the following four types of records:

1. School records to see how the child is functioning in this important context? Does the child have any developmental or learning problems? Does the child have any behavioral or conduct problems at school? How are they doing socially with their peers? Have any problems emerged postabuse or exacerbated by the abuse?

2. Forensic abuse records. What were the details of the abuse? How extensive was the abuse? What was the child's relationship to the abuser? Were there any unusual features to the child's allegation (e.g., fantastical details). What has happened to the perpetrator? Is the child safe? Did the child have problems recounting the abuse? Did the nonoffending parent support the child? How was the child's experience of their testimony?

3. Medical records. Was the child physically harmed by the abuse and if so are these problems receiving proper medical attention? Does the child have any other medical problems and is the management of these being compromised by the child's psychological functioning (e.g., the child has Type II diabetes and is overeating postabuse)?

4. Mental health records. What treatments, by whom, and for what has the child received? Are any of these ongoing and need to be coordinated? What diagnoses has the child been given in the past and do these seem reasonable? Have the treatments the child received been reasonable and evidence-based? How have the children responded to therapy—have they been cooperative; do they generally complete homework, and attend sessions?

Interview with guardian (nonoffending parent). The purpose of this part of the assessment is twofold: One is trying to understand more about past history and current functioning of the child, but one is also trying to get an understanding of the strengths and weaknesses of the guardian. If the guardians have their own set of problems (e.g., is an active alcoholic) this can impact the child's functioning and impact the child's involvement with therapy. Key questions include: What do you see as the child's current strengths and weaknesses? What changes did you see in the child while they were being abused? How is the child doing in school? How is the child doing socially? How is the child's basic health? Do you see the child having problems such as bedwetting, being sad, being nervous and afraid, sleeping, loss of appetite? How are you doing? How did the abuse affect you?

Interview with the child. This varies a lot depending on the child's age. Obviously it is very different interviewing a 3-year-old versus a 13-year-old. However, the first stage of the interview is spent on developing rapport. One cannot just charge in and "get down to business" and start asking questions. One has to engage the child and to get the child comfortable with the interviewer. Time is usually spent talking about fun things—the child's favorite foods or past birthday. The interviewer needs to be very positive and reinforcing. Usually in age-appropriate language the interviewers then explain what they are going to do today and the child's role. The interviewer may provide crayons and coloring books so the children can play while they are talking. The interviewer also needs to be careful and watch if the child is bored, stressed, or tired and take appropriate breaks.

The interviewers are trying to gain most of the same information that they are also getting from the nonoffending guardian—but from the child's perspective. The interviewer is also viewing the children's behavior as a sample—what does the clinician see in the children—do they appear to be highly anxious or comfortable—do they appear to be happy or sad, and so on.

Collateral contact with teacher. Teachers, especially experienced teachers can be excellent sources of information. They can spend 7 or so hours a day with a child and see the child with their peers and thus have the potential to more clearly observe deviants from normative behavior at a certain age.

Testing with guardian. Parents or guardians are "informants" regarding children in their care and as such can fill out testing about their observations regarding their child. The Child Behavior Checklist (Achenbach, 1991) is often given and there are three versions of this test: one that the child fills out; one that the child's teacher fills out; and one that the parent fills out.

Testing with child. There are a number of tests that a child can complete, again depending on their age. Sometimes there are versions of adult tests for adolescents or children. One of the most frequently given adult tests is the Minnesota Multiphasic Personality Inventory. There is an adolescent version of this for children often known as the MMPI-A. There are depression inventories for children, PTSD report scales, and so on.

CONCLUSIONS AND INFORMING SESSION

All this assessment information needs to be compiled and conclusions need to be made. Often there is an informing session where the guardian is first told of these results and then the child is brought in. This is a critical step in treatment planning. The guardian needs to know what was ruled out and why and what diagnoses or problems were ruled in and why. Treatment options and priorities need to be discussed. A key consideration in this is: What problems, if any, are impairing the child's functioning? What problems, if any, are causing the child pain or discomfort? What problems, if any, are causing others pain or problems functioning? In the usual case, treatment is voluntary and the child's guardian needs to consent to treatment, and some providers want the child to assent to treatment. Assent is the notion that although the children's cognitive development is not such that they can give fully informed consent, they do have a general understanding of their problems and what their treatment will entail and they agree to this.

EVIDENCE-BASED TREATMENT

Next, actual treatment begins if the child has any treatment needs and the guardian consents to treatment. The quality of treatment unfortunately can vary tremendously.

We all want treatment that is effective, efficient, and safe. Unfortunately there is evidence to suggest that both in medical and in mental health service delivery this is not always the case (Institute of Medicine, 2001). In mental health, treatments that have been studied scientifically and found to be effective are called *evidence-based treatments* or sometimes *empirically supported treatments* These interventions generally have been studied in randomly controlled trials and found to have superior effects to some control group (often a no-treatment control). Sometimes the standards are more rigorous and there have to be at least two studies in two different settings before a treatment is considered "evidence-based."

Unfortunately it has been the case that service providers choose to deliver therapies for other reasons then their demonstrated effectiveness in scientific studies. Some therapists may choose a therapy because "it sounds like it should work"; or because they have been to a workshop and a charismatic workshop leader presented cases in which the therapy worked; or because they have been trained in a certain model of therapy (e.g., psychoanalytic) and they might not know how to deliver any other therapy. On the other hand, to be fair, sometimes the research literature is not all that clear: Some studies show a therapy to have strong effects; others do not. Some studies have problems, for example, small sample sizes or were conducted by researchers who have some vested interest in the therapy working (this is called the *therapist allegiance effect*). So, it gets complicated.

An additional complication is that outcome research on psychotherapeutic effectiveness often has not been conducted all that well. Notice in a sentence earlier we talked about a therapy being "safe," that is, that no problematic side effects occur during the course of therapy (these are called *iatrogenic effects*—negative effects caused by therapies themselves). This is a wonderful ideal but often not investigated by outcome research protocols in psychotherapy. Notice also we mentioned that we generally want treatments to be efficient—for example, to be as quick as possible or low-cost as possible. Again, unfortunately, there has been little research into what are the most efficient treatment alternatives: Is an antidepressant medication more or less efficient than a course of cognitive behavior therapy? Is reading a good self-help book for depression more efficient that group therapy? These are key questions and more research is needed.

However, we again know some key information. There are resources that attempt to review the literature and help the clinician more easily identify these. In physical medicine, for example, there are the Cochrane Reviews (2014), which distill randomly controlled trials of the treatments of a wide variety of medical problems. The prestigious Institute of Medicine (IOM; 2001) also periodically comes out with reports on reviews of the literature. For example, the IOM recently reviewed all the research and found that after looking at all the controlled trials for both medications and psychotherapies, the only treatment that can be called evidence-based for PTSD is cognitive behavior therapy. This is vitally important as this therapy is relevant because PTSD is one of the most common diagnoses for sexually abused children.

The American Psychological Association (APA) also convened a committee to identify all the empirically supported treatments. These often are known as *the Chambless report* after the chair of the committee (Chambless et al., 1998). Table 9.1 contains the most recent Chambless report.

An inspection of this table reveals four conclusions:

1. Most of the **empirically supported therapies** come from one school of therapy— cognitive behavior therapy.
2. Many disorders do not have an empirically supported therapy—that is, although there are hundreds of disorders in the *DSM-5* (American Psychiatric Association, 2013) there are many "orphaned disorders" such as antisocial personality or dissociative disorder where no therapy has been shown to be effective in randomly controlled scientific studies.
3. Even though cognitive behavior therapy is the school where the vast majority of evidence-based therapies are derived, cognitive behavior therapy actually involves a number of techniques such as contingency management, exposure therapy, irrational belief disputation, behavioral activation, and systematic desensitization (O'Donohue & Fisher, 2008, 2009). To know how to intervene on all these problems requires a sophisticated therapist who has a wide skill set.
4. Often if therapists want to remain evidence-based, they do not have many choices—only one or in some rare cases two therapies are evidence-based for a particular problem.

Consider This

Why would it be important to use (whenever possible) treatment approaches identified on the Empirically Supported Treatment list? What are some risks with using interventions *not* on the list?

TREATMENT PROTOCOLS FOR CASES OF SEXUAL AND PHYSICAL ABUSE

Trauma-Focused Cognitive Behavioral Treatment (CBT)

Ester Deblinger of the Medical University of New Jersey has done the most work and has the most publications on evidence-based treatment for the problems of sexually

Table 9.1 Empirically Supported Treatments

Disorder	Well-Established Treatments	Citation for Efficacy Evidence
Anxiety and stress	Cognitive behavior therapy for panic disorder with and without agoraphobia	Barlow, Craske, Cerny, and Klosko (1989)
		Clark et al. (1994)
	Cognitive behavior therapy for generalized anxiety disorder	Butler and Booth (1991)
		York, Borkovec, Vasey, and Stern (1987)
	Exposure treatment for agoraphobia	Trull, Nietzel, and Main (1988)
	Exposure/guided mastery for specific phobia	Bandura (1969)
		Öst, Fellenius, and Sterner (1991)
	Exposure and response prevention for obsessive-compulsive disorder	van Balkom et al. (1994)
	Stress Inoculation Training for Coping with Stressors	Saunders et al. (1996)
Depression	Behavior therapy for depression	Jacobson et al. (1996)
		McLean and Hakstian (1979)
	Cognitive therapy for depression	Dobson (1989)
		DiMascio et al. (1979)
	Interpersonal therapy for depression	Elkin et al. (1989)
Health problems	Behavior therapy for headache	Blanchard, Andrasik, Ahles, Teders, and O'Keefe (1980)
		Holroyd and Penzien (1990)
	Cognitive behavior therapy for bulimia	Agras, Schneider, Arnow, Raeburn, and Telch (1989)
		Thackwray, Smith, Bodfish, and Meyers (1993)
	Multicomponent cognitive behavior therapy for pain associated with rheumatic disease	Keefe et al. (1990)
		Parker et al. (1988)
	Multicomponent cognitive behavior therapy with relapse prevention for smoking cessation	Hill, Rigdon, and Johnson (1993)
		Stevens and Hollis (1989)
Problems of childhood	Behavior modification for enuresis	Houts, Berman, and Abramson (1994)
	Parent training programs for children with oppositional behavior	Walter and Gilmore (1973)
		Wells and Egan (1988)
Marital discord	Behavioral marital therapy	Azrin et al. (1980)
		Jacobson and Follette (1985)
Sexual dysfunction	Behavior therapy for female orgasmic dysfunction and male erectile dysfunction	LoPiccolo and Stock (1986)
		Auerbach and Kilmann (1977)

(*continued overleaf*)

Table 9.1 (*continued*)

Disorder	Probably Efficacious Treatments	Citation
Anxiety	Applied relaxation for panic disorder	Öst (1988)
	Applied relaxation for generalized anxiety disorder	Barlow, Rapee, and Brown (1992)
		Borkovec and Costello (1993)
	Cognitive behavior therapy for social phobia	Heimberg et al. (1990)
		Feske and Chambless (1995)
	Cognitive therapy for OCD	van Oppen et al. (1995)
	Couples communication training adjunctive to exposure for agoraphobia	Arnow, Taylor, Agras, and Telch (1985)
	Exposure treatment for PTSD	Foa, Feske, Murdock, Kozak, and McCarthy (1991)
		Keane, Fairbank, Caddell, and Zimering (1989)
	Exposure treatment for social phobia	Feske and Chambless (1995)
	Stress Inoculation Training for PTSD	Foa, Rothbaum, Biggs, and Murdock (1991)
	Relapse prevention program for obsessive-compulsive disorder	Hiss, Foa, and Kozak (1994)
	Systematic desensitization for animal phobia	Kirsch, Tennen, Wickless, Saccone, and Cody (1983)
		Öst (1978)
	Systematic desensitization for public speaking anxiety	Kirsch et al. (1983)
		Öst (1978)
	Systematic desensitization for social anxiety	Paul and Shannon (1966)
Chemical abuse and dependence	Behavior therapy for cocaine abuse	Higgins and Budney (1993)
	Brief dynamic therapy for opiate dependence	Woody, McLellan, Luborsky, and O'Brien (1990)
	Cognitive-behavioral relapse prevention therapy for cocaine dependence	Ball, Carroll, and Rounsaville (1994)
	Cognitive therapy for opiate dependence	Woody et al. (1990)
	Cognitive behavior therapy for benzodiazepine withdrawal in panic disorder patients	Ball, Otto, Pollack, and Rosenbaum (1994)
		Spiegel et al. (1993)
	Community Reinforcement Approach for alcohol dependence	Azrin (1976)
		Hunt and Azrin (1973)
	Cue exposure adjunctive to inpatient treatment for alcohol dependence	Drummond and Glautier (1994)
	Project CALM for mixed alcohol abuse and dependence (behavioral marital therapy plus disulfiram)	O'Farrell, Cutter, and Floyd (1985)
		O'Farrell, Cutter, Choquette, Floyd, and Bayog (1992)
	Social skills training adjunctive to inpatient treatment for alcohol dependence	Eriksen, Björnstad, and Götestam (1986)

Table 9.1 (*continued*)

Disorder	Probably Efficacious Treatments	Citation
Depression	Brief dynamic therapy	Gallagher-Thompson and Steffen (1994)
	Cognitive therapy for geriatric patients	Scogin and McElreath (1994)
	Reminiscence therapy for geriatric patients	Arean et al. (1993)
		Scogin and McElreath (1994)
	Self-control therapy	Fuchs and Rehm (1977)
		Rehm, Fuchs, Roth, Kornblith, and Romano (1979)
Health problems	Behavior therapy for childhood obesity	Epstein, Valoski, Wing, and McCurley (1994)
		Wheeler and Hess (1976)
	Cognitive behavior therapy for binge eating disorder	Telch, Agras, Rossiter, Wilfley, and Kenardy (1990)
		Wilfley et al. (1993)
	Cognitive behavior therapy adjunctive to physical therapy for chronic pain	Nicholas, Wilson, and Goyen (1991)
	Cognitive behavior therapy for chronic low back pain	Turner and Clancy (1988)
	EMG biofeedback for chronic pain	Flor and Birbaumer (1993)
		Spence, Sharpe, Newton-John, and Champion (1995)
	Hypnosis as an adjunct to cognitive-behavior therapy for obesity	Bolocofsky, Coulthard-Morris, and Spinier (1984)
		Wilfley et al. (1993)
	Interpersonal therapy for binge eating disorder	
	Interpersonal therapy for bulimia	Fairburn, Jones, Peveler, Hope, and O'Connor (1993)
	Multicomponent cognitive therapy for irritable bowel syndrome	Lynch and Zamble (1989)
	Multicomponent cognitive behavior therapy for pain of sickle cell disease	Gil, Williams, Keefe, and Beckham (1996)
	Multicomponent operant behavioral therapy for chronic pain	Turner and Clancy (1988)
		Turner, Clancy, McQuade, and Cardenas (1990)
	Scheduled, reduced smoking adjunctive to multicomponent behavior therapy for smoking cessation	Cinciripini et al. (1994)
		Cinciripini et al. (1995)
	Thermal biofeedback for Raynaud's syndrome	Freedman, Ianni, and Wenig (1983)
	Thermal biofeedback plus autogenic relaxation training for migraine	Blanchard, Theobald, Williamson, Silver, and Brown (1978)
		Sargent, Solbach, Coyne, Spohn, and Segerson (1986)
Marital discord	Emotionally focused couples therapy	Johnson and Greenberg (1985)
	Insight-oriented marital therapy	Snyder and Wills (1989)
		Snyder, Wills, and Grady-Fletcher (1991)

(*continued overleaf*)

Table 9.1 (*continued*)

Disorder	Probably Efficacious Treatments	Citation
Problems of childhood	Behavior modification of encopresis	O'Brien, Ross, and Christophersen (1986)
	Cognitive-behavior therapy for anxious children (overanxious, separation anxiety, and avoidant disorders)	Kendall (1994) Kendall et al. (1997)
	Exposure for simple phobia	Menzies and Clarke (1993)
	Family anxiety management training for anxiety disorders	Barrett et al. (in press)
Sexual dysfunction	Hurlbert's combined treatment approach for female hypoactive sexual desire	Hurlbert, White, Powell, and Apt (1993)
	Masters and Johnson's sex therapy for female orgasmic dysfunction	Everaerd and Dekker (1981)
	Zimmer's combined sex and marital therapy for female hypoactive sexual desire	Zimmer (1987)
Other	Behavior modification for sex offenders	Marshall, Jones, Ward, Johnston, and Barbaree (1991)
	Dialectical behavior therapy for borderline personality disorder	Linehan, Armstrong, Suarez, Allmon, and Heard (1991)
	Family intervention for schizophrenia	Falloon and Pederson (1985) Randolph et al. (1994)
	Habit reversal and control techniques	Azrin, Nunn, and Frantz (1980) Azrin, Nunn, and Frantz-Renshaw (1980)
	Social skills training for improving social adjustment of schizophrenic patients	Marder et al. (1996)
	Supported employment for severely mentally ill clients	Drake, Mueser, Clark, and Wallach (1996)

Source: From Chambless et al. (1998).

abused children. Her focus is on their anxiety disorders, particularly PTSD as this is the most common problem of these children. Deblinger's protocol (Cohen, Mannarino, & Deblinger, 2006) is summarized by the word PRACTICE. It first entails psychoeducation and teaching the nonoffending parents child management and parenting skills. This includes teaching effective communication, basic information about child abuse, what common behavioral reactions are to abuse, and teaching parents how to manage their child's behavior. Next are relaxation techniques. Children are taught focused breathing, muscle relaxation, and visual imaging. Next the therapy targets affective expression and regulation; this entails teaching both parents and children how to manage emotional reactions when they are reminded of the traumatic event, how to self-soothe, and how to express emotions in a healthy way. The next component of the protocol is cognitive coping and processing. This is an attempt to assist the adults and children recognize their thoughts, feelings, and behaviors about the traumatic event and help them to stop attributing those feelings to events in everyday life. The next component is trauma narrative and processing. This stage uses exposure techniques to the traumatic events and work to decrease the frequency of inaccurate or unhelpful thoughts about the traumatic event as well as anxiety reactions to stimuli similar to the event. The next component of the protocol is in vivo exposure. This involves gradual exposure to help the abused children deal with reminders of the traumatic event in their environment and how to control their emotional reactions to them. The next step is conjoint parent/child sessions. This is where the families work together to improve communication by discussing the traumatic events in a healthy way. The final step in the protocol is enhancing personal safety and future growth. This focuses on training on safety, healthy sexuality, and interpersonal relationships. This also teaches how to apply these new skills to future stressors and future reminders of the traumatic event.

It is beyond the scope of this book to describe this diverse set of techniques in any detail. The interested reader is referred to Fisher and O'Donohue (2006) for a more detailed account of the evidence-based assessments and treatments for nearly 70 disorders. Also, O'Donohue and Fisher (2008) have much more detailed descriptions of these techniques. Finally, youtube.com has many demonstrations of these techniques that are quite interesting. Just type in, for example, "systematic desensitization" or "exposure therapy" in the search function and enactments of these treatment techniques are shown.

Problems in Contemporary Health Care Delivery

We do not want to leave the reader with the impression that this assessment and treatment process occurs with ease and universal regularity. It can be said that there are many problems that occur in actual service delivery to the sexually abused children. Increasingly researchers are also studying this problem: How can we increase the likelihood that any child who needs services actually gets high-quality services in a timely manner? Crossing the Quality Chasm (IOM, 2001) is a classic report that was a wake-up call for Americans as it depicted many problems in the U.S. health care system. These also apply to health care delivery to the sexually abused child. Here is a brief description of some of the main problems:

Access. Many factors contrive to cause problems in accessing services. Services can cost money and poor individuals or individuals without services simply do not have these funds. In addition, there may not be professionals in close proximity to where the sexually abused child lives. Folks who live in rural or frontier areas may simply have no professionals or qualified professionals within a few hours' drive.

Safety. Safety has been a particular concern with medications. Medications—even psychotropic medications such as antidepressants—often have serious side effects (Antonuccio, Danton, DeNelsky, Greenberg, & Gordon, 1999). In fact, after years of being given to children fairly indiscriminately, antidepressants now have what are called *black box warnings*, which tell parents that there is evidence to show that among serious side effects of antidepressant usage in children is an increased likelihood of suicide. A prominent researcher has concluded that the randomly controlled trials show that cognitive behavior therapy and antidepressant medications show approximately equivalent effectiveness but psychotherapy is safer—it shows much fewer side effects.

Cost. Therapy can be quite costly. For example, protocols for cognitive behavior therapy for PTSD or depression often last between 12 and 18 one-hour sessions. Professionals can charge around $100 an hour. Thus, to be treated for even one of these disorders may cost $1,200 to $1,800 and maybe more if the case is more difficult or when the assessment phase is also considered. There are too few steps being made to drive down the cost of therapy to make it more affordable (Cummings & O'Donohue, 2011).

Effectiveness. We have already discussed this. There is unfortunately a large number of therapists who are still not delivering evidence-based assessments and therapies.

Efficiency. There is an additional question of how to most efficiently treat a problem. That is, how to get the most "bang for the buck" or how to do this most quickly or in a way that is less disruptive for the client. One innovation is stepped care (O'Donohue & Draper, 2011), in which, when appropriate, the client is given options for their treatment, some of which are cheaper, easier, and less disruptive—and all of which have evidence for the effectiveness. For example, here are eight stepped care options for the treatment of depressions.

1. Watchful waiting (when the problem just occurred and is mild—one is waiting a brief amount of time to see if the problem spontaneously remits).
2. Psychoeducation. The patient is given a brief pamphlet or a website to see if they can self-manage the problem. The content may cover practical ways to gain increased social support; how exercise can help; and how increasing positive events in one's life has ameliorative effects. Again, this is most appropriate when the problem is mild.
3. Bibliotherapy. Some folks like reading self-help books. For depression David Burns's book *Feeling Good* (Burns, 1999) has been extensively studied and found to be effective for adult depression. The book costs around $10 and through amazon.com can be sent in a few days to any U.S. address.
4. E-health. There are increasingly available treatment options on the web that can be self-administered. Australia has been a leader in this and its beacon sites (www.beacon.anu.edu.au) have been studied and are effective and low cost.

5. Group therapy. This can be lower cost than individual therapy for obvious reasons—the therapist time cost is spread over many clients. In general the outcome research shows clients like this format (although not all do) and that group therapy generally is as effective as individual therapy.

6. Individual therapy. This is the therapist's "hammer"—most therapists think in terms that this is the "go to" or even only mode of intervention. It has its advantages but two disadvantages are: (1) it is relatively expensive and (2) it is not available for all. That is, when we examine the incidence of disorders in the United States we simply cannot provide individual psychotherapy to everyone with the number of therapists we have.

7. Medication. This often needs a psychiatrist to prescribe. Currently there is a shortage of psychiatrists and therefore it can take months to gain an appointment and get a prescription. In addition, medications can be expensive and have a wide range of side effects.

8. Inpatient therapy. This is the most expensive and most intrusive option for the patient. However, at times, such as when the patient is seriously suicidal, it can be the best option.

The basic idea then in stepped care is for the therapist and the client (or if a child the client's guardian) to jointly see what step is best for the client. This again depends on a number of factors, including the severity of the problem, what options are available, cost, and patient preference.

Continuity of care. Sometimes care is not continuous. That is, there are gaps or breaks in care that do not serve the client well. In general if the patient has been treated in an inpatient unit, one wants a fairly immediate transition to outpatient therapy. However, it can be the case that "Murphy's law" happens and there are no outpatient therapists available.

Equitability. This is the notion that certain variables ought not to influence the quality of treatment one receives. It seems unfair that poor folks get poorer (or no) treatment than richer folks; or that folks who live in cities get better treatment than folks who live in rural settings; or that minorities get poorer treatments than those in the majority culture. However, this seems to be the case.

Patient-centered. Finally, therapy is best when it is patient-centered, meaning that the patient's needs and preferences are given priority, instead, for example, of the provider's. Providers, on the whole, would like to work bankers' hours and have their weekends off. If then clinics are open only during these hours, the treatment delivery system can then be said to be "provider-centric" rather than "patient-centered. Changing hours so that patients can more easily access treatment, making treatment more affordable, making it more local, giving the patient choice, and improving the transparency of the process are all steps that make health care delivery more patient-centered.

CONCLUSIONS

One can see that providing high-quality treatment for the problems of a sexually abused child is quite complex and challenging. For those of you looking for careers in this field there is a lot of need for creativity and research on the extent to which creative solutions actually achieve these ends. If you end up being a health care consumer, caveat emptor—let the buyer beware. Be an educated consumer who asks questions and becomes informed about what assessments and treatments are being offered, why certain diagnoses were ruled in or ruled out, the psychometrics of assessments used, and the safety, effectiveness, and costs of any treatments being proposed. There are many good therapists out there, but as *Crossing the Quality Chasm* shows, this quality is far from universal.

STUDY QUESTIONS

1. Why is the idea of "treatment for the sexually abused child" essentially a meaningless phrase?

2. Discuss the causes of variability in the aftereffects of child sexual abuse for child functioning.

3. Which mental health diagnoses are sometimes associated with having been sexually abused?

4. What are some reasons that a sexually abused child might recover without significant psychological harm?

5. Name some of the reasons that assessment of the psychological adjustment of child sexual abuse victims can be difficult.

6. What are reliability and validity in the assessment of psychological functioning? Name some types of each.

7. What does it mean when a treatment technique is not considered an "empirically supported treatment?"

8. Name some empirically supported treatment techniques for specific problems as identified by the Chambless report.

9. Name some problems the chapter discusses related to access to contemporary health care delivery.

10. If you are put in a position to find interventions for a child who has been sexually abused, think through the numerous difficulties that you must be prepared to handle. Write a short guide outline for the things you will need to think about and understand.

GLOSSARY

construct validity The accuracy of inferences or assumptions regarding the construct.

content validity Whether the measure contains the right sort of items and the extent to which it comprehensively covers the domain.

discriminant validity The ability to make accurate inferences about the construct without error being added by other constructs.

empirically supported therapies Treatment approaches that have shown, in the scientific literature, some consistency in their helpful effects for certain populations and certain problems.

interrater reliability The degree to which two people giving the same assessment to the same person agree with each other.

predictive validity The extent that the measure can be used to make inferences about other points of time. For example, does it help us to understand prognosis?

reliability The consistency or repeatability of a measurement.

sensitivity The probability of a positive test among clients with the problem.

specificity The probability of a negative result in clients without the problem.

split-half reliability The degree to which the first half and last half of an assessment agree with each other.

test-retest reliability The degree to which an assessment done twice yields similar results.

validity The accuracy of inferences made from a measurement.

REFERENCES

Achenbach, T. M. (1966). The classification of children's psychiatric symptoms: A factor-analytic study. *Psychological Monographs: General and Applied, 80*(7), 1–37. doi:10.1037/h0093906

Achenbach, T. M. (1991). *Integrative guide to the 1991 CBCL/4–18, YSR, and TRF Profiles.* Burlington: University of Vermont.

Ackerman, P. T., Newton, J. E., McPherson, W. B., Jones, J. G., & Dykman, R. A. (1998). Prevalence of post traumatic stress disorder and other psychiatric diagnoses in three groups of abused children (sexual, physical, and both). *Child Abuse & Neglect, 22*(8), 759–774.

Agras, W. S., Schneider, J. A., Arnow, B., Raeburn, S. D., & Telch, C. F. (1989). Cognitive-behavioral treatment with and without exposure plus response prevention in the treatment of bulimia nervosa: A reply to Leitenberg and Rosen. *Journal of Consulting and Clinical Psychology, 57*(6), 778–779.

American Psychiatric Association. (2013). *Diagnostic and statistical manual of mental disorders* (5th ed.). Arlington, VA: American Psychiatric Publishing.

Antonuccio, D. O., Danton, W. G., DeNelsky, G. Y., Greenberg, R. P., & Gordon, J. S. (1999). Raising questions about antidepressants. *Psychotherapy and Psychosomatics*, 68(1), 3–14. doi:10.1159/000012304

Arean, P. A., Perri, M. G., Nezu, A. M., Schein, R. L., Christopher, F., & Joseph, T. X. (1993). Comparative effectiveness of social problem-solving therapy and reminiscence therapy as treatments for depression in older adults. *Journal of Consulting and Clinical Psychology*, 61(6), 1003.

Arnow, B. A., Taylor, C. B., Agras, W. S., & Telch, M. J. (1985). Enhancing agoraphobia treatment outcome by changing couple communication patterns. *Behavior Therapy*, 16(5), 452–467.

Auerbach, R., & Kilmann, P. R. (1977). The effects of group systematic desensitization on secondary erectile failure. *Behavior Therapy*, 8(3), 330–339.

Azrin, N. H. (1976). Improvements in the community-reinforcement approach to alcoholism. *Behaviour Research and Therapy*, 14(5), 339–348.

Azrin, N. H., Besalel, V. A., Bechtel, R., Michalicek, A., Mancera, M., Carroll, D., ... Cox, J. (1980). Comparison of reciprocity and discussion-type counseling for marital problems. *American Journal of Family Therapy*, 8(4), 21–28.

Azrin, N. H., Nunn, R. G., & Frantz, S. E. (1980). Habit reversal vs. negative practice treatment of nervous tics. *Behavior Therapy*, 11(2), 169–178.

Azrin, N. H., Nunn, R. G., & Frantz-Renshaw, S. (1980). Habit reversal treatment of thumbsucking. *Behaviour Research and Therapy*, 18(5), 395–399.

Ball, S. A., Carroll, K. M., & Rounsaville, B. J. (1994). Sensation seeking, substance abuse, and psychopathology in treatment-seeking and community cocaine abusers. *Journal of Consulting and Clinical Psychology*, 62(5), 1053.

Ball, S. G., Otto, M. W., Pollack, M. H., & Rosenbaum, J. F. (1994). Predicting prospective episodes of depression in patients with panic disorder: A longitudinal study. *Journal of Consulting and Clinical Psychology*, 62(2), 359.

Bandura, A. (1969). Social-learning theory of identificatory processes. *Handbook of Socialization Theory and Research*, 213, 262.

Barlow, D. H., Craske, M. G., Cerny, J. A., & Klosko, J. S. (1989). Behavioral treatment of panic disorder. *Behavior Therapy*, 20, 261–282.

Barlow, D. H., Rapee, R. M., & Brown, T. A. (1992). Behavioral treatment of generalized anxiety disorder. *Behavior Therapy*, 23(4), 551–570.

Blanchard, E. B., Andrasik, F., Ahles, T. A., Teders, S. J., & O'Keefe, D. (1980). Migraine and tension headache: A meta-analytic review. *Behavior Therapy*, 11(5), 613–631.

Blanchard, E. B., Theobald, D. E., Williamson, D. A., Silver, B. V., & Brown, D. A. (1978). Temperature biofeedback in the treatment of migraine headaches: A controlled evaluation. *Archives of General Psychiatry*, 35, 581–588.

Bolocofsky, D. N., Coulthard-Morris, L., & Spinier, D. (1984). Prediction of successful weight management from personality and demographic data. *Psychological Reports*, 55(3), 795–802.

Borkovec, T. D., & Costello, E. (1993). Efficacy of applied relaxation and cognitive-behavioral therapy in the treatment of generalized anxiety disorder. *Journal of Consulting and Clinical Psychology*, *61*(4), 611.

Burns, D. D. (1999). *Feeling good: The new mood therapy*. New York, NY: Avon Books.

Butler, G., & Booth, R. G. (1991). Developing psychological treatments for generalized anxiety disorder. In R. M. Rapee & D. H. Barlow (Eds.), *Chronic anxiety, generalized anxiety disorder, and mixed anxiety depression* (pp. 187–209). New York, NY: Guilford Press.

Cinciripini, P. M., Lapitsky, L., Seay, S., Wallfisch, A., Kitchens, K., & Van Vunakis, H. (1995). The effects of smoking schedules on cessation outcome: Can we improve on common methods of gradual and abrupt nicotine withdrawal? *Journal of Consulting and Clinical Psychology*, *63*(3), 388.

Cinciripini, P. M., Lapitsky, L. G., Wallfisch, A., Mace, R., Nezami, E., & Van Vunakis, H. (1994). An evaluation of a multicomponent treatment program involving scheduled smoking and relapse prevention procedures: Initial findings. *Addictive Behaviors*, *19*(1), 13–22.

Chambless, D. L., Baker, M. J., Baucom, D. H., Beulter, L. E., Calhoun, K. S., Crits-Christoph, P., ... Woody, S. R. (1998). Update on empirically validated therapies, II. *Clinical Psychologist*, *51*, 3–16.

Clark, D. M., Salkovskis, P. M., Hackmann, A., Middleton, H., Anastasiades, P., & Gelder, M. (1994). A comparison of cognitive therapy, applied relaxation and imipramine in the treatment of panic disorder. *British Journal of Psychiatry*, *164*(6), 759–769.

The Cochrane Library. (2014). Chichester, England: Wiley. www.cochrane.org

Cohen, J. A., Mannarino, A. P., & Deblinger, E. (2006). *Treating trauma and traumatic grief in children and adolescents*. New York, NY: Guilford Press.

Cummings, N. A., & O'Donohue, W. T. (2011). *Understanding the behavioral healthcare crisis: The promise of integrated care and diagnostic reform*. New York, NY: Routledge/Taylor & Francis.

DiMascio, A., Weissman, M. M., Prusoff, B. A., Neu, C., Zwilling, M., & Klerman, G. L. (1979). Differential symptom reduction by drugs and psychotherapy in acute depression. *Archives of General Psychiatry*, *36*(13), 1450–1456.

Dobson, K. S. (1989). A meta-analysis of the efficacy of cognitive therapy for depression. *Journal of Consulting and Clinical Psychology*, *57*(3), 414.

Drake, R. E., Mueser, K. T., Clark, R. E., & Wallach, M. E. (1996). The course, treatment, and outcome of substance disorder in persons with severe mental illness. *American Journal of Orthopsychiatry*, *66*(1), 42–51.

Drummond, D. C., & Glautier, S. (1994). A controlled trial of cue exposure treatment in alcohol dependence. *Journal of Consulting and Clinical Psychology*, *62*(4), 809.

Elkin, I., Shea, M. T., Watkins, J. T., Imber, S. D., Sotsky, S. M., Collins, J. F., ... Parloff, M. B. (1989). National Institute of Mental Health treatment of depression collaborative research program: General effectiveness of treatments. *Archives of General Psychiatry*, *46*(11), 971–982.

Epstein, L. H., Valoski, A., Wing, R. R., & McCurley, J. (1994). Ten-year outcomes of behavioral family-based treatment for childhood obesity. *Health Psychology*, *13*(5), 373.

Eriksen, L., Björnstad, S., & Götestam, K. G. (1986). Social skills training in groups for alcoholics: One-year treatment outcome for groups and individuals. *Addictive Behaviors*, *11*(3), 309–329.

Everaerd, W., & Dekker, J. (1981). A comparison of sex therapy and communication therapy: Couples complaining of orgasmic dysfunction. *Journal of Sex & Marital Therapy*, *7*(4), 278–289.

Fairburn, C. G., Jones, R., Peveler, R. C., Hope, R. A., & O'Connor, M. (1993). Psychotherapy and bulimia nervosa: Longer-term effects of interpersonal psychotherapy, behavior therapy, and cognitive behavior therapy. *Archives of General Psychiatry*, *50*(6), 419–428.

Falloon, I. R., & Pederson, J. (1985). Family management in the prevention of morbidity of schizophrenia: the adjustment of the family unit. *British Journal of Psychiatry*, *147*(2), 156–163.

Fergusson, D. M., McLeod, G. H., & Horwood, L. (2013). Childhood sexual abuse and adult developmental outcomes: Findings from a 30-year longitudinal study in New Zealand. *Child Abuse & Neglect*, *37*(9), 664–674. doi:10.1016/j.chiabu.2013.03.013

Feske, U., & Chambless, D. L. (1995). Cognitive behavioral versus exposure only treatment for social phobia: A meta-analysis. *Behavior Therapy*, *26*(4), 695–720.

Fisher, J. E., & O'Donohue, W. (2006). *Practitioner's guide to evidence-based psychotherapy.* New York, NY: Springer.

Flor, H., & Birbaumer, N. (1993). Comparison of the efficacy of electromyographic biofeedback, cognitive-behavioral therapy, and conservative medical interventions in the treatment of chronic musculoskeletal pain. *Journal of Consulting and Clinical Psychology*, *61*(4), 653.

Foa, E. B., Feske, U., Murdock, T. B., Kozak, M. J., & McCarthy, P. R. (1991). Processing of threat-related information in rape victims. *Journal of Abnormal Psychology*, *100*(2), 156.

Foa, E. B., Keane, T. M., Friedman, M. J., & Cohen, J. A. (Eds). (2008). *Effective treatments for PTSD: Practice guidelines from the International Society for Traumatic Stress Studies.* New York, NY: Guilford Press.

Foa, E. B., Rothbaum, B. O., Riggs, D. S., & Murdock, T. B. (1991). Treatment of posttraumatic stress disorder in rape victims: A comparison between cognitive-behavioral procedures and counseling. *Journal of Consulting and Clinical Psychology*, *59*(5), 715.

Freedman, R. R., Ianni, P., & Wenig, P. (1983). Behavioral treatment of Raynaud's disease. *Journal of Consulting and Clinical Psychology*, *51*(4), 539.

Friedrich, W. N., Urquiza, A. J., & Beilke, R. L. (1986). Behavior problems in sexually abused young children. *Journal of Pediatric Psychology*, *11*(1), 47–57.

Fuchs, C. Z., & Rehm, L. P. (1977). A self-control behavior therapy program for depression. *Journal of Consulting and Clinical Psychology*, *45*(2), 206.

Gallagher-Thompson, D., & Steffen, A. M. (1994). Comparative effects of cognitive-behavioral and brief psychodynamic psychotherapies for depressed family caregivers. *Journal of Consulting and Clinical Psychology*, *62*(3), 543.

Gil, K. M., Williams, D. A., Keefe, F. J., & Beckham, J. C. (1990). The relationship of negative thoughts to pain and psychological distress. *Behavior Therapy*, *21*(3), 349–362.

Heimberg, R. G., Dodge, C. S., Hope, D. A., Kennedy, C. R., Zollo, L. J., & Becker, R. E. (1990). Cognitive behavioral group treatment for social phobia: Comparison with a credible placebo control. *Cognitive Therapy and Research*, *14*(1), 1–23.

Higgins, S. T., & Budney, A. J. (1993). Treatment of cocaine dependence through the principles of behavior analysis and behavioral pharmacology. In L. S. Onken, J. D. Blaine, & J. J. Boren (Eds.), *Behavioral treatments for drug abuse and dependence.* NIDA Research Monograph Series no. 137 (pp. 97–121). Rockville, MD: National Institute on Drug Abuse.

Hill, R. D., Rigdon, M., & Johnson, S. (1993). Behavioral smoking cessation treatment for older chronic smokers. *Behavior Therapy, 24*(2), 321–329.

Hiss, H., Foa, E. B., & Kozak, M. J. (1994). Relapse prevention program for treatment of obsessive-compulsive disorder. *Journal of Consulting and Clinical Psychology, 62*(4), 801.

Holroyd, K. A., & Penzien, D. B. (1990). Pharmacological versus non-pharmacological prophylaxis of recurrent migraine headache: A meta-analytic review of clinical trials. *Pain, 42*(1), 1–13.

Houts, A. C., Berman, J. S., & Abramson, H. (1994). Effectiveness of psychological and pharmacological treatments for nocturnal enuresis. *Journal of Consulting and Clinical Psychology, 62*(4), 737.

Hunt, G. M., & Azrin, N. H. (1973). A community-reinforcement approach to alcoholism. *Behaviour Research and Therapy, 11*(1), 91–104.

Hurlbert, D. F., White, L. C., Powell, R. D., & Apt, C. (1993). Orgasm consistency training in the treatment of women reporting hypoactive sexual desire: An outcome comparison of women-only groups and couples-only groups. *Journal of Behavior Therapy and Experimental Psychiatry, 24*(1), 3–13.

Institute of Medicine. (2001). *Crossing the quality chasm: A new health system for the 21st century.* Washington, DC: National Academies Press.

Jacobson, N. S., Dobson, K. S., Truax, P. A., Addis, M. E., Koerner, K., Gollan, J. K., ... Prince, S. E. (1996). A component analysis of cognitive-behavioral treatment for depression. *Journal of Consulting and Clinical Psychology, 64*(2), 295.

Jacobson, N. S., & Follette, W. C. (1985). Clinical significance of improvement resulting from two behavioral marital therapy components. *Behavior Therapy, 16*(3), 249–262.

Johnson, S. M., & Greenberg, L. S. (1985). Emotionally focused couples therapy: An outcome study. *Journal of Marital and Family Therapy, 11*(3), 313–317.

Keefe, F. J., Caldwell, D. S., Williams, D. A., Gil, K. M., Mitchell, D., Robertson, C., ... Helms, M. (1990). Pain coping skills training in the management of osteoarthritic knee pain-II: Follow-up results. *Behavior Therapy, 21*(4), 435–447.

Keane, T. M., Fairbank, J. A., Caddell, J. M., & Zimering, R. T. (1989). Implosive (flooding) therapy reduces symptoms of PTSD in Vietnam combat veterans. *Behavior Therapy, 20*(2), 245–260.

Kendall, P. C. (1994). Treating anxiety disorders in children: Results of a randomized clinical trial. *Journal of Consulting and Clinical Psychology, 62*(1), 100.

Kendall, P. C., Flannery-Schroeder, E., Panichelli-Mindel, S. M., Southam-Gerow, M., Henin, A., & Warman, M. (1997). Therapy for youths with anxiety disorders: A second randomized clinical trial. *Journal of Consulting and Clinical Psychology, 65*(3), 366.

Kirsch, I., Tennen, H., Wickless, C., Saccone, A. J., & Cody, S. (1983). The role of expectancy in fear reduction. *Behavior Therapy, 14*(4), 520–533.

Linehan, M. M., Armstrong, H. E., Suarez, A., Allmon, D., & Heard, H. L. (1991). Cognitive-behavioral treatment of chronically parasuicidal borderline patients. *Archives of General Psychiatry*, *48*(12), 1060–1064.

LoPiccolo, J., & Stock, W. E. (1986). Treatment of sexual dysfunction. *Journal of Consulting and Clinical Psychology*, *54*(2), 158.

Lynch, P. M., & Zamble, E. (1989). A controlled behavioral treatment study of irritable bowel syndrome. *Behavior Therapy*, *20*(4), 509–523.

Marder, S. R., Wirshing, W. C., Mintz, J., McKenzie, J., Johnston, K., Eckman, T. A., … Liberman, R. P. (1996). Two-year outcome of social skills training and group psychotherapy for outpatients with schizophrenia. *American Journal of Psychiatry*, *153*(12), 1585–1592.

Marshall, W. L., Jones, R., Ward, T., Johnston, P., & Barbaree, H. E. (1991). Treatment outcome with sex offenders. *Clinical Psychology Review*, *11*(4), 465–485.

McLean, P. D., & Hakstian, A. R. (1979). Clinical depression: Comparative efficacy of outpatient treatments. *Journal of Consulting and Clinical Psychology*, *47*(5), 818.

Menzies, R. G., & Clarke, J. C. (1993). The etiology of childhood water phobia. *Behaviour Research and Therapy*, *31*(5), 499–501.

Nicholas, M. K., Wilson, P. H., & Goyen, J. (1991). Operant-behavioural and cognitive-behavioural treatment for chronic low back pain. *Behaviour Research and Therapy*, *29*(3), 225–238.

O'Brien, S., Ross, L. V., & Christophersen, E. R. (1986). Primary encopresis: Evaluation and treatment. *Journal of Applied Behavior Analysis*, *19*(2), 137–145.

O'Donohue, W. T., & Draper, C. (2011). *Stepped care and e-health: Practical applications to behavioral disorders*. New York, NY: Springer.

O'Donohue, W. T., & Fisher, J. E. (2008). *Cognitive behavior therapy: Applying empirically supported techniques in your practice* (2nd ed.). Hoboken, NJ: Wiley.

O'Donohue, W. T., & Fisher, J. E. (2009). *General principles and empirically supported techniques of cognitive behavior therapy*. Hoboken, NJ: Wiley.

O'Farrell, T. J., Cutter, H. S., Choquette, K. A., Floyd, F. J., & Bayog, R. D. (1992). Behavioral marital therapy for male alcoholics: Marital and drinking adjustment during the two years after treatment. *Behavior Therapy*, *23*(4), 529–549.

O'Farrell, T. J., Cutter, H. S., & Floyd, F. J. (1985). Evaluating behavioral marital therapy for male alcoholics: Effects on marital adjustment and communication from before to after treatment. *Behavior Therapy*, *16*(2), 147–167.

Öst, L. G. (1978). Fading vs systematic desensitization in the treatment of snake and spider phobia. *Behaviour Research and Therapy*, *16*(6), 379–389.

Öst, L. G. (1988). Applied relaxation vs progressive relaxation in the treatment of panic disorder. *Behaviour Research and Therapy*, *26*(1), 13–22.

Öst, L. G., Fellenius, J., & Sterner, U. (1991). Applied tension, exposure *in vivo*, and tension-only in the treatment of blood phobia. *Behaviour Research and Therapy*, *29*(6), 561–574.

Parker, J. C., Frank, R. G., Beck, N. C., Smarr, K. L., Buescher, K. L., Phillips, L. R., … Walker, S. E. (1988). Pain management in rheumatoid arthritis patients. *Arthritis & Rheumatism*, *31*(5), 593–601.

Paul, G. L., & Shannon, D. T. (1966). Treatment of anxiety through systematic desensitization in therapy groups. *Journal of Abnormal Psychology, 71*(2), 124.

Randolph, E. T., Eth, S., Glynn, S. M., Paz, G. G., Leong, G. B., Shaner, A. L., … Liberman, R. P. (1994). Behavioural family management in schizophrenia. Outcome of a clinic-based intervention. *British Journal of Psychiatry, 164*(4), 501–506.

Rehm, L. P., Fuchs, C. Z., Roth, D. M., Kornblith, S. J., & Romano, J. M. (1979). A comparison of self-control and assertion skills treatment of depression. *Behavior Therapy, 10*(4), 429–442.

Ryle, G. (1949). *The concept of the mind.* New York, NY: Barnes & Noble.

Sargent, J., Solbach, P., Coyne, L., Spohn, H., & Segerson, J. (1986). Results of a controlled, experimental, outcome study of nondrug treatments for the control of migraine headaches. *Journal of Behavioral Medicine, 9*(3), 291–323.

Saunders, T., Driskell, J., Johnston, J., & Salas, E. (1996). The effects of stress inoculation training on anxiety and performance. *Journal of Occupational Health Psychology, 1*(2), p. 170–186.

Sbraga, T., & O'Donohue, W. (2003). Post hoc reasoning in possible cases of child sexual abuse: Symptoms of inconclusive origins. *Clinical Psychology: Science and Practice, 10*(3), 320–334. doi:10.1093/clipsy/bpg029

Scogin, F., & McElreath, L. (1994). Efficacy of psychosocial treatments for geriatric depression: A quantitative review. *Journal of Consulting and Clinical Psychology, 62*(1), 69.

Snyder, D. K., & Wills, R. M. (1989). Behavioral versus insight-oriented marital therapy: Effects on individual and interspousal functioning. *Journal of Consulting and Clinical Psychology, 57*(1), 39.

Snyder, D. K., Wills, R. M., & Grady-Fletcher, A. (1991). Long-term effectiveness of behavioral versus insight-oriented marital therapy: A 4-year follow-up study. *Journal of Consulting and Clinical Psychology, 59*(1), 138.

Spence, S. H., Sharpe, L., Newton-John, T., & Champion, D. (1995). Effect of EMG biofeedback compared to applied relaxation training with chronic, upper extremity cumulative trauma disorders. *Pain, 63*(2), 199–206.

Spiegel, D. A., Roth, M., Weissman, M., Lavori, P., Gorman, J., Rush, J., & Ballenger, J. (1993). Comment on the London/Toronto study of alprazolam and exposure in panic disorder with agoraphobia. *British Journal of Psychiatry, 162*, 788–789; discussion, 790–794.

Stevens, V. J., & Hollis, J. F. (1989). Preventing smoking relapse, using an individually tailored skills-training technique. *Journal of Consulting and Clinical Psychology, 57*(3), 420.

Telch, C. F., Agras, W. S., Rossiter, E. M., Wilfley, D., & Kenardy, J. (1990). Group cognitive-behavioral treatment for the nonpurging bulimic: An initial evaluation. *Journal of Consulting and Clinical Psychology, 58*(5), 629.

Thackwray, D. E., Smith, M. C., Bodfish, J. W., & Meyers, A. W. (1993). A comparison of behavioral and cognitive-behavioral interventions for bulimia nervosa. *Journal of Consulting and Clinical Psychology, 61*(4), 639.

Trull, T. J., Nietzel, M. T., & Main, A. (1988). The use of meta-analysis to assess the clinical significance of behavior therapy for agoraphobia. *Behavior Therapy, 19*(4), 527–538.

Turner, J. A., & Clancy, S. (1988). Comparison of operant behavioral and cognitive-behavioral group treatment for chronic low back pain. *Journal of Consulting and Clinical Psychology, 56*(2), 261.

Turner, J. A., Clancy, S., McQuade, K. J., & Cardenas, D. D. (1990). Effectiveness of behavioral therapy for chronic low back pain: A component analysis. *Journal of Consulting and Clinical Psychology*, 58(5), 573.

Walter, H. I., & Gilmore, S. K. (1973). Placebo versus social learning effects in parent training procedures designed to alter the behavior of aggressive boys. *Behavior Therapy*, 4(3), 361–377.

Wells, K. C., & Egan, J. (1988). Social learning and systems family therapy for childhood opposi-tional disorder: Comparative treatment outcome. *Comprehensive Psychiatry*, 29(2), 138–146.

Wheeler, M. E., & Hess, K. W. (1976). Treatment of juvenile obesity by successive approximation control of eating. *Journal of Behavior Therapy and Experimental Psychiatry*, 7(3), 235–241.

Wilfley, D. E., Agras, W. S., Telch, C. F., Rossiter, E. M., Schneider, J. A., Cole, A. G., ... Raeburn, S. D. (1993). Group cognitive-behavioral therapy and group interpersonal psychotherapy for the nonpurging bulimic individual: A controlled comparison. *Journal of Consulting and Clinical Psychology*, 61(2), 296.

Wilson, S. A., Becker, L. A., & Tinker, R. H. (1995). Eye movement desensitization and repro-cessing (EMDR) treatment for psychologically traumatized individuals. *Journal of Consulting and Clinical Psychology*, 63(6), 928.

Wood, J. M., & Lilienfeld, S. O. (1999). The Rorschach inkblot test: A case of overstatement? *Assessment*, 6(4), 341–351. doi:10.1177/107319119900600405

Woody, G. E., McLellan, A. T., Luborsky, L., & O'Brien, C. P. (1990). Psychotherapy and coun-seling for methadone-maintained opiate addicts: Results of research studies. *NIDA Research Monograph*, 104(9), 9–23.

van Balkom, A. J., van Oppen, P., Vermeulen, A. W., van Dyck, R., Nauta, M. C., & Vorst, H. (1994). A meta-analysis on the treatment of obsessive compulsive disorder: A comparison of antidepressants, behavior, and cognitive therapy. *Clinical Psychology Review*, 14(5), 359–381.

Van Oppen, P., De Haan, E., Van Balkom, A. J., Spinhoven, P., Hoogduin, K., & Van Dyck, R. (1995). Cognitive therapy and exposure in vivo in the treatment of obsessive compulsive disorder. *Behaviour Research and Therapy*, 33(4), 379–390.

York, D., Borkovec, T. D., Vasey, M., & Stern, R. (1987). Effects of worry and somatic anxiety induction on thoughts, emotion and physiological activity. *Behaviour Research and Therapy*, 25(6), 523–526.

Zimmer, D. (1987). Does marital therapy enhance the effectiveness of treatment for sexual dys-function? *Journal of Sex & Marital Therapy*, 13(3), 193–209.

Understanding the Law

PART

III

Understanding the Law

10

Understanding What It Is to Be an Expert Witness

GOALS OF THIS CHAPTER:

1. To understand aspects of the law related to expert testimony.
2. To be prepared for the possibility of offering expert testimony.
3. To learn about how professional forensic interviews may be evaluated.

M ental health professionals (and others) can be asked (or even required) to serve as an expert witness in a legal procedure. This chapter discusses the main issues involved in this role. In order to understand how a mental health professional can perform this role well, first it is necessary to understand some basics about the American legal system. Note that we only discuss the legal system in the United States because legal systems vary significantly across nations, thus our discussion may have little relevance for functioning in the legal system of other nations.

BASIC INFORMATION AND THE LEGAL SYSTEM IN THE UNITED STATES

The legal system is always changing. This adds complexity as what we are attempting to understand and often even to function in, is a bit of a moving target. The American legal system is based on the Constitution of the United States. This is the foundational legal document. The Constitution can change through amendments, although this is a relatively rare occurrence and it is a very complicated process. However, as you have heard, the words of the Constitution may at times be somewhat ambiguous or their exact relevance for some legal issue or set of facts is unclear (e.g., is there a right to privacy in the Constitution?—when the Supreme Court ruled in Roe v. Wade allowing abortions, it decided that there is). Thus, the major function of the Supreme Court is to rule on cases in which someone is arguing that there is something in the Constitution that a prior legal decision has not properly considered (the Supreme Court is an appellate court—it hears requests for appeals of prior legal decisions). When the Supreme Court makes a ruling (which is very often not unanimous—the Supreme Court Justices are divided on the issue, which shows how complex and ambiguous the issues often are), the law of the land can then be changed as a result of the decision (as in Roe v. Wade, which overturned the state laws—now considered unconstitutional—outlawing abortions).

Other (lower) appellate courts are also making decisions that change the way laws are interpreted. And the major way laws change is that elected officials pass new laws. This also gets more than a little complex because there are many bodies that can pass laws (city, county, state, federal legislatures). So, "what laws are relevant, and what these laws exactly say" is a bit of a complex matter and a matter that can change over time. That is why God in his infinite wisdom invented lawyers. They are supposed to understand and keep abreast of all these issues and changes.

The legal system is complex. Part of this complexity is due to the first issue that we have just discussed, that is, the legal system is always changing. But part of the reason is also that there really are multiple legal systems. The Constitution gave certain powers to the federal government but many powers to the states. In turn, state constitutions retained some of these powers given to them by the U.S. Constitution but gave others to other more local jurisdictions (literally, "saying of the law"). So counties and cities also have their own set of laws. Thus, when there is a legal issue that comes up, one needs to find out if this is a federal matter, a state matter, a county matter, or a city matter. For example, many times the possession of child pornography is prosecuted as a federal offense as there are federal laws against it and federal agencies often have the budget to investigate and prosecute this. Thus, even though there may be state laws, these may become irrelevant to a particular proceeding because the charge is a federal one heard in federal court. In contrast, in general, child custody in divorce proceedings is a state matter—not a federal one. Sexual harassment claims, on the other hand, are again federal matters, as these usually are considered violations of federal rules regarding fair employment.

Finally, part of the difficulty is that each state or each city may, through how they write their laws, introduce a lot of variability in the legal matter. For example, each state has written laws regarding how custody should be decided. However, the problem is that each state has defined this differently. Most states, but not all, use the concept of "best interest of the child" (Tolle & O'Donohue, 2012). However, most states define what is the "best interests of the child" in very different ways—some recognize that the child's spiritual development matters—some do not; some state that the child's social development matters—some do not. The bottom line is that when mental health professionals are professionally involved in a case they should attempt to understand what kind of court is relevant—federal, state, and so on. The variance across jurisdictions makes it tough for researchers to develop uniform procedures—say a uniform method to conduct a child custody evaluation—as it may be more or less consistent with 50 jurisdictions.

The American legal system is **adversarial**. This means that there are multiple sides—usually two but there can be more and they disagree with one another. If there were no disagreements or if the two sides could compromise they would not need to be in court. The basic process going on is something along the lines of—"We are in a disagreement over *x* (and, perhaps, *y* and *z* ...). Each of us will do basically three things: (1) we will present, in the context of relevant law, why we think we are right; (2) we will criticize the other side's case that they are right, and, finally, (3) we will rebut the other side's criticisms of our case." So there is a lot going on as both sides are doing all three things.

In general, the issues in the disagreement can be divided into two broad camps—**legal issues**—what the law says, and **factual issues**—what actually happened. Let us use a fictitious example to illustrate this. Suppose there is a criminal matter and a father is being charged with sexually abusing his 4-year-old child. Suppose further the prosecution is alleging that on a certain date in Los Angeles, California the father abused the child by rubbing ointment in a prurient manner on the child's genitals. Suppose further that the state law says child abuse consists of "physical contact with a child for the purpose of sexual gratification." Now the issues in the case might be two: The factual issues will be what did the father actually do: Did he even rub ointment on the child's genitals? But secondly the prosecution has to prove all elements of the crime according to the law: That not only is it factually true that the father rubbed ointment on the child's genitals, but he did so for his sexual gratification. The defense may construct their defense by saying, the father did rub ointment, but he was doing it as a responsible caretaker and not for sexual gratification and thus, the legal burden is not met by the prosecution. In addition, the defense may say, the prosecutor has not shown that the child clearly said it happened in California so there may be an additional legal issue of jurisdiction: Why are we here in Los Angeles trying this case when it is not clear that even if a crime occurred it occurred in this jurisdiction? There is a half-humorous adage in the law: If attorneys have the law on their side, they should pound on the law; and if attorneys have the facts on their side, they should pound on the facts; and if attorneys have neither the law nor the facts on their side, then they should pound on the table.

There is another important concept in this case: Laws also often dictate who has the *burden of proof*. We all know that in criminal matters it is the prosecution that has this burden: The prosecution's case is presented first as they have the legal burden of proving beyond a reasonable doubt that the crime did occur. If they fail to do this, the defense may not even need to put on their case—they can move to ask the judge to dismiss because the "state has not met their burden of proof."

A final issue on this complexity of the law: Not only are there many jurisdictions (federal, state, city) but there are many different kinds of courts. The best known is the criminal court (where guilt regarding the commission of some crime is decided). There is also family court—where family issues like custody and guardianship are decided. This type of court is also called *civil court*. There are also appellate courts (where one side is disputing a prior court's ruling). Many states also have specialized trial courts that hear cases related to a very specific area of the law. These courts can include probate courts, juvenile courts, traffic courts, drug courts, and small claims courts. So, one can start to see the complexity of the legal system. We turn next to a discussion of some key terms that are generally useful to know.

Expert witness. This designation is in contrast to a material witness. A **material witness** is often what you see on television. They come in to answer questions regarding what they have directly experienced—"I saw the blue truck run a red light and hit the red car." **Expert witnesses** on the other hand are there to educate the trier of fact (the judge if it is a *bench trial* and the jury if it is a jury trial). The basic premise is that there is a technical matter that is beyond the average layperson's ability to know or understand. The expert's job is to educate the jury members on these issues so they are in a position to do their job and render a verdict on the ultimate legal issue at hand. Mental health experts may come in and tell the jury what diagnoses they have given to key parties to the dispute. They may come in to answer questions about the status of a theory or technique used in the case, for example, how well a forensic interview was conducted, or present the results of their work, for example, to testify regarding the results of their child custody report or presentencing evaluation. Note how each of these matters is rather technical and goes beyond the general knowledge of the average layperson. Thus, the need for an expert.

Voir dire (Latin for "telling the truth"). Before experts can testify for an attorney the judge first needs to find that they indeed are experts in a relevant matter. This phase is called voir dire. Usually the experts have submitted their vita or resume but the lawyer then asks questions about their education, their publications, their clinical work, and so on. The lawyer must also define a scope of expertise: Is the expert an expert in the treatment of sexually abused children (but not forensic interviewing of them)? Is the expert an expert in this topic as well as the treatment of sexual offenders? In addition, the attorney must show that this kind of opinion is legally permissible and relevant to the case. The judge can hear questions from the other side contesting this expertise or attempting to limit it and then the judge makes a decision about the admissibility of the expert.

There are actually three issues going on here: *admissibility* (whether the expert can even testify); *scope* (how many issues can the expert testify on); and *weight* (how strong is the expert). In general the testimony of one expert who has, for example, published 10 books on the subject is going to have more weight than one who just took a 1-week training on the issue—both can be experts (because they know more than the average layperson) but one's testimony is probably going to have more weight with the trier of fact.

Subpoena. This is an order usually signed by a judge that compels someone to do something—to produce records, to come at a certain time and place to testify, and so on.

Deposition. A deposition occurs when the lawyers ask questions to witnesses before the actual trial or hearing. A basic rule is that attorneys should not ask questions that they do not already know the answer to. The deposition's major function is to ask potential witnesses questions to commit them to certain answers. The witness—if actually called in the trial or hearing then when asked the same question—should then give the same answer. If not, the attorney can confront them with their prior answer and **impeach** them (i.e., cast doubt on their credibility) by then reading from the deposition transcript and showing their inconsistency. Depositions are not done in front of the judge, and are usually done in one of the lawyer's offices. Lawyers representing all interested parties are usually present as well as a court reporter who records all questions and answers verbatim and thus creates a firm record.

Transcripts. The written document of the testimony from a trial or hearing.

Ultimate opinion. Experts are not allowed to give an ultimate opinion as this is the job of the judge or jury. Experts are not there to do the same job as the ultimate trier of fact—the judge or jury needs to decide, for example, if the person is guilty or not guilty. Thus, an expert should not and cannot say, "In my expert opinion the defendant is guilty." The expert can give relevant testimony to issues that greatly impact this decision, for example, "The forensic interviews were so flawed in this case due to leading questions, that the child's allegations may have been a product of the suggestiveness of these interviews."

Appeal. Sometimes an expert is involved in an appellate proceeding. Basically, an attorney (who often are specialists in appeals) is saying some previous legal decision or proceeding was so unsound that its result should be thrown out. This is harder than commonly portrayed on television. The adage is that everyone is entitled to a fair trial, not a perfect one. The errors have to be somewhat egregious (called *reversible error*) for appeals to be granted.

Sentencing phase. After someone is found guilty there usually is another proceeding, sometimes several months in the future, where the judge hears evidence relevant to his or her pronouncing a sentence. There may be probation and parole reports, testimony of victims or their families, testimony from treatment providers, and even testimony from the person to be sentenced.

Direct testimony, cross-examination, *and redirect testimony.* Direct testimony are the answers to questions from the lawyer who calls the expert. Cross-examination is the questions from and answers to any lawyers representing any other side. Redirect questioning then is simply the first lawyer asking more questions after cross. There then can be recross until all lawyers are done. It is important that witnesses do not just go on the stand and talk. Their testimony is always in response to a question.

Expert reports. Experts can be asked to prepare a report detailing their opinions. Usually they list what materials they reviewed, what methods they used to generate their opinions, and then their opinions. These reports, if used, then usually must be given to the other side a few weeks before the trial or hearing so the other side has time to examine them and perhaps retain their own expert to evaluate this. Also jurors are not expected just to read the report. The way the judicial system works is that experts opinions are generated through questions about the report.

Objections. Lawyers may raise objections to the questions or answers of other lawyers or the experts on the stand. They are essentially saying, either the question or the answer was legally improper in some way. Judges then may hear from the other side and then render their decision by saying "Sustained" (if they agree) or "Overruled" (when they do not). Objections can be, for example:

Relevance (the question was not legally relevant to the case).

Asked and answered (lawyers cannot repeat the same question).

Compound questions (lawyers are supposed to ask simple questions, not complex questions, such as, "Was he wearing a hat, walking with a limp, and shivering?").

Lack of foundation. Lawyers must establish a basis before they ask certain other questions. For example, they must first establish that the experts were given materials, that they reviewed them, and that they prepared a report, before they ask a question such as "What opinions were contained in your report?"

Nonresponsive. If experts are asked how long they went to school and they start answering a different question, for example, where they went to school, the other lawyer can object that the answer is nonresponsive to the question.

There are other numerous objections, although these are some of the most common. Basically as an expert you just have to wait when you hear an objection for the judge to rule and then follow the judge's instructions.

Opening the door. There is a rule that if you are not asked a question on direct you cannot be asked about this matter on cross. However, if you are asked or if you do mention this matter then you have "opened the door" to this issue and the other side then can ask questions about it. An example will help. Suppose you are a defense witness and the defendant has some prior convictions that the defense attorney does not want in the record. They will not want the defendant's past history to be part of your opinion or part of their questioning of you. They will not ask questions like "He has had a normal past, hasn't he?" However, you also will need to restrict your answer so you do not open the door. For example, if you say "I did a complete psychological evaluation of the subject including his past history, in order to form my opinions about his psychological status," this may open the door to his criminal history.

Hearsay. Hearsay refers to something you did not directly observe but rather got from a third party. Material witnesses cannot testify to hearsay (I heard Bob say that he saw the defendant with a gun). Expert witnesses have more latitude regarding this (I read his treatment psychiatrist's report who said that in December 2013 he was successfully treated for depression) but not unlimited latitude.

ADVICE FOR THE EXPERT WITNESS

To further understand the role and proper function of an expert witness we discuss some general advice that others have found useful in preparing to be an expert witness. The following is patterned after O'Donohue, Benuto, and Cirlugea (2013).

Tips for Preparing for Your Testimony

Know the specifics of the case. A common question you can ask the lawyer early on is, "On what issues would you like me to opine (give an opinion)?" Listen carefully and ask clarifying questions to make sure that you and the attorney have the same understanding of keywords or phrases (e.g., "risk," "profile," "probability of reoffending," "psychopathy," "suggestibility," "effective therapy," "personality testing," "child's best interest"). You may then need to give the attorney feedback on whether you can opine on these issues. There are a variety of reasons why you may be unable to opine on a particular question. You may state that you cannot opine for various reasons including: (1) You do not believe that it is within your expertise. You may believe that a different type of expert is needed. For example, you may believe that a pediatrician is better qualified to opine on what you see as a medical issue. (2) The issue may be within your expertise but you may not have formed a clear opinion. Perhaps you have not had sufficient contact with the client, or the information you have gained thus far is ambiguous. For example, it is unethical to diagnose someone without having professional contact, but a lawyer may want you to give an opinion whether someone is suffering from PTSD. If you have not had any professional contact, but rather just read their records or had someone else tell you about what they observed, you simply cannot make the diagnosis ethically and thus you cannot give an opinion on this issue. (3) You may believe that it is inappropriate for you to give an opinion on a particular issue. Let us say the attorney is asking you to give an opinion regarding custody and you have treated the juvenile involved for, say, a major depressive episode (but you have not conducted a custody evaluation). You might need to say that you cannot render an opinion because your role was as a therapist for a particular problem, not a custody evaluator. You can and should negotiate what you think are reasonable issues on which you can opine. (4) You may believe that testifying is precluded by confidentiality duties. You may need a release of information before you testify and if you cannot get one, and if you are subpoenaed (basically ordered by the court to testify) you will be in a bind. (5) You may believe that it is not in your client's best interest for you to testify. If the lawyer is representing your client, you may need to explain this to him or her. (6) Logistically, it may be impossible for you to testify—you may be out of town on vacation or attending a conference that day. Sometimes the procedure can be continued to accommodate your schedule.

Determine what information you need to form a sound opinion and to work with the attorney to get this information: Do you need certain records or materials (e.g., school records, arrest records, treatment records)? Do you need to have clinical contact or more clinical contact with the client to conduct further testing or interview—gather more clinical information relevant to the issues on which you will opine? Give a timeline for when this can be completed (ask the attorney if there are any set dates already) as well as a budget to be certain the attorney who retained your services is willing to pay for your professional time. Do you need to meet with collaterals or even the attorney to obtain more information? The heuristic some experts use is that they want all relevant information so that if the other side poses a question such as "Doctor, if I represent that this document says *x*, and given that you have testified that you have not reviewed this document, could reviewing this document potentially alter the opinion on issue *y* that you are giving here" the expert can say no. That is, the expert wants to review all materials that are potentially relevant to any issue the expert will be asked to opine on. The expert will generally want to gather all reasonable and practical clinical information as well as to be able to conduct clinical procedures generally accepted to form an opinion about *y*. In addition, it is important to ask the attorneys if they want a written report. There are advantages associated with a written report—it helps the experts organize their thoughts; it makes clear what the experts' opinions are and why the experts have come to these; and it can be a guide for the attorneys for their direct examination when the expert is on the stand. However, most attorneys regard written reports as having one significant disadvantage. It allows the other side to see their expert's opinions and have a chance to prepare to cross-examine their expert or call their own expert to rebut their expert's opinion(s). The other major disadvantage is financial: It takes more of the expert's time and thus the cost associated with hiring an expert will be greater.

All conclusions of an expert must be made "within a reasonable degree of psychological certainty." It is unclear exactly what this phrase means, but can be interpreted as meaning that you're not merely guessing about what you're saying, presumably, it's based on good science—maybe even the best science—and solid evidence.

Make sure you understand the question to which you're responding and do not respond until you understand the question. (Attorneys sometimes use complex wording or embed some true and some untrue assertions in one question.) Ask the attorney to rephrase the question as many times as necessary until you understand what is being asked.

Remember, your role is to educate the trier of fact (the judge or the jury). You are not in court to advocate for one side or another. You have expertise that can help the trier of fact make certain key legal decisions. Think of your role as that of an educator. Tell the judge or jury about relevant research findings in ways that are readily understandable. You can describe these studies in a bit of detail so the judge and jury can see their strengths as well as their limitations. Be fair. Feel free to talk about limitations to these studies or results that have been inconsistent with the general trend. Your job is to be informative and even-handed. This will serve you best in the short term as well as the long term. Good lawyers (and most lawyers are good) want fair experts, not what are called "whores." When you are giving a clinical opinion, "This person meets diagnostic criteria for major depressive episode," state the reasons you came to this conclusion. For example, "One of the most common ways of assessing depression is through the use of a 30-item self-report test called the Beck Depression Inventory. The person's BDI score was 25, which is regarded as moderately depressed. In my clinical interview I also found he met these specific diagnostic criteria x, y, z ... contained in the *DSM-5.* I had seen that his primary care doctor also gave him this diagnosis earlier this year and put him on an antidepressant. I also interviewed his spouse who confirmed the depressive symptoms, etc." Just because you are an expert does not mean you can just throw out unsubstantiated opinions—give the rationale underlying your opinions and demonstrate that you have been fair, comprehensive, and reasonable.

During the initial contact, ask the attorneys what their "theory of the case" is. This will help you understand the context for your testimony. You might also give the attorneys feedback on how your opinions help and/or do not help them with this theory. This may be useful for the attorneys and they may revise their theory of the case. On the other hand, it may become clear that the attorney may not want to call you.

Get all financial agreements ironed out before beginning any work on a case. Do you require a retainer (i.e., upfront payment)? What is your hourly rate for such work—does this differ by activity—reviewing documents, report writing, clinical contact, testifying? Are there any limits to the sum that can be paid to you and can you complete your work well within any such limits? As an aside, opposing counsel will often ask you about these financial arrangements during your testimony. Often, the other side might want to suggest to the jury (this tactic does not work as well in bench trials with an experienced judge) that your opinion is not due to the facts and evidence you reviewed—but simply due to the fact that you are being paid. Do not worry too much about this. All professionals involved in the court are being paid. You are not an exception.

Know that scheduling, like war, is hell. Remember that dates and times the lawyers are giving you are their best estimates and these rarely turn out to be accurate. Cases often get continued (legalese for rescheduled). Prior motions, evidence, and testimony take longer or shorter than the estimate and it can be your turn to testify hours or days before or later than the estimate you were given. Sometimes the issues resolve (e.g., a last minute plea bargain is worked out) and you will not need to testify at all. Your court appearance will be cancelled. Sometimes these issues resolve at the last minute. I have been involved in cases in which the morning before I was to board a flight, the attorney called and said that I no longer needed to come. In another child custody case, I traveled to another state the previous day, arrived the next day at the courtroom, found that the parties were in conference, and ultimately was informed that they had resolved the issue. Prepare for delays and unexpected schedule changes.

When you are actually testifying on the stand, first make sure you understand each question. It is perfectly legitimate for you to say that you do not understand the question or want a key term in the question clarified. Sometimes it is the lawyer's strategy to get you to answer a vague question or use a vague term and then later use it against you. Ponder each question for a bit to make sure you understand it. This pause is also useful in that it can give the other side a chance to raise an objection to the question.

Some lawyers and judges want you to try to give only yes and no answers. Material witnesses are generally confined to yes and no answers. Experts generally have more latitude to explain their answers. For example, an attorney may ask you the question "Is your client cured of the mental health issues you treated him for?" and want a yes or no answer. If you feel you can answer it this way, do so. However, if you feel the need to explain your answer some or even a lot, then do so (or attempt to do so—it ultimately depends on the judge's decision). You may say, "I can't give a simple yes or no answer because it is more complex. We don't really have a good definition of 'cure' in our field since there is often relapse. Furthermore my client made differential progress toward resolving the three problems I treated him for." Usually, judges will let you give this sort of more prolonged answer because they believe it best conveys the necessary information. Lawyers may not like this, as they thought that if the answer was to be confined to yes or no, you would have to answer in the negative and it is this answer the attorney wanted before the judge or jury.

Give clear, substantive answers. Do not be wishy-washy or give too many "on the one hand and on the other hand answers." (Remember Harry Truman's reactions to economists giving these kinds of answers—he only wanted to listen to one-handed economists). These answers are generally not very educational for the trier of fact. If, for example, the vast majority of more than 100 studies show how suggestible children are under certain conditions, say this; do not say, "well, some studies show the suggestibility effect, some studies don't." Although literally true, this is misleading, as the vast majority show the suggestibility effect.

Be organized. Know where information is in your report. Give information in a coherent manner (e.g., give your educational background chronologically).

A small matter, but you may ask for a break at any time. If you have been on the stand for a couple hours you may feel fatigued and that your answers are not as sharp as they initially were. Ask the judge for a break. In general, judges accommodate such requests.

Do not let your answers wander. An objection is "nonresponsive." For example, if you are asked, "How old are you?" a responsive answer is "40." A nonresponsive answer is, "Well, my mother and father met in Pittsburgh and dated for over two years before becoming married and then it was another two years before my mother became pregnant with me." Make sure each sentence you say is relevant to answering the question.

Do not be afraid to say you do not know when you do not know (although some lawyers prefer you to say "I don't recall"). Also, clearly label any estimate in your answer as an estimate. For example, if an attorney asks when you took a workshop on relapse prevention and you cannot recall the exact date (a common occurrence) your answer can simply be "I don't recall"—because you do not. Or you can answer, "I don't recall the exact date, but I estimate it was in late 2011." If you give a wrong answer, that is, if you do not label it as an estimate and say " January 2012" and then the opposing attorneys see on your vita that you said it was September 2011, they can point out this discrepancy in their next question. "But, doctor, on your vita you say it was September 2011, but here today under oath you say in was January 2012, which was it?" The next set of questions can have the same tone, "So doctor, which is inaccurate—your vita or your testimony?" "So doctor, you obviously make mistakes, isn't that correct?"

Do not get emotional. Especially do not get defensive. You may feel that the lawyers are attacking you (and sometimes they are) but remember that is their job. Testimony and legal work in general is not a love fest. You may also feel that the lawyer is being disrespectful. Lawyers are not supposed to roll their eyes at your answers, and if the other lawyers are good, they will object and point this out to the judge and the judge will admonish the attorneys not to do this again. In addition, sometimes lawyers will have certain strategies of which you should be aware. For example, an attorney may mischaracterize your prior testimony. Do not agree to an attorney's summary if it is incorrect or incomplete. Your job is also not to be a "nice person" and just let things slide like you might do in a social situation. If an attorney says, "But doctor, you have already testified that the client is cured, and thus why are you recommending him for continued treatment?" State (if true), "I never testified that he is cured. That mischaracterizes my prior testimony. I did testify that he has improved significantly but this is different than cured."

Watch for tricks. Probably the worst gambit I have experienced was during voir dire. The opposing side asked me a rather long series of questions about books that I read. They asked questions like "Doctor, have your read Brown and Smith's *Handbook of the Treatment of Sexual Abusers?* Doctor, have you read Jones and Haley's *Evidence-Based Treatment of the Juvenile Offender?*" He asked about a dozen or so books, none of which I had read (or even had heard of). To all of these questions, I said, "No, I haven't read that book." To the jury it must have sounded like I had not read a lot of key books in the field. Because I had not heard of these books, I subsequently looked them up and found that none of these even existed! Thus, if I answered "Yes, I had read the book," the lawyer's next question would have been something along the lines of, "Really, what if I tell you this book doesn't exist?" My credibility would have been significantly diminished.

OTHER MISCELLANEOUS ISSUES

The opposing attorney may want to meet with you before you testify. Generally, attorneys do not like to ask questions in the courtroom unless they know how you are going to answer. Check with the attorney who is retaining you before having any such meetings to determine if this is permissible (generally it is). Clarify who will pay for this time well in advance of the meeting.

All email, correspondence, and so on you have with the attorney may be subpoenaed. Be careful what you say in print. Some lawyers prefer telephone conversations for this reason.

Wear professional attire (e.g., suit and tie for men, skirt and blouse for women). Most courtrooms are formal and this shows respect to the court.

As always feel free to consult with your colleagues, especially colleagues who have a lot of forensic experience. In an unusual case, you might also need to consult your attorney on any especially complicated legal issue.

Bring all records that are subpoenaed. There is usually a list, so respond in writing if some of these are unavailable. Conversely, do not bring any records that have not been subpoenaed. In many courts, opposing counsel has the right to review such documents and question you on any documents you have brought to court.

Meet all deadlines. The lawyer needs time to prepare or time to send your report to the judge or opposing side (who in turn needs to read it). If your do not meet a deadline your report may not be admitted into evidence and you may be putting other people in a bind.

Prepare to be ignored. The lawyer who is calling you may have dozens or even hundreds of other cases (public defenders often have 200 to 300 cases). They may call you at the last minute (never a good situation) or may get materials to you and then turn their attention to other cases only to refocus on you a few weeks or days before the legal proceeding. But if you need to talk to the lawyers retaining you, do not hesitate to contact them.

Decide if you need any charts, visual aids, or other materials. For example, defense lawyers have made charts of all the inconsistencies found in children's allegations of their abuse. It is best to avoid jargon, but if you decide to use it, explain clearly what each and every technical term means. Have empathy for the judge or jury—they are not mental health professionals so explain terms like DSM-5, "pedophilia," "relapse prevention," actuarial assessment, validity, reliability, and empathy. Many of these words may have a colloquial meaning, but remember we are using them in a technical context and these meanings, if you are to be understood properly, need to be explained.

AN EXAMPLE OF AN EXPERT REPORT USED AS EVIDENCE

In cases of child sexual abuse, a common part of the investigative process is a forensic interview of a child witness or alleged victim. As described in Chapter 4, regarding child memories and the practices that can make them more or less accurate, such forensic interviews must be done carefully and must refrain from certain problematic ways of asking questions. However, who will make the determination of the degree to which an interview is free from those problems, or is not? Who will determine whether the interview was done well? Because these issues are complex and well beyond the scope of an average person's knowledge or training, expert witnesses are needed to answer these questions.

To establish expertise, a professional will need to demonstrate to the court that they have the needed training and experiences to be able to offer well-informed opinions. In the case of evaluations of forensic child interviews, such evaluators usually have to demonstrate that they have an education that has given them access to the important literature, that they have experiences that will inform their opinions, and (often) that they have some form of peer acknowledgment of their status as expert. This peer acknowledgment can come from things such as peer-reviewed publications in scientific professional journals. Being peer-reviewed means that other professionals have had the chance to criticize your scientific or scholarly work (before publication) and the work has withstood the criticism. Furthermore, the method by which you come to your conclusions must be described. If that method has also withstood peer evaluation, it may be viewed as yielding stronger evidence.

One tool used by qualified professionals to determine the quality of an interview of a child witness is the Protocol for Evaluating Forensic Interviews of Children, or PEFIC (Fanetti, O'Donohue, & Bradley, 2006). PEFIC training teaches reviewers to look for (1) certain problematic styles of questioning and (2) the presence of certain important assessments, which should be done by an interviewer. Each of the things assessed by the

PEFIC, or biasing factors, has been demonstrated in the scientific literature as something to control or consider. These include:

Questioning Style

- **Rapport**. The interviewer is required to ensure that enough interpersonal relationship exists to allow the child to provide answers to questions.
- **Leading questions**. It is not allowed to ask questions that suggest an answer or provide certain important forensic details, not already given by the child.
- **Disconfirmation**. Interviewers are not allowed to indicate that they believe a child is answering incorrectly.
- **Inappropriate reinforcement**. An interviewer is allowed to reinforce general participation in the interview, but not for certain types of responses or answers.
- **Repeated questions**. Interviewers are not allowed to repeat questions, unless they have provided a good reason, such as "I did not hear what you said."
- **Integrated response confusion**. Interviewers must pay attention to not only what children say, but also how they say it. Saying, "Yeah," but with a questioning tone, is not an affirmative response.
- **Encouraging speculation**. An interviewer is not allowed to suggest that a child should guess about answers.
- **Conformity press**. An interviewer is not allowed to mention other children's ideas, other adults' ideas, other evidence, or even the child's previous statements (even if they conflict with the current statement).
- **Response class bias**. An interviewer is not allowed to refocus a child away from discussion of some people toward others or away from some details toward others.

Important Assessments

- **Outside contamination**. The interviewer must assess for the possibility that previous interviews or conversations about the alleged events have occurred. This allows an assessment for the possibility of retroactive interference as described in Chapter 4.
- **Role and purpose**. An interviewer must assess the degree to which the child understands what the interview is designed to do and what the child's role is in the interview.
- **Threats and bribes**. An interviewer must assess for the possibility that the children have experienced threats about how they answer questions, or are offered bribes. These threats or bribes can be either explicit or implicit.
- **Truth meaning**. An interviewer must assess the degree to which the child understands what it means to tell the truth.

- **Truth importance.** An interviewer must assess the degree to which the child understands the importance of telling the truth in the courtroom setting.
- **Right of "I Don't Know."** An interviewer must assess the degree to which children understand that they can say, "I don't know" when they are unsure.
- **Authority pleasing.** An interviewer must assess the degree to which a child believes important people will be pleased or satisfied by a certain specific answer, and the extent to which it affected what the child said.
- **Appropriate use of open-ended questions.** An interviewer must assess the degree to which open-ended questions ("Can you tell me what your remember about that day?") are used versus closed-ended questions ("Did he also touch you on your rear?"). Research has shown that closed-ended questions result in more erroneous answers.

An expert witness may be asked to evaluate an interview based on the above set of criteria and issue a report. A good report will provide details about (1) what materials were reviewed and when, (2) the intentions and limitations of the review, (3) the scientific basis for the review and the way it was conducted, (4) a detailed description of each point of analysis and the observations made, and (5) a summary of the observations and the conclusions drawn from them. The following is a section of an actual forensic interview evaluation (with identifying information changed). It was pulled from observations made of an interview regarding the PEFIC section "Leading Questions." This level of specificity and explanation is required for the entire interview, and for each individual point of evaluations.

Time Code: c. 9:57:10

Interviewer: "And how come you wouldn't want to go to Mike's?"

Analysis: At this time in the interview, the child had not indicated that he did not want to go to Mike's home. Although it is understandable that the interviewer assumed this, it is a leading question. In order for the question to be appropriate, the child would have had to state this idea before it is included in the question.

Time Code: c. 10:00:54

Interviewer: "Uh huh. So when Mike put his mouth on your penis, where were you when that happened? Like were you in a car, or outside, or in a house or something else?"

Analysis: This is a particularly problematic leading question because it contains very important forensic details and the child has not said anything about anybody putting a mouth on a penis. The first mention of this (in the interview) comes from the interviewer.

Furthermore, the question is about location. It is phrased as assuming that the first part of the question (in fact) happened. To answer it, the child would need to accept the first assertion. Finally, multiple-choice questions are a problematic choice in forensic interviews. They may be an option as a way to describe the type of answer being solicited, but they usually present one choice which is important. Because children are more likely to pick a presented choice than to verbalize an absent choice, it becomes unclear whether the verbalization is the product of the offered choices or a recollection of experienced events. Even more problematic is the possibility that, once verbalized, the selected choice can be integrated into the child's subsequent recollections.

Here is another selected evaluation point from a different interview. This excerpt is related to the PEFIC factor, "Outside Contamination."

Time Code: c. 10:47:35

Child: ... "Well, actually that's all the story my momma told me."
Interviewer: "What story did your mom tell you?"
Child: "About girl parts. But I still don't know the story."
Analysis: This is a particularly straightforward statement about the possibility of coaching, but it goes without follow-up by the interviewer. It is unclear even what this child means about what her mother told her about. This is a serious oversight of a fairly easy assessment. Coaching by parents is common (though not helpful). When the child directly mentions it, it becomes imperative to assess exactly what happened. This was not done so this factor cannot be ruled out as a potential source of contamination or bias.

An interviewer that is assessing for the occurrence of child sexual abuse should be prepared to use the best available interviewing techniques as provided by their training. In this way, they should be prepared for thorough evaluations, by others, of their interviews with a critical purpose. Having your work evaluated should not be intimidating, but rather it should be expected. Knowing how an evaluation is going to be done is the best way to prepare your work to withstand scrutiny. We would encourage those who wish to be forensic interviewers to become familiar with (1) the best available interviewing methods and (2) the most commonly used postinterview evaluations done by experts hired by defense experts.

Finally, interviewers should also remember that evaluators examining their work are not free from scrutiny of their evaluations. These post-hoc experts must also use the best available knowledge and procedure to produce scientifically valid conclusions. The degree to which their technique has been scientifically studied is every bit as important as is the degree to which the interviewing technique has been scientifically studied. In other words, do not be afraid to find an expert who can challenge the technique used by other experts.

STUDY QUESTIONS

1. What does it mean to say that the U.S. legal system is adversarial?
2. Discuss the concepts of admissibility, scope, and weight when evaluating expert testimony.
3. What are subpoenas and depositions? How might an expert witness encounter them?
4. What is the difference between direct testimony and cross-examination?
5. What is an "ultimate opinion" and why are experts often forbidden to make one?
6. What is an "objection" to questions in court? Discuss several reasons that might be used to justify an objection.
7. The chapter details several tips to use when preparing for testifying in court as an expert witness. Outline and detail them.
8. Name the point of evaluation described in the Protocol for Evaluating Forensic Interviews of Children (PEFIC).

GLOSSARY

admissibility of expert testimony Judicial determination about whether an expert can testify.

appeal In some cases, legal judgments can be reconsidered by an appeals court to determine if a convicted person was, in fact, allowed all of their due process rights. Errors that involve defendant rights that were not provided for are called *reversible errors* because an appeals court can reverse the verdict and retry the case.

cross-examination Opposing attorneys can question expert witnesses to establish the boundaries of their observations or conclusions.

deposition Lawyers ask questions to witnesses, under oath, before the actual trial or hearing. Usually held outside of courtrooms.

direct testimony Testimony provided by a witness related to their observations, conclusions, or opinions. For expert witnesses, this is conducted by the attorney that secured their testimony.

expert reports Expert witnesses are usually required to file written reports that detail their observations or conclusions. This forms the actual evidence. Expert testimony is used to provide verbal clarity to judges and juries about the substance of the report.

expert witness Educate the trier of fact about issues beyond the average layperson's ability to know or understand.

hearsay Testimony as to what other people have said. This is usually not allowed in court. Experts may be allowed to testify to the reports of others, but do not have universal latitude.

impeachment of expert testimony A tactic used to discredit an expert witness in the eyes of the court, perhaps to pointing to conflicting answers or answers countered by other experts with greater weight.

material witness Answer questions in court regarding what they have directly experienced.

objections Attorneys may pose objections to specific testimony, but are required to justify the objection with specific reasons. A judge will determine whether the objection has merit—that is, is sustained—or if it does not have merit—that is, is overruled.

opening the door A potential error in testimony. Opening the door allows opposing attorneys to ask questions that they would otherwise not be allowed to introduce. For example, an opposing attorney would not be able to ask personal questions of an expert—unless the expert first introduces the specific topic in direct testimony. This is a good reason to keep answers short and to-the-point when testifying.

PEFIC Protocol for Evaluating Forensic Interviews of Children. A standardized evaluation system used to review the quality of forensic interviews based on known biasing factors.

scope of expert testimony Judicial determination about the range of things an expert can discuss.

subpoena An order usually signed by a judge that compels someone to do something— to produce records, to come at a certain time and place to testify, and so on.

transcripts Official documentation of the answers and responses provided within a courtroom proceeding. Usually collected by court reporters specially trained to transfer verbal discussion to written form as it occurs.

ultimate opinion Usually an expert opinion on the guilt or innocence of the defendant. This is usually expressly not allowed, because it usurps the right of the jury, or judge, to make the ultimate decision.

voir dire For expert witnesses, a way to question a witness to establish that they are, in fact, an expert on a specific issue.

weight of expert testimony Judicial determination about the strength of the expert. Determinations can be made in contrast to different experts, especially if they provide conflicting testimony.

REFERENCES

Fanetti, M., O'Donohue, W., & Bradley, A. (2006). A method for evaluating forensic interviews of children (PEFIC). *American Journal of Forensic Psychology*, *24*(3), 1–23.

O'Donohue, W., Benuto, L., & Cirlugea, O. (2013). Analyzing child sexual abuse allegations. *Journal of Forensic Psychology Practice*, *14*(3), 296–314.

Tolle, L., & O'Donohue, W. (Eds.). (2012). *Improving the quality of child custody evaluations*. New York, NY: Springer.

11

An Overview of the U.S. Legal System

GOALS OF THIS CHAPTER:

1. To understand the different types of legal cases people may encounter.
2. To understand the functions of different players in the judicial system.
3. To understand the basic procedures people may experience in the judicial system.

Regardless of what future career you decide on, if you decide to work in social services, law enforcement, for probation, or for any other area in which you have frequent contact with children and their families, you are likely to have contact with the law and with courts. Whether you work for the courts or just have frequent contact with the courts, it is very important for you to have a general understanding of how the legal system functions.

Contrary to what you see on television, much of what goes on in courtrooms is not high drama, it is not exciting, and it is not surprising. Lawyers on both sides spend many hours working, investigating, and planning so they know what to expect in court. Judges expect the lawyers who appear before them to be well prepared. Among the important functions of judges is their interaction with jurors. Jurors take time out of their busy lives to serve on juries. Judges want to ensure that trials run smoothly so jurors can return to their daily responsibilities as soon as possible. Surprises can and do happen but it is the expectation of the judges and the lawyers that those surprises are rare.

If you are working in a field that has frequent contact with the court system you need to be familiar with the expectations of the judges and the lawyers that you do your job efficiently and effectively. You also need to understand the system so you can explain it to the children and families with whom you work. In order for you to fully understand how the legal system works, you need to understand some of the history and how the legal system has evolved to where we are today.

The idea of legal evolution is very important. Contrary to what many people think, laws are not fixed. They are not static. Instead laws change, sometimes rapidly, to address changes in society. The only thing that remains the same about the U.S. legal system is its goal—to protect people's access to justice and defend the rights of every person. It is safe to say that every person who works in the legal system believes in the importance of ensuring the system works—even if they do not always agree on how it is supposed to work.

The fact that the legal system is always changing and the fact that the people in the system do not agree on how the system should work is actually one of the best parts of the U.S. legal system. The ability for people to argue about the system and how the system should work is one of our legal system's greatest attributes—it is what allows the system to change with the times. It is why a **constitution** that was written nearly 250 years ago, before cars, before television, and before the Internet, still works today.

Other chapters in this book discuss what happens to children when they become involved in the court system, either in juvenile delinquency courts or in dependency courts. At the end of this chapter we discuss some specific laws that affect children. Children, especially teenagers, often engage in conduct that can get them into significant legal trouble. Many kids and teenagers underestimate the seriousness of their conduct because either their friends are doing the same thing or they think they will not get into serious trouble because of their age. Nothing could be further from the truth. The reason you need to be familiar with some of these crimes is so you can use your contacts with kids to teach them about the consequences of their actions as well as to try to keep them safe. Sometimes keeping them safe will mean explaining to them how much trouble they can get into, and sometimes it will mean calling the authorities or making a report as a mandated reporter. You have to use your good judgment to decide.

FUNDAMENTALS OF THE U.S. LEGAL SYSTEM

In the Declaration of Independence the first 13 colonies declared their independence from England. When this country was first formed the 13 colonies were governed by the Articles of Confederation. The Articles of Confederation were drafted in 1776 and formally adopted in 1781.

During the time this country was formed there were two main schools of thought—there were the Federalists and the anti-Federalists. The **Federalists** wanted a structured, centralized government. The **anti-Federalists**, having just gotten rid of

English rule, wanted a looser organization of states. The Articles of Confederation were originally believed to strike a balance between these two competing schools of thought. This original plan allowed for one house of Congress to have the authority to regulate money and military. One of the significant flaws in the Articles of Confederation is that Congress had no enforcement ability.

In other words, Congress could declare a war and order troops to go fight the war, but if no troops arrived there was nothing Congress could do. Congress could obtain a loan from a foreign country but when it came time to repay that loan, Congress could not force the states or the people to pay the loan back.

Other problems with the Articles of Confederation included the fact that there was no president, no centralized government (other than a powerless Congress), no courts, and no way to levy and collect taxes. There was no way to fund a central government. The Articles of Confederation did not refer to the 13 states as a country, government, or a nation. Rather, it said "[t]he said States hereby severally enter into a firm league of friendship with each other." The fact that the 13 colonies did not consider themselves a country made it virtually impossible for the colonies to work with other countries.

After much debate and several drafts the U.S. Constitution was finalized in 1788 and went into effect on January 1, 1789. The Constitution as we know it today provides for three branches of government: the executive, the judiciary, and the legislative. Each branch has specific, delegated powers. With the passage of the Constitution the anti-Federalists essentially lost the intellectual argument over whether there should be a centralized, federal government or a loose alliance among the several states. The anti-Federalists believed that the broad powers of the government infringed on both individual liberties and states' rights.

Even most anti-Federalists would probably agree that absent a centralized federal government, the United States would not exist in its current form today because the country would not have been able to successfully fight subsequent wars or prosper economically in a global economy. Many anti-Federalist arguments influence our everyday lives in this country. The anti-Federalists may have lost the battle over a single, centralized government but the intellectual struggle between Federalists and anti-Federalists continues to the present day. Anytime Congress debates legislation over new laws or new taxes or when federal courts rule on whether they have jurisdiction, lawmakers and the courts have to consider Federalism and anti-Federalism.

The Constitution may not be as decentralized as the anti-Federalists of the 1780s may have wanted, but it attempts to strike a balance between Federalist and anti-Federalist principles. Either in government or history classes you probably read that the federal government is one of limited, delegated powers. Any power not expressly given by the

Constitution to the federal government (Congress, the president, and the court) remains with the individual states.

Understanding the constant tension between the desire to have a centralized government (Federalism) and the desire to protect the rights of both the states and the individuals (anti-Federalism) is key to understanding why and how laws get passed, why some cases end up in some courts and other cases end up in others, and some of the reasons why the laws are constantly changing and evolving.

STATE LAW AND FEDERAL LAW

The Constitution grants specific, limited powers to the federal government. Because of this states are free to make many of their own laws. For example, in Chapter 12, which discusses mandated reporters, there are examples of how different states have included different professions in the mandated reporter statutes. Another chapter discusses how different states have defined the term *minor*. Both of those are general examples of the rights of states to make their own laws.

Because both the states and the federal government have the right to make their own laws, it is called a dual sovereign system. Sovereign means the ability to rule a specific area, such as a state. Sovereignty also includes the right to make laws.

Dual sovereignty is important in the criminal justice system because of the Fifth Amendment, which states that a defendant in the criminal justice system has the right not be prosecuted by the same sovereign twice. This is referred to as the **double jeopardy** clause.

Some crimes can be prosecuted in both state and federal court. It is possible for someone to be prosecuted for the same crime in state court and again in federal court. This is because the double jeopardy clause only prevents the same sovereign from prosecuting someone twice. For example, bank robbery is both a state and federal crime. If a person committed a bank robbery in Wyoming the state of Wyoming could prosecute that person. The same person could also be prosecuted in federal court by the U.S. government.

Dual prosecutions are common in some jurisdictions, less so in others. On the one hand it makes sense that both the state and the federal government seek justice under their laws. On the other hand, it can be seen as a waste of resources to prosecute the same person in two different jurisdictions for the same conduct.

Consider This

If U.S. citizens were not protected against double jeopardy, how might multiple trials with multiple juries ultimately work against the defendant? What other ramifications might also ensue?

CIVIL VERSUS CRIMINAL COURTS

Courts hear cases. Cases are usually disputes between two parties. Sometimes a case comes to court when there is no dispute—sometimes two parties cannot figure out what the law requires in a particular situation and they go to court to ask the court to tell them.

All cases fall into one of two categories. There are criminal cases and there are civil cases. A civil case can be about many different things. A civil case could come to court because someone was hurt in a car accident and they are seeking to recover damages (money) from the person who hit them. A civil case could involve two foreign governments who have a dispute over who has rights over a river. Civil cases generally, but not always, involve disputes over money. Juvenile dependency is considered a civil case, as are family law cases. Although these cases sometimes involve questions about money, they also involve determinations about where a child should live or how a divorce is going to be settled.

Broadly stated, anyone can bring a civil case. Assuming you have a reason you can walk into a lawyer's office and hire the lawyer to sue a person, a government, or a corporation. Criminal cases are very different. Only the government can file a criminal case.

The one thing that sets criminal cases apart is that if a person is convicted in a criminal case they could go to jail. Only the government has the power to bring a case where the issue is whether a person should go to jail.

Different parts of the government have the power to bring a criminal case. In state court cases are frequently brought by the district attorney's office in a particular county. Most states have some form of a state prosecutor or a state attorney general who can bring a case anywhere in the state. Often lawyers in the city attorney's office prosecute certain crimes such as illegal camping inside a city.

At the state level prosecutors work with police, sheriffs, and state agencies to investigate and enforce the laws. For example, in most states it is illegal to work as a contractor without a license. Someone who works without a license can be subject to civil or criminal penalties. A homeowner who hired an unlicensed contractor could civilly sue the contractor and recover money. If the homeowner thought the contractor should go to jail the only thing the homeowner could do about that is file a report with law enforcement. The claim would be investigated and ultimately someone at the district attorney's office would decide whether a criminal case should be filed.

One important thing to understand about criminal cases is that a criminal case can only be dismissed by whichever branch of the government that made the decision to file the case.

So, using the example of the homeowner and the unlicensed contractor again, if homeowners filed a civil suit, then decided not to go forward for whatever reason, they can dismiss the case. The case would be over and nothing more would happen. Maybe the homeowner learned something about the unlicensed contractor that made the homeowner not want to sue the contractor anymore, like the contractor had a large family and the lawsuit was placing a heavy financial strain on the family. Or the contractor had subsequently obtained his contractor's license.

If the same homeowner had filed a police report and the district attorney's office filed criminal charges against the contractor, there is nothing the homeowner can do to prevent the criminal case from going forward. The homeowners can call the district attorney and explain they wish to dismiss the case, but the district attorney does not have to do so. Many states have victim's rights laws that require the district attorney to listen to what a crime victim wants, but no state has a law that requires the district attorney to actually do what the victim wants.

It makes sense if you think about it that the district attorney or other government agency has complete discretion to decide whether to bring and/or dismiss criminal charges. If they did not have such discretion the entire criminal justice system could be motivated by personal vendettas. If there were two businesspeople who got into a dispute over a contract, one could have the other businessperson prosecuted and potentially sent to jail, until the other businessperson agreed to whatever the first businessperson wanted.

Or think of the following scenario: A 20-year-old is texting on his phone while driving. He is not paying attention, crosses the center lane, and hits an oncoming car. The driver of the other car is killed. In almost every state the district attorney would charge this as a form of negligent homicide or manslaughter. The teenager very well could go to prison, in some states for a long time. Penalties for manslaughter vary greatly across the United States from a year or less in county jail to more than 20 years in prison. But say the family of the driver who died thinks the 20-year-old should be subject to the death penalty for killing their loved one. To family members whose lives are forever changed because they have lost a loved one such a sentence may seem just. But sentences like the death penalty are reserved for only the most heinous and callous of crimes—a negligent act by a young adult is not comparable to a premeditated and intentional murder. Under this circumstance it also makes sense that the district attorney has the discretion not to follow the wishes of the victims or their family. It is the job of the district attorney to serve and protect society as a whole, but not any specific person or group of people within society.

In the federal government the most common agency that files criminal charges is the U.S. Attorney's office. The U.S. Attorney's office works with a broad range of law enforcement agencies to investigate and prosecute crimes. Common examples are the Federal Bureau of Investigation (FBI), the Drug Enforcement Administration (DEA), the Department of Homeland Security, and the Bureau of Alcohol, Tobacco, Firearms, and Explosives (ATF). The actual number of federal agencies who investigate crimes is enormous; an entire book could be written just describing each of those agencies and their responsibilities.

STATE VERSUS FEDERAL JURISDICTION

In civil cases determining whether a case should be filed in state court or federal court is often complicated. There are a few basic rules although these rules have lots of exceptions. Federal courts have jurisdiction, or the ability to hear a case, when the case involves a federal law. Think of the Affordable Care Act, the ACA. The ACA was passed by Congress and it is a federal law. That means that any lawsuit about the ACA has to be heard in federal court.

Pursuant to Article III, Section 2 of the U.S. Constitution, federal courts also have jurisdiction over disputes between the states. Say Nebraska wanted to sue South Dakota for some reason. It would be unfair for Nebraska if the case were in South Dakota. Similarly it would be unfair for South Dakota if the case were in Nebraska. Therefore the case will always be in federal court.

At the beginning of this chapter there was a discussion about federalism and the problems presented by the Articles of Confederation when this country was first formed. One of the problems posed by the Articles of Confederation was that the federal government had no power to resolve disputes between the states. If Nebraska and South Dakota had different economic policies and those policies hurt the other state, society would need a way to reconcile those policies for the good of the country. By giving federal courts the ability to hear disputes between the states, the founders of the Constitution ensured that this country could move forward and work as a single united country instead of a loose coalition of states that frequently fought with each other.

Determining the proper jurisdiction (state court or federal court) in a civil case is difficult. Lawyers often think there are tactical advantages to filing in one court or the other. Lawyers, even those who have spent years practicing law, make mistakes about whether a civil case should be filed in state court or federal court.

In a criminal case, issues of where the case should be filed are frequently much simpler. Generally speaking the FBI, DEA, ATF, and other federal agencies only investigate federal crimes and those criminal cases are filed in federal court. Similarly, state law enforcement typically investigates violations of state law and those cases are filed in state court.

Things become a little more complicated when law enforcement investigates a crime that can be prosecuted in both state court and federal court. Drug crimes are a great example. All states, as well as the federal government, have laws prohibiting drug trafficking. Technically both the state and the federal government could file charges against the same drug dealers. The drug dealers would have to defend themselves in both courts and, if convicted, could serve two separate prison sentences. As discussed earlier, this does not violate the prohibition against double jeopardy because the state government and the federal government are separate sovereigns.

Although dual prosecutions are possible they are relatively rare. More commonly the U.S. Attorney's office and a local district attorney's office work together to decide which case should be prosecuted where. As a general rule the larger and therefore more serious cases are prosecuted in federal court. For example, in a drug case, while the U.S. Attorney's office could decide to prosecute people who grew eight marijuana plants in their backyard, the resources of the federal government are better spent investigating and prosecuting a marijuana grow involving 5,000 plants.

There are some cases that can only be brought in state court or federal court. Drunk driving, domestic violence, and assault and battery are all examples of cases that generally can only be filed in state court. Income tax fraud, bankruptcy fraud, and securities violations are examples of crimes that typically only the federal government has the authority to prosecute. Words such like "typically" and "generally" are used because there are so many exceptions in the law that it is impossible to state anything with an absolute certainty.

THE PROFESSIONAL PARTIES

In both state and federal court the professional parties are all lawyers. With some narrow exceptions, generally in family law cases, only lawyers are allowed to represent other people in court. Only lawyers can become judges.

Lawyers spend years in school. After they finish their undergraduate degree they go to law school. Most law schools are 3-year programs although there are some night school programs that require 4 years. Much of the curriculum is set by the American Bar Association. In other words, for much of the time law students are in school they have little say in what classes they take. They are all required to take Contracts, Civil Procedure, Evidence, Criminal Law, Torts (a **tort** is traditionally defined as a civil wrong that causes another person damage. Personal injury and medical malpractice are common examples of torts but there are many other kinds.). Constitutional Law, and Property Law are a few of the courses that law students are required to take. At some point law students are allowed to take electives, courses more narrowly focused on the area of law that student may want to practice.

Just as it is important for you, someone who is likely to have frequent contact with the court system, to understand how the courts work, it is important for lawyers to understand the basics of all areas of the law. Because the law developed and evolved along with society the areas of the law are not discrete. In other words, in a civil case there might be issues regarding property, contracts, and torts. In white collar crimes the lawyers have to understand contract law to understand the transactions underlying the alleged crimes.

Most future judges spend many years working as lawyers. Sometimes future judges decide at a very young age that they want to become a judge. These future judges often make a concerted effort to work in as many different areas of the law as possible. They might work as a prosecutor for a few years, then as a criminal defense lawyer, and later as a civil litigator. Regardless of what areas they practiced as a lawyer, most judges are expected to know all areas of the law.

While both lawyers and judges know more about the law than the average person, no judge or lawyer knows everything about the law. What they do know is how to find the answer. Most lawyers and judges are extremely good researchers and they spend hours researching—lawyers are trying to find arguments to help their clients and judges are trying to determine what the correct result is in any given case.

Civil Attorneys

In the United States all lawyers, once they pass the bar exam, are allowed to practice civil or criminal law. Because the law is so complicated most lawyers specialize in either a civil or criminal practice. The lawyers who focus on civil practice specialize even further. They practice in family law, business litigation, estate planning, personal injury, and the list could go on and on.

A **civil lawyer** can represent a private party, an individual, or a business. Civil lawyers also represent the government. For example, most school districts have lawyers who represent them in negotiations to buy more property to build a new school. The possible situations in which civil lawyers are involved are almost endless.

Prosecutors

Prosecutors are lawyers who work for the government, usually the U.S. Attorney's office or the district attorney's office, and all they do is prosecute crimes. Every prosecutor's office is structured differently but there are some common features.

When lawyers first become prosecutors they start prosecuting less serious crimes, usually misdemeanors such as drunk driving or very minor drug possession cases. Over time they work their way up to prosecuting more serious and more complex cases.

In some offices, prosecutors work very closely with law enforcement officers investigating cases. This is very common for federal prosecutors or U.S. Attorneys. Imagine a federal investigation in which the FBI is involved. Very early on in the FBI agents' investigation they will start consulting with one or two members of the local U.S. Attorney's office. The attorney will help direct the investigation and advise the FBI agents. These investigations are structured this way for a few reasons: (1) If the case goes to court the prosecutor will want certain evidence. If the prosecutor is involved in the case early on they can direct the FBI agents to look for the evidence they want. (2) Federal cases are often very complicated and the investigation can go on for many years. A prosecutor needs to be involved to aid in the drafting of search warrants or to develop the legal theories that will form the basis of the case.

District attorney's offices are generally structured very differently largely because of the types of cases district attorneys prosecute in state court. In the typical state court case the process starts when law enforcement is contacted. Think of a fight at a local bar. Two people get into a fight. The police are called. They investigate, interview witnesses, and make a decision that one person should be arrested. At some point they go back to the police department and write reports. Those reports get forwarded to the district attorney. The district attorney decides whether to prosecute the case. The time frame in which these decisions are made is very short, frequently just a few days.

Many of the cases you are likely to be involved with may require more investigation but still be in state court. For example, in a child molestation case, once law enforcement learns of the allegations there are many different steps they can take depending on a variety of factors. If law enforcement has reason to believe a child is in danger they will do everything in their power to remove the child from the home as soon as possible. The need to protect the child will take priority over gathering evidence or conducting a lengthy investigation prior to making an arrest.

On the other hand, if the authorities believe the suspect is a distant family member, someone the child has infrequent contact with, or someone the parents can keep away from the child, the investigation may be lengthier. For example, there was a case a few years ago in which two young sisters were being inappropriately touched by their Bible study teacher. The parents became aware of the situation and contacted law enforcement. The Bible study teacher frequently came to the family home and worked with the sisters in the living room. Law enforcement decided the best way to build a case against the teacher was to catch him making admissions on tape.

The family kept their regular meeting time with the teacher. When the teacher arrived he went in the living room and waited for the sisters. What he did not know was that before he got there, law enforcement had installed multiple listening devices in the living room and there was a police officer hiding in the closet! The dad came into the living room and confronted the teacher about the allegations involving the two sisters. During the conversation with the father, the teacher made several statements that showed he was guilty.

Law enforcement has a lot of authority on how to investigate a case when they know the victim is safe. In this instance the investigation took several weeks, longer than many investigations in state court. The officers were able to develop evidence that was helpful in the eventual prosecution of the Bible study teacher.

Defense Attorneys

The other lawyers in the criminal justice system are defense attorneys. Anyone who is accused of a crime is constitutionally entitled to be represented by an attorney. In 1963 the U.S. Supreme Court issued a decision in a case entitled *Gideon v. Wainwright* (372 U.S. 335) in which the court held that if people who are accused of a crime cannot afford to hire their own lawyer, a lawyer will be appointed to represent them at public expense. In making this decision, the court was interpreting the Sixth Amendment of the United States, which guarantees, among other things, that all people accused of crimes have the right to a speedy and public jury trial. The court ruled that in order for the constitutional right to a trial to be meaningful, people had to be represented by lawyers. In light of how complicated the legal system is this makes sense. The average person does not spend years and years in law school learning how to defend themselves in court.

As a result of the Supreme Court's decision in *Gideon* all states have some kind of public defender's office. In some locations there is a formal public defender's office. In other counties, often smaller and more rural counties, private lawyers have contracts with the county to work as public defenders.

In federal court there are federal public defenders who do the same thing as a state public defender, only federal public defenders exclusively practice in federal court.

There are also private criminal defense attorneys. Under the constitution, any person who can afford to retain a private criminal defense attorney has the absolute right to do so. The government cannot interfere in the person's decision about which lawyer they want to hire.

The U.S. Constitution divides the federal government into three distinct branches: the executive (the President), the legislative (Congress), and the judiciary (the courts). The government is divided this way to create a system of checks and balances so no one branch of government becomes too powerful. The role of a criminal defense lawyer is very similar. It is the job of a defense attorney to provide checks and balances on the power of prosecutors and law enforcement.

The job of criminal defense attorneys is, first and foremost, to make sure that their client's constitutional rights are being protected. The vast majority of prosecutors and law enforcement officers are well meaning and would not intentionally violate a criminal defendant's constitutional rights. Defense attorneys and prosecutors often genuinely disagree about what the Constitution requires in a particular circumstance. There are also rare examples of cases where prosecutors and/or law enforcement bent the rules because they believed a particular set of circumstances justified their actions. Defense attorneys work to make sure that the rules are not bent. Most defense attorneys believe that the best way to protect every member of society's constitutional rights is to make sure no one's rights are violated.

The Role of the Court

The judge serves many important roles. In many cases judges are actively involved in cases for many months, sometimes even years, before a trial.

In a criminal case if law enforcement officers want to get a search warrant, that search warrant has to be reviewed and signed by a judge. The judge makes a determination that the officers have probable cause to believe a crime has been committed and evidence relating to that crime will be located in a particular place. By reviewing search warrants before they are served, judges are making sure law enforcement agencies are complying with the requirements of the Fourth Amendment. The Fourth Amendment of the U.S. Constitution states that the people of this country have the right to be secure in their homes, papers, and things and that they shall be free of unreasonable searches and seizures.

As proceedings in a criminal case move forward the judge decides bail amounts, when motions have to be filed, when trial will start, and what can and cannot be said at trial.

Many people are suspicious about why and when courts prevent certain evidence from being heard at a trial. Over the course of history our society has developed a large number of rules about when evidence is and is not admissible in court. Those rules generally serve two purposes. The first purpose is to prevent a party to a lawsuit, be it civil or criminal, from illegally obtaining evidence. The justice system exists to preserve and uphold the law—it would make no sense if that same system allowed evidence to be used in court that was obtained illegally or in violation of the Constitution.

The second purpose is to make sure that the evidence presented to a jury is reliable. As a general rule witnesses are only allowed to testify to things they have personal knowledge about, something they saw or heard. They cannot testify to what they heard someone else say or what someone else wrote. If witnesses were allowed to testify to things they did not know about, the results of both criminal and civil trials would be unreliable. In order for the justice system to work society must have confidence that the results are reliable.

The court is actively involved in civil cases at many different points in the proceedings. Prior to trial the parties can file many different kinds of motions. The motions can seek to do any number of things from forcing one side to produce certain evidence to dismissing an entire case. The judge decides all of these motions.

When a case finally goes to trial, judges explain their role to the jury. They often tell jurors that jurors are the judges of the facts and the judge is the judge of the law. What this means is the judge, after listening to the lawyers from both sides, decides what law should apply. The jury decides what the facts are and how the facts apply to the law. U.S. Supreme Court Chief Justice John Roberts likened the role of a judge to that of an umpire at a baseball game—a judge's job is to call balls and strikes. While deciding what the law requires in a particular circumstance is harder than determining if a pitch is a ball or a strike, it is a good analogy to summarize the role of the court.

Perhaps the most important part of Chief Justice Roberts' baseball analogy about the role of judges is more subtle. Umpires are independent. They are not influenced by either team. The independence of judges, the fact that they cannot be aligned with any side in a legal case, is very important. Judges are neutral. Because they are not an advocate for one side or the other and they are not being paid by one side or the other, their only goal is to ensure the law is accurately and fairly applied. Just as an umpire has no interest in the result of a baseball game, judges have no interest in the result of a case—they just want the rules to be followed.

BURDENS OF PROOF

There are four common *burdens of proof* in the U.S. justice system: probable cause, preponderance of the evidence, clear and convincing evidence, and beyond a reasonable doubt.

Probable cause is a low evidentiary standard, the lowest used in the law. This standard is only used in very limited circumstances. A court can issue a search warrant if there is probable cause to believe a crime was committed. A person can be arrested based on probable cause. Probable cause is really just another way of saying, given all the facts and circumstances it is reasonable to believe this person committed a crime.

A preponderance of the evidence is the standard that governs most civil cases. In order for the jury to find for one side over the other they have to decide that the preponderance of the evidence supports that side. Over the years people have tried many different ways to describe exactly what this means. One common description is to say that a preponderance of the evidence is 50% plus a feather—its ever so slightly more than being equal.

Clear and convincing evidence is a medium-level burden of proof. It is more than a preponderance of the evidence, meaning it is more than 50% but there is no specific percentage that defines clear and convincing. Unlike other evidentiary standards, it is very difficult to precisely define clear and convincing evidence because exactly how this evidentiary standard is defined changes based on the circumstance in which it is being used.

One good example of clear and convincing evidence is how it can be used in juvenile dependency proceedings. In a different chapter we discussed the juvenile dependency system and the fact that courts may remove a child from a home if there is probable cause to believe a child is being abused or neglected. In the 1980s the U.S. Supreme Court decided a case involving the New York state's statute regarding when parental rights can be terminated. In that case the court decided if the state wants to terminate the parents' parental rights forever based on the abuse of neglect, the state must present clear and convincing evidence that a nurturing parent-child relationship no longer exists (*Santosky v. Kramer* [1982], 455 U.S. 745). The rationale behind this is complicated but essentially the court said that parents have a constitutional right to care for their children. In order to end this right, the state, in this case New York, must provide more than a preponderance of the evidence to terminate this important constitutional right. More evidence was required in order to balance out the risk that the state might be wrong about recommending that parental rights be terminated.

To find a defendant in a criminal case guilty, every juror must agree the defendant is guilty *beyond a reasonable doubt.* A common jury instruction defining "beyond a reasonable doubt" goes something like this: Beyond a reasonable doubt is not beyond all doubt. Proof beyond a reasonable doubt is proof that leaves you with an abiding conviction of the truth of the charges. The evidence need not eliminate all possible doubt because everything in life is open to some possible or imaginary doubt (California Criminal Jury Instructions, CalCrim 103, 2006). Beyond a reasonable doubt is the highest burden of proof required in the law. Because the penalties in a criminal case can be severe and life altering, society has decided that prior to imposing those penalties, prosecutors must present a lot of evidence to prove a person is guilty of a crime.

BASIC PROCEDURE IN CIVIL CASES

Civil cases are started when one party decides to sue another. This person is a plaintiff. The person hires a lawyer and the lawyer drafts what is called a *complaint.* A complaint is a legal document that is filed with the court. The complaint includes a description of what happened, and the facts the plaintiffs believe they will be able to prove at trial. The complaint also contains an explanation of how the plaintiff believes the facts violated the law. A complaint can be very simple and allege one violation of the law, or can be very lengthy and allege potentially hundreds of violations of the law.

Once the complaint is written it is filed in court and served on the defendant. Service is the formal legal process that notifies the defendant that they are being sued. Depending on the nature of the case defendants are served by process servers (people whose job it is to serve legal documents), sheriff's deputies, or the U.S. Marshall's service. After the defendant receives the complaint they have a specific amount of time to file a document in court. The defendant has several options for the kind of document they wish to file in response to the complaint, the most common of which is an answer.

In juvenile dependency court, as well as some other areas of the law, a case is started by the filing of a petition. The opposing party is not necessarily required to file an answer or other document responding to the petition.

Once these initial documents have been filed the parties begin a process called *discovery.* Discovery is the time when the parties find out what evidence the other side has. Discovery can come in many forms. Lawyers serve written discovery, which requests evidence and documents be turned over and they ask the other side to admit certain things.

Parties and witnesses can be required to attend a deposition. A deposition is a formal legal proceeding, usually held at one of the lawyer's offices. During the deposition the witness is placed under penalty of perjury and asked questions. The answers to these questions can later be used at trial.

The lawyers for both sides have a specific length of time to complete the discovery process. How long they have depends on what the case is about and whether they are in state or federal court. It is common for the case to end up in court during the discovery process because the lawyers often disagree about what evidence they have to produce to the other side during the discovery process.

Once discovery is over the case goes to trial. Trials can last a few days, a few months or, in rare cases, a few years. The length of the trial is usually determined by how complex the issues are that the jury has to decide.

During the entire time a civil case is pending both sides have the opportunity to file motions before the court. These motions can ask for all kinds of things from requiring one side to produce evidence to dismissing the case. The parties are also able to negotiate while the case is pending. The majority of civil suits are resolved through negotiation and never go to trial.

BASIC PROCEDURE IN CRIMINAL CASES

Procedures in federal criminal cases are standard throughout the United States. Procedure and terminology in state court criminal proceedings varies widely from state to state. While the terminology may vary, the process by which a criminal case is moved through the court system is fairly similar.

Pretrial Proceedings

Although criminal investigations can take days, weeks, months, and sometimes even years, a criminal case formally starts when a complaint or an indictment is filed. A complaint in a criminal case is similar to a complaint in a civil case. The prosecutor is the plaintiff and files a complaint that sets forth the laws the defendant allegedly broke. There are generally very few facts in a criminal complaint in state court—the only requirement is that there be enough information for a criminal defendant to know what crimes they are alleged to have committed.

In some states, as well as federal court, prosecutors generally file indictments instead of complaints. An indictment is very similar to a complaint with one important difference. An indictment is issued by a grand jury.

A grand jury is made up of ordinary citizens. In order to protect the members of the grand jury they meet in secret and generally their identities cannot be found out. A grand jury is comprised of at least 16 and not more than 23 jurors. When the grand jury is deciding whether to issue an indictment, the prosecutor appears before them and presents evidence of the crime. A defendant does not have the right to appear before a grand jury. The grand jury members decide whether there is probable cause to believe a crime has been committed. If they do, they can vote to issue an indictment. The vote to indict does not have to be unanimous but it does have to be a majority of the grand jurors.

Depending on a number of factors either shortly before an indictment or complaint is filed or shortly after, the defendant is arrested or notified that they must appear in court on a specific date and time.

Defendants can be arrested when there is no complaint or indictment filed. If law enforcement has probable cause to believe a crime has been committed the officer can arrest a person on the spot.

Once people have been arrested they generally have the right to bail out of jail. Each state sets its own rules regarding bail. Generally speaking the more serious the crime, the higher the bail is to get out of jail. For very serious crimes, such as murder, often a defendant does not have the right to bail.

In jurisdictions that proceed by way of a criminal complaint, defendants usually have the right to a hearing to determine whether there is enough evidence to go forward with a trial. This is often called a *preliminary hearing*. The evidentiary standard at this hearing is the very low probable cause standard.

Trial

The right of a criminal defendant to a speedy, public, and fair trial is one of the cornerstones of our constitutional rights. The first step in a trial is the selection of a jury. In a criminal case, a jury must consist of 12 jurors. The jurors must be selected at random. The process used to select the jury must be a system that is race- and gender-neutral. Lists of prospective jurors can be pulled from voter registration, telephone directories, motor vehicle records, customer mail lists, and utility company lists.

The actual trial process is the same in both criminal and civil trials. During jury selection the judge, and in some jurisdictions, the lawyers, ask questions of the prospective jurors. The questions are intended to find out whether the prospective jurors know anything about the case or have any biases that would prevent them from acting in a fair and impartial manner.

After the jury is selected the jurors are sworn. The jurors are also given some preliminary instructions. Two particularly important instructions that are given in virtually every case is the instruction not to discuss the facts of the case with anyone while the trial is in process and not unless all jurors are present. This means that when jurors go home at night they cannot discuss the case with their family, they cannot give an interview with the news media, and they cannot discuss the case with two other jurors over lunch. They have to wait until all of them have heard all the evidence in the case and all of the jurors are in the jury deliberation room discussing the case. These instructions are very important because the purpose of the jury system is to make sure the verdict reflects the independent judgment of each individual juror who heard and considered all the facts and evidence presented in court.

Jurors are also instructed they are not to investigate the facts of the case, conduct any experiments, or do any research on their own about the facts or the law. Lawyers and judges work very hard to make sure that only properly reliable evidence is shown before a jury. Similarly they work very hard to make sure the jury is instructed on the law that applies to the particular issues the jury is being asked to decide. A very small change in the facts can sometimes cause a very big change in what law applies—because of this and because jurors are not experts on the law it is important for them to only consider the law that the judge decides is appropriate.

After the jurors are sworn and receive some preliminary jury instructions the lawyers give opening statements. Lawyers are allowed to explain what they expect the evidence to show during the trial. The lawyers are not allowed to argue or try to persuade the jury to believe one side or the other.

During the course of the trial both sides are allowed to call witnesses. Witnesses are people who witnessed a particular event or who have knowledge about the issue at trial. Particularly in criminal trials, there are few limitations about how many witnesses each side can call. The parties are also allowed to call expert witnesses. An expert witness is any witness with special training and knowledge that will assist the jurors in making their decision.

After all of the witnesses have testified the lawyers are allowed to give closing arguments. Now the lawyers can argue and try to persuade the members of the jury to side one way or the other. The plaintiff or the prosecutor always has the burden of proof so they get to argue first. The defense argues second and then the plaintiff is allowed to rebut—to argue only those points that were raised in the defense's closing argument.

Either before or after the closing arguments the judge will instruct the jury on the law. The judge reads to the jurors all of the law they will need in order to reach their decision. In most jurisdictions the court sends a written copy of the relevant law back into the jury deliberation room.

Once the arguments are over the jurors are allowed to retire to deliberate. There is no limit on how long a jurors can consider a case before reaching their verdict. If the jurors have questions about the facts or the law they can send a note to the court with their question. Before answering the question the judge has to consult the lawyers for both sides.

Juries can either reach a verdict or they can hang. If a jury hangs it means they cannot reach a decision. Hung juries are more common in criminal cases than civil cases because of the requirement that criminal juries reach a unanimous decision.

Once the jurors have made their decision they are discharged, which means they have fulfilled their jury service and are free to go. This is also the first time the jurors are allowed to talk about the case with people other than their fellow jurors.

CRIMINAL SENTENCES

The kinds of sentences a criminal defendant can receive upon conviction of a crime are extremely varied. Every state has unique sentencing rules. Federal crimes also have very specific sentencing rules. Generally speaking, if people are convicted of a misdemeanor they cannot be sentenced to more than one year, usually in county jail. Under some circumstances it is possible for a person to be convicted of a felony and not be sentenced to prison or jail.

Depending on the jurisdiction, judges have varying amounts of authority to decide a criminal sentence. During the 1980s and 1990s there was a movement toward the imposition of mandatory minimum sentences both by Congress as well as by many state governments. In cases where there is a mandatory minimum the judge generally has no ability to give a defendant a lesser sentence even if the judge believes a lesser sentence is appropriate. The future of mandatory minimums, especially in many drug crimes, is uncertain. Over the past 5 or 6 years there has been increasing criticism of these laws and it seems likely that many of them may be changed.

COLLATERAL CONSEQUENCES OF FELONY CONVICTIONS

Many felony convictions can carry very serious noncriminal consequences. Many of the people you work with might have to deal with these consequences on a daily basis.

Almost every state and the federal government has a system of sex offender registration laws. Every jurisdiction has a list of sex crimes; if people have been convicted of one of those crimes, they have to register as a sex offender. In some states registerable crimes are limited to very serious sex offenses. In other states crimes that you may not even think of as a sex crime can require registration. For example, in California a person convicted of indecent exposure can be ordered to register as a sex offender. (Indecent exposure could include conduct such as sun bathing in the nude where other people could see the sunbather.)

In some states sex offenders are required to register for the rest of their lives, while other states only require registration for a certain number of years. The number of years people are required to register is often reflective of how serious a sex crime for which they were convicted.

There are many other kinds of registration that can be required in some states on conviction of a certain offense. Gang registration for known gang members, drug offender registration, and arson registration are some of the more common types of registration.

All of the registration laws have the same purpose—to help law enforcement. It is easier for law enforcement to keep an eye on known offenders if they know where they live. Whether these registration laws are the best way to help law enforcement is an open question. Think of the case of Jaycee Dugard, the young woman who was held captive for nearly 19 years by registered sex offender Phillip Garrido. Parole and probation regularly visited Garrido's home where Dugard was held. Unfortunately, given the enormous caseloads most parole and probation officers find themselves trying to manage, they had neither the time nor the resources to properly investigate.

Felony convictions can also carry a number of other collateral consequences such as the loss of the right to vote, the right to bear arms, the right to run for public office, and the right to sit on a jury. Collateral consequences are not the same in every state so it is important to know the laws in the state in which you live.

When you are working with children and families it is important to understand the unwritten collateral consequences—the things that happen to people convicted of felonies that are not necessarily required by law. For example, it is very hard for people who have felonies on their records to get jobs. In many states, people who have been convicted of felonies cannot receive welfare or other public assistance. Not only do you need to understand these additional hurdles, you need to be able to inform people, particularly the young people who will be looking to you as an authority figure. Hopefully, if they understand that committing a crime can and likely will ruin their future, they might think twice.

CRIMES CHILDREN SHOULD KNOW ABOUT

There are some laws children and young adults are prone to breaking, in large part because they do not know their conduct is illegal and, in some circles, their conduct is socially acceptable. These crimes can have very serious consequences that can affect a person for the rest of their life.

Sexting

It seems like everyone has a cell phone these days. Teenagers and young adults appear to be constantly texting each other. Some people also engage in sexting, the practice of sending sexually explicit texts or photos to another person. In almost every state sexting, by an adult or a minor, is illegal even if the person who received the text message wanted to receive the message. In many states a person who is convicted of sexting can be required to register as a sex offender.

A few states have started amending sex registration laws that apply to sexting. Florida changed their law in 2011 so minors do not have to register, at least on their first sexting conviction. The problem with many sexting and sex registration laws is that they were written before it was common for everyone, including young people, to have a cell phone. The laws regarding sexual communications were originally intended to catch predators—not young people engaging in youthful but probably harmless indiscretions. Although it appears other states may relax their criminal laws as well as their sex offender registration laws, such changes take time.

A lot of minors and young adults think sexting is socially acceptable. Whether it is acceptable among certain peer groups, it is frequently illegal. There are countless stories in which young people across the country have been prosecuted for such conduct. If you work with minors or young adults, informing them of this potentially serious crime that could require them to register as a sex offender for the rest of their lives could make an enormous difference.

Child Pornography Laws

Everyone would agree that the laws preventing the production and distribution of child pornography is a good thing. But again, most of these laws were written decades ago, before smartphones with cameras and minors had smartphones. Child pornography laws are another area that has yet to change in order to keep up with technology and society. A 16-year-old boy who takes naked pictures of himself has probably violated the federal statute preventing the production of child pornography. That statute carries a mandatory minimum 15-year sentence in federal prison. It is unlikely any federal prosecutor would ever prosecute such conduct, but it is important for people to understand how potentially serious such conduct can be.

Equally as serious is if the same 16-year-old boy takes naked pictures of his girlfriend and later emails them to other people. Cases like this have been prosecuted all around the country, most frequently in state courts where the penalties are lower than in federal court. In almost all of these cases the defendant was required to register as sex offender.

The issue is not whether these laws are right or wrong. Society has to decide if these laws should remain as they are or if they should be changed. What is most important is your ability to warn young people about how conduct they think is okay is actually very serious and could impact them for the rest of their lives.

VICTIMS' RIGHTS

Many states have a crime victims' bill of rights. Such laws protect the privacy of a crime victim as well as allowing the victims to be heard in court and, in some cases, receive money to cover their losses.

All crime victims have the right to recover money to compensate them for their injuries. Some newer laws have made it easier for a child to recover damages. Masha's Law, 18 USC 2255, is a federal statute that allows any child who was the victim of certain sex crimes to presumptively recover $250,000. The purpose of the presumptive minimum recovery is so the children do not have retain experts to establish how much money they lost and hopefully limit whether the victim would have to testify and recount their molestation.

CONCLUSION

If you decide to work in the social services you will almost invariably have a lot of contact with the justice system. You will be in a position to do a tremendous amount of good to serve the children and the families who are involved in the system. In order to help these people, among the things you need to know is how and why the courts work.

Children who are involved in court proceedings for one reason or another are often scared and confused. They likely will be looking to you to help them understand. You need to be able to explain to them what is happening and why. It may well be impossible to adequately explain such a complex system to very young children, but as most kids get older they will be able to understand the basics of our legal system.

You are also in the position to warn children about the consequences of their actions. If you can prevent just one minor from ending up a defendant in the criminal justice system just by repeating hundreds of times to hundreds of minors the consequences of sexting or taking naked pictures, it will have been worth your time and effort.

STUDY QUESTIONS

1. What were the Articles of Confederation? And what were some flaws?
2. Describe the differences between Federalist ideas and anti-Federalist ideas.
3. What is the double jeopardy clause of the Constitution?
4. What is the difference between a civil trial and a criminal trial?
5. What is the difference between criminal cases of federal and state jurisdiction? How does this affect the concept of double jeopardy?
6. List and describe the four standards of a "burden of proof" discussed in the chapter.
7. Outline the basic procedures in a civil case.
8. Outline the basic procedures in a criminal case.
9. What is the difference between a criminal complaint and an indictment?
10. Describe some of the collateral consequences of a felony conviction.

GLOSSARY

anti-Federalists Wanted a looser organization of states.

beyond a reasonable doubt/burden of proof Proof that leaves you with an abiding conviction of the truth of the charges. The evidence need not eliminate all possible doubt because everything in life is open to some possible or imaginary doubt.

civil cases Often involving money, these are expressly not related to the determination of criminal responsibility.

civil lawyer Can represent a private party, an individual, or a business. Civil lawyers sometimes also represent the government.

clear and convincing evidence burden of proof More evidence than "preponderance," but very difficult to precisely define clear and convincing evidence because exactly how this evidentiary standard is defined changes based on the circumstance in which it is being used.

Constitution Binding document that delineates the branches of government, the limits of federal government, and the right of the states and of individuals.

criminal cases These cases involve the accusation of specific violations of identified criminal code or law.

defense attorney A lawyer who specializes in defending people against accusations of criminal misconduct.

double jeopardy Individuals cannot be tried twice by the same power for the same crime.

Federalists Wanted a structured, centralized government.

grand jury A panel of citizens tasked with hearing evidence to determine whether to issue an *indictment* in a criminal case.

judge A presumptively neutral specialist in law who is tasked with ensuring that trials proceed with fairness and within the boundaries set by the constitution of the United States and/or individual states.

jurisdiction Specific authorities have influence and decision-making power only as granted by laws related to areas of specific influence.

jury A panel of 12 citizens, chosen at random and passing voir dire questioning, tasked with listening to evidence to determine whether the evidence meets the burden of proof required to affect a conviction, or if not then an acquittal.

preponderance of the evidence burden of proof "50% plus a feather" or "ever so slightly more than being equal."

probable cause burden of proof Another way of saying that, given all the facts and circumstances, it is reasonable to believe this person committed a crime.

prosecutors Lawyers who work for the government, usually the U.S. Attorney's office or the district attorney's office, and all they do is prosecute crimes.

public defender A publically funded defense attorney who works to help people fight criminal prosecution, even if the defendant cannot afford to pay for services.

tort A civil wrong that causes another person damage.

CHAPTER

12

❖⟩——

Mandated Reporters

GOALS OF THIS CHAPTER:

1. To become familiar with the general rules and purposes of mandated reporting.
2. To become familiar with the special duties and obligations of mandated reporters.
3. To become familiar with the expected procedures during a mandated report and the events that might follow.

Over the past 200 years views on the role of children in our society have changed dramatically. Gone are the days when children toiled in factories 16 hours a day. As our views about children have changed our laws have evolved. The first dramatic shift toward protecting children was the passage of child labor laws. Beginning in the 1960s states began passing mandated reporter laws. By 1967 all 50 states had some version of a mandated reporter statute. These early laws were passed in large part due to the efforts of the media and special interest groups.

In 1974 Congress enacted the Child Abuse Prevention and Treatment Act (**CAPTA**). Since then CAPTA has been amended and reauthorized on multiple occasions. CAPTA broadly expanded the protection of children. CAPTA has no federal mandatory reporting provision but requires states to pass their own mandatory reporting provisions in order to receive federal grants. The grants allow states to obtain funds to investigate and prosecute child abuse. There are also grants available for treatment and prevention programs. Many of the grants are available to nonprofit agencies as well as Indian Tribes (Child Welfare Information Gateway, 2011).

Around 1990 the federal government passed a mandated reporter law that covered federal land such as military bases and national parks as well as federal buildings.

Mandated reporter statutes vary greatly from state to state. Some states have a short list of people who are required to report, while other states have a very long list of people who are required to report. Some states have broadened the laws to cover all adults who have reasonable cause to suspect abuse or neglect. In the early days of mandated reporter laws the initial trend was toward requiring every adult to report suspected abuse or neglect. In the late 1970s more than half of the states had universal reporting requirements. Since then many states have backed away from universal reporting requirements and adopted lists of people who are required to report suspected abuse or neglect.

The purpose of this chapter is to explain the more common elements of mandated reporter laws including who is covered by those laws, what the laws require, and what happens after a report is made. At their core, all mandated reporter laws have the same goal—to protect children.

BASIC LEGAL PRINCIPLES

This chapter talks about a lot of different laws. In order to understand those laws and how they affect mandated reporters you need to know some basics about the legal system.

In this chapter the term **jurisdiction** is used frequently. The term can have different meanings depending on how it is used. For example, before judges can hear a case, they must determine whether they have jurisdiction over a case. In this sense, jurisdiction means the legal authority to hear whatever the case is about and jurisdiction over the people involved. Issues involving jurisdiction can become extremely complicated. A simplified way to summarize jurisdiction would be to say state courts can only hear cases that involve state laws. Federal courts can only hear cases that involve federal laws. There are many, many exceptions to this general principle. Jurisdiction can also be used to refer to places. Each state in the United States is its own jurisdiction. Guam, the U.S. Virgin Islands, and Puerto Rico are all their own jurisdictions. Many states are organized by county. Each county is also a jurisdiction.

There are two main ways laws come to exist. Some laws are *statutes* or black letter law. Other law is called *case law*. **Statutary laws** are voted on and passed by the legislature or some other elected body. **Case law** refers to how judges interpret statutes. Case law evolves over time as laws and facts change. One judge interprets a law under one set of facts. A later judge has to interpret the same law while faced with a different set of facts and the later judge is required to rule in a manner that is not inconsistent with the first judge's ruling. Statutes and case law are treated equally—the only difference is how they come to exist.

This chapter is devoted to a discussion of mandated reports and the legal standard to trigger a mandated report. The term *legal standard* means that point at which the law requires action. The most common legal standard requiring a mandated reporter to report suspected child abuse or molestation is when the mandated reporter has **reasonable**

cause to believe a child is being abused or molested. This is a low standard. Think about it in comparison to burdens of proof in court. In a criminal case a prosecutor must prove that the accused is guilty "beyond a reasonable doubt." Reasonable doubt is frequently defined as when a juror has an abiding conviction in the truth of the charges. Compare that to "more likely than not," which is the burden of proof when money is at issue. "More likely than not" has been described as 50% plus a feather or 50% plus a peppercorn. "Reasonable cause to believe" is lower than "beyond a reasonable doubt" and it is lower than "more likely than not."

There are lots of different ways to define "reasonable cause to believe." A common definition is that state of affairs when a reasonably prudent person would believe a certain event may have occurred. For example, you see your dog walk into the house. The dog's paws are muddy and wet. It is January. It is reasonable to believe that it was raining outside. There are other possible answers that are equally reasonable. Maybe someone left a hose turned on and the dog walked through the water. Maybe the dog stepped into his water bowl before walking into the house. In order for there to be reasonable cause to believe an event has occurred you do not have to eliminate all other reasonable explanations.

The law recognizes something called **legal privileges**. Legal privileges protect certain communications. Legal privileges exist to encourage people to freely communicate with members of certain professions and inside of certain relationships. For example, we want people to be able to honestly and openly communicate with their doctors, otherwise doctors cannot provide accurate medical advice. In order to make people feel more comfortable disclosing private, personal details the law prohibits doctors from divulging the information they learn from their patients for nonmedical purposes. Similarly for hundreds of years courts have recognized that the things people tell their priest, rabbi, or other spiritual leader in confidence are private. Members of the clergy are legally prohibited from disclosing confidential communications in many circumstances. People who are married have a privilege not to disclose marital communications. There is also the privilege against self-incrimination contained in the **Fifth Amendment** to the U.S. Constitution. This privilege means that a person who is accused of a crime cannot be forced to talk about the crime for which they are accused. Another way of saying this is a person cannot be forced to be a witness against themselves.

Consider This

Why is it important to remove the "option" of reporting child abuse from certain types of professional people? What might happen (did happen) when these reports were left to the discretion of each professional?

WHO IS A MANDATED REPORTER?

People commonly defined as mandated reporters include doctors, nurses, dentists, psychologists, psychiatrists, social workers, day care workers, members of the clergy, teachers and school employees, members of law enforcement, or any other person with the responsibility to care for a child. Many of the people on this list are in contact with children on a daily basis, while others have much less frequent contact with children. States vary in how they define who is a member of law enforcement. The definition of law enforcement always includes police or sheriff and frequently also includes parole and probation officers.

Some states include people in other occupations who may not necessarily come to mind when you think of who would be a mandated reporter. For example, Alaska and Illinois both include people who process or produce visual or printed materials (Alaska Stat. §§47.17.020; 47.17.023 and Illinois Comp. Stat. Ch. 325, §5/4; Ch. 720, §5/11–20.2). While people who print photos or work on movies may not immediately come to mind as people who should be mandated reporters, their inclusion on the list makes a lot of sense as people working in such occupations are in a very good position to come across images of child pornography or other exploitation of children.

American Samoa, Arizona, Arkansas, Colorado, Guam, Louisiana, Massachusetts, Missouri, Nevada, New Hampshire, New York, Pennsylvania, South Carolina, and West Virginia all have statutes that specifically include Christian Scientists as mandated reporters. Some Christian Scientists do not believe in modern medical care and will not allow their children to be treated by traditional health care practitioners such as doctors and nurses. These mandated reporter statutes may be at odds with the freedom of religion clause in the First Amendment of the U.S. Constitution. Whether the First Amendment is violated by these mandated reporter statutes does not appear to have been addressed by the courts.

Whether it is constitutionally sound to single out the members of a certain religion, many of the jurisdictions that did so likely acted in response to a number of high profile cases that occurred some years ago. According to the *New York Times* between 1980 and 1990 seven parents who practiced Christian Science in the United States were prosecuted on charges of neglect—some of those charges alleged that the neglect caused the death of a child ("Christian Scientists Found Liable in Death," 1993). Around the same time several families won large monetary judgments against certain members of the Christian Science religion. In later civil suits the parents of the dead children alleged that their children died because their parents relied on the advice of the church and failed to seek medical attention for these children because of the teachings of Christian Scientists.

Montana, North Dakota, and Northern Mariana Islands all have mandated reporter statutes that specifically refer to religious healers (Montana Ann. Code §41-3-201, North Dakota Cent. Code §50-25.1-03, Northern Mariana Islands Commonwealth Code Tit. 6, §5313). Tennessee has a broad statute concerning religious healers—the Tennessee statute defines a mandated reporter as any practitioner who relies solely on spiritual means for healing (Tennessee Ann. Code §§37-1-403; 37-1-605). All of these statutes have the same intent as the statutes that focus on members of certain religions.

Other states have included on their lists of mandated reporters members of certain occupations not because the primary function of their job is not to care for or observe children, but because their jobs come into frequent contact with children. For example, Illinois includes animal control officers, people who work for the Department of Agriculture Bureau, school board members, and the Chicago Board of Education (Illinois Comp. Stat. Ch. 325, §5/4; Ch. 720, §5/11–20.2). Animal control officers and people who work for the Department of Agriculture have frequent contact with adults and children in their homes or on their farms. These people are in an ideal position to observe possible abuse or neglect because of the nature of the contact they have with the public.

Society continues to grapple with whether there should be universal mandated reporter requirements. At the time of writing this book only New Jersey and Wisconsin had universal mandated reporting requirements. There are good arguments both for and against universal reporting requirements. One argument in favor of requiring all adults to report suspected abuse or neglect is that all members of society should be responsible for protecting children. Some form of this argument was what many states relied on in passing universal reporting requirements. An argument against universal mandated reporting is the idea that people will not report because they assume someone else has or will report the suspicious conduct.

Research in the area shows that child abuse and neglect is underreported. One of the results of CAPTA, the 1974 federal law, was the creation of the Office on Child Abuse and Neglect and the National Clearinghouse on Child Abuse and Neglect Information. These organizations, along with many others, maintain information on the rates of reporting of child abuse. The reporting rates of abuse or neglect do not appear to be affected by whether a state has a universal reporting requirement.

A study reported in *American Pediatrics* concluded that primary care providers underreport by at least 20% in cases of suspected physical child abuse (Sege et al., 2011). Another study found that 65% of social workers, 53% of doctors, and 58% of physicians assistants were not reporting all cases of suspected abuse (Delaronde, King, Bendel, & Reece, 2000).

In recent times changes to mandated reporter laws have occurred in response to events in the media. For example, in response to the sexual abuse allegations made against some Catholic priests, some states amended their laws to include members of the clergy among those who are mandated reporters. Other high-profile child sex abuse scandals have prompted states to rethink their laws and attempt to modify the mandated reporting statutes accordingly.

The portion of mandated reporting laws that define which members of our society are legally required to report suspected abuse or neglect are a work in progress. As society's norms change our laws change as well. The definition of who is and who should be a mandated reporter is evolving and will continue to evolve. Most states have a child abuse prevention agency. If you are unsure if you are a mandated reporter under the laws of your state you can contact state agencies for more information. People who are not mandated reporters can still report suspected child abuse or neglect. Most states have some form of confidential reporting allowing private citizens to make reports to child protective services while protecting their identity.

Consider This

Why are some people mandated reporters, but not all people? What might happen if all people were mandated reporters? What burden might this place on people untrained or unable to understand when abuse has occurred?

WHAT TRIGGERS A REPORT?

The specific language for what conduct a mandated reporter is required to report varies from state to state. Generally speaking a mandated reporter is required to report when that person knows or has reasonable cause to suspect a child has been abused or neglected or is subject to conditions that would likely result in abuse or neglect.

When a mandated reporter has actual knowledge that a child is being abused or neglected a mandated reporter's actions are simple and clear-cut. The mandated reporter does not need to make any decisions—you have to report the suspected abuse or neglect. In real life it is uncommon for a mandated reporter to know for certain that a child is the victim of abuse or neglect. It is far more common for a mandated reporter to suspect abuse or neglect. Many mandated reporters find themselves trying to determine whether they have reasonable cause to suspect a child is in physical or emotional danger.

What constitutes reasonable cause can be difficult to define not only from a legal perspective but also from the perspective of someone who is a mandated reporter. It is hard to know exactly when to report suspected child abuse. The issue is further complicated when trying to determine what exactly is child abuse.

A general definition of child abuse would include physical abuse, sexual abuse, neglect, and willful cruelty. *Willful cruelty* is a term used by some states to describe emotional abuse. If a child's emotional well-being is being harmed because of emotional abuse by a parent or other caregiver, that abuse is sufficient to trigger a report. Willful cruelty is a lot like being intentionally and recklessly mean to a child. A thoughtless comment by a tired parent is not willful cruelty. Willful cruelty is often a pattern of demoralizing or demeaning behavior directed at a child over a period of time. If you know or have reasonable cause to suspect a child is the victim of willful cruelty you have to make a report.

Determining whether a report of physical abuse or neglect is required is often more simple than determining whether a report of sexual misconduct is legally required. Any time you suspect a child is being physically abused or neglected, a report is mandated. There are obvious signs of abuse such as changes in demeanor and unexplained or illogical physical injuries. Children who are always hungry or dirty might be being subjected to neglect.

Suspected incest and molestation should always be reported regardless of the age of the child involved. Consensual sexual conduct poses a greater difficulty. No state allows young children to engage in consensual sexual conduct. Different states have different laws defining at what age mandated reporters are required to report suspected consensual conduct between minors. Many states define mandatory reporting requirements differently than the age of consent.

For example, in California a person has to be 18 years old to legally consent to engage in consensual sexual conduct. However, if there are two children both 13 or younger who engaged in consensual conduct, there is no indication the relationship exploits either child, and it appears the touching was not sexually motivated, a mandated report is probably not required (*In re Jerry M.*, 1997, citing *Planned Parenthood Affiliates v. Van de Kamp*, 1986). However, if the conduct is consensual but one child is 14 and the other 16, a mandated reporter is required to report. If a child is 14 or 15, their partner is under the age of 21, and there is no evidence of exploitation, the conduct is not reportable. If a child is 16 or 17 they can engage in consensual sexual conduct with any person their age or older and no report is required. If that were not complicated enough the law requires a report if anyone under the age of 18 is suspected of engaging in sodomy, oral copulation, or penetration by a foreign object regardless of whether they consented.

The California statutory scheme is extremely complicated. Many other states have equally complicated laws. It is also important to remember that laws change. Sometimes even dramatic changes in the laws are not widely reported in the news so mandated reporters may not know about a significant development for several months. It is also unlikely a mandated reporter will have sufficient details about a suspected abusive situation to make a determination as to whether a report is required. It is impossible to make a perfect decision when you have imperfect information. You have to make a decision based on what you reasonably suspect and as a mandated reporter, you have to be mindful of your duty to follow and enforce the law. This means in most instances it is better to err on the side of caution and make a report.

Determining when to report suspected abuse can be complicated. Some abused children report their abuse to a trusted adult, often a teacher or other authority figure. As a society we do not want to believe that people would intentionally harm a child. Many people have preconceived notions about how a child should act when they report abuse and when they believe a child would make the report. For example, years ago it was believed that any child who was being abused would report the abuse at the first possible opportunity. We now know that is not true. Some children do report sexual abuse immediately, other children do not report abuse for many years, and still others never make a report. Often, allegations of sexual abuse arise when parents are battling over who should get custody of the children in a nasty divorce. On rare occasions children make up fantastic reports of abuse or neglect as a cry for help. Your job as a mandated reporter is to make a report when you have a reasonable cause to suspect a child is being harmed. It is impossible to give a precise definition of when there is reasonable cause to believe a child is being abused. You have to rely on your good judgment.

Reasonable cause is a low standard to trigger a report. The standard is intentionally low to encourage reporting of suspected abuse and to assist mandated reporters. Mandated reporters do not have to have actual knowledge of abuse, and they do not have to see physical injuries or wait for a child to make a complaint. The system is intended for mandated reporters, those people who often have significant contact with children, to be able to act on their well-founded suspicions. Mandated reporters are not expected to act as investigators—they are not expected or required to try to figure out whether or not a crime has occurred. As we discuss later, there is no penalty for making a report that turns out to be unfounded. There are penalties for failing to make a report.

WHAT MANDATED REPORTERS ARE REQUIRED TO REPORT

Specifically, what is required in a report to law enforcement varies greatly from state to state. Most states have toll-free hotlines that mandated reporters can call. California, Colorado, Florida, Illinois, Indiana, Iowa, Louisiana, Maine, Massachusetts, Minnesota, Mississippi, Missouri, Nebraska, New Mexico, New York, North Carolina, Pennsylvania, and Vermont require mandatory reporters to provide their names and contact information when making a report. This information can be provided either during the initial report or as part of a written report (Child Welfare Information Gateway, 2012).

Most jurisdictions have statutes that protect the identity of the reporter from the alleged abuser. In addition, all states have laws that protect abuse and neglect records although almost all of these laws have exceptions. Normally the custodial parent can access these records, so long as the custodial parent is not the one accused of the abuse or neglect. Family law courts and juvenile dependency courts also frequently have ways to access these records. When the courts access these records it must be done for the protection and benefit of the child.

WHAT IS ABUSE AND NEGLECT?

Although Chapter 5 is devoted to definitions of abuse and neglect, child abuse can be broadly defined as the physical, emotional, or sexual abuse of a child. Literally anyone who has contact with children could commit child abuse. Child neglect is more specific. Only a person who has an obligation to care for a child can neglect that child. The laws of each state more specifically define who has the legal obligation to care for a child. Generally speaking parents or guardians of a child, other members of the child's household, those exercising supervision over a child for any part of a 24-hour day, or members of the child's household or the family.

There are countless ways a child could be neglected. These can include: failure to supervise a child; failure to provide basic provisions, such as food, shelter, and clothing; failure to provide medical care when the child is sick or injured; exposing a child to criminal activity or drugs; failing to protect a child from abuse from another person; and providing a child with drugs or alcohol. It is often difficult for mandated reporters to determine when to report neglect. The line between poor parenting and neglect is often blurry. There is no bright line rule to help you decide when you must make a report.

If you are faced with a situation where you are trying to decide if you should report a case of suspected neglect, there are several factors that can help you make a decision. Think about this: Most neglect is chronic and it gets worse over time. Houses that are so filthy that a child has nothing clean to sleep on, no clean clothes to wear, or no clean dishes to eat on, do not develop overnight.

If a child's living conditions are such that it affects their well-being, a report should be made. If you have regular contact with a child who is being neglected your awareness of the situation will likely develop over time. Children go to school dirty on occasion—either they leave the house dirty or they get dirty on the way to school. But when a child appears in the same dirty and disheveled state day in and day out you should have a legitimate concern about how well that child is being cared for. If you know a child has no clean clothes, that even when there is food in the house there are no clean dishes, there are animal droppings on the floor inside the home, the child has no shampoo or soap, or other facts that affect the child's well-being, a report should be made.

Other indicators of neglect can include if a young child is not being adequately supervised. Children who are left out to play near traffic, kids who regularly wear clothes that are inappropriate for the weather, or who are left alone all might be suffering from neglect. Normally evidence of neglect appears in multiple aspects of a child's life. It is not just that the child comes to school dirty, they are also hungry and not being properly supervised at home. In many neglectful scenarios, the parents do not mean to be harmful to their child. Sometimes the fact that a reporter believes that the parents are doing their best prevents them from reporting neglect. In order to fulfill their legal obligation, mandated reporters must remember the intent of the parent is irrelevant. There is a place for consideration of the parents' intent later on in the process when child protective services (CPS) and the juvenile office is working with the family.

Every state allows some form of **corporal punishment**. Mandated reporters have their own views about whether they believe in corporal punishment or would ever use it. Most statutes that allow for corporal punishment require that the corporal punishment be reasonable under the circumstances. Few statutes provide a clear definition of what "reasonable under the circumstances" means.

Some experts in the field have proposed a four-part test to evaluate "reasonable under the circumstances":

1. What is the age, size, and health of the child?
2. What is the reason the discipline was exercised?
3. What was the disciplinary act?
4. Was there any resulting injury from the discipline?

An example of the application of these four criteria is: A 13-year-old child was told by his parents to make sure he came home before curfew. He came home late. His parents took away all of his screen time. In response the 13-year-old snuck out of the house, stole the family car, and crashed it. His father spanks his bottom. The analysis would be: The child is old enough to understand the purpose of the discipline. He has no special health concerns and his parents are well within their rights to discipline a child exhibiting this behavior. The placement of the spanking is in an appropriate area for such discipline and there was no resulting injury.

Compare this to a 3-year-old who refused to clean up her room. Her parents made her stand outside for hours in the freezing cold with no jacket. This child is not old enough to understand the discipline. There is little point in disciplining a child so young over not cleaning her room because it is not clear a 3-year-old fully understands the concept of why her room should be clean. The child is young enough that she could be injured by being exposed to the cold while improperly dressed.

Every case a mandated reporter encounters is different. No book could ever possibly come up with every scenario a mandated reporter might face. In the end mandated reporters are going to have to rely on their own good judgment about whether they should report specific conduct.

Consider This

Why is it important for jurisdictions to have some formal way to determine the difference between acceptable corporal punishment and child abuse? What might happen if that standard did not exist?

PRIVILEGED OR CONFIDENTIAL INFORMATION

As mentioned earlier, legal privileges protect certain communications. You may have heard about the spousal privilege, the priest-penitent privilege, or the psychotherapist-patient privilege. Almost all states recognize two spousal privileges. One spousal privilege makes it unlawful to force one spouse to testify against another spouse. This privilege has many exceptions; the most noteworthy for our purposes is that in instances of abuse, including child abuse, this exception frequently does not apply. The other spousal privilege is also referred to as the *marital communication privilege*. This privilege makes it unlawful to force a spouse to disclose something said by the other spouse. In cases of suspected abuse and neglect most states will not allow this privilege to be invoked.

The priest-penitent privilege originally came about to protect communications that occur in confidence. While this privilege is widely affirmed, most jurisdictions are very strict about how they define the confidential communication (Child Welfare Information Gateway, 2012). For example, a Catholic person inside a confessional speaking to a priest would almost certainly qualify but if the same person had the same conversation with a priest at a café the privilege would not apply. New Hampshire, North Carolina, Oklahoma, Rhode Island, Texas, West Virginia, and Guam require mandated reporters to report suspected child abuse or neglect regardless of whether the information necessitating the report was gained because of a priest-penitent relationship.

Another common privilege is the attorney-client privilege. The attorney-client privilege is extremely broad and covers almost every conversation attorneys have with their client. This privilege is almost always upheld, even in cases of child abuse or neglect. The most commonly recognized exception to this privilege is when the clients clearly communicate to their lawyer that they are going to cause harm to another person in the future. Such a statement of future harm has to be clear and credible. In other words, a statement by clients to their lawyer that they are so frustrated with their teenage child who just crashed the family car that they are "going to kill that kid when they get home" on its own would probably be a protected communication and would not be reportable. The client would have to make additional statements that evidence an actual plan to engage in such conduct for privilege to be denied.

HOW DO MANDATED REPORTERS MAKE A REPORT?

All states have hotlines that mandated reporters can call to make a report. Additionally, many states allow mandated reporters to simply make a police report. Some jurisdictions require that a mandated reporter make the report to child protective services—a report made to local law enforcement does not comply with this law. Some states require certain kinds of reports be made directly to law enforcement. Remember the Alaska law requiring people who print photos or videos to be mandated reporters. The Alaska law Alaska Stat. §§ 47.17.020; 47.17.023 specifically requires that any person providing, either commercially or privately, film, photo, or other visual or printed materials who observes matter depicting a child engaged in sexually exploitive conduct to immediately report the observation to the nearest law enforcement agency rather than CPS.

Except in extreme situations where the mandated reporter is gravely concerned about the health and safety of a child, it is preferable to make a report to child protective services. Child protective services is generally in the best position to conduct a proper investigation of suspected abuse or neglect.

There is good reason to require all mandated reporters to report suspicion of abuse and neglect to one central location. In most states, the hotline is located in one place and the information is disseminated to local branches, or CPS offices, which investigate the reports. In any child abuse or neglect investigation, the background and history of CPS with the family or child is an important consideration. If a family has a history of involvement with CPS this information is crucial to investigators when a new report is received. For example, if a report comes in that a child has suspicious bruises and that family has never had contact with CPS before, that case might be handled differently than if the same report came in but there had been five reports made about the same child in the past 12 months. CPS maintains a history of each child and each family with which it has contact. The level and speed of intervention by CPS is often determined based on these histories.

Local law enforcement rarely has access to CPS histories. Most research supports the argument that when abuse and neglect occurs, the abuse and neglect are chronic. It is generally not an isolated situation but rather something that exists over a long period of time and tends to get worse. The histories maintained by CPS allow the child welfare system to review a new report in context, alongside other prior reports regarding the same child or the same family. Case workers are trained to review the files to look for escalation in abuse or neglect and to act accordingly.

In addition, requiring all mandated reporters to call the same centralized hotline means that if a family moves around any prior information about a family follows them—at least within the same state. In other words, if a family moves from Austin to Dallas it is important that prior reports of abuse and neglect regarding a child follows that family to its new home.

In many states, people who work for CPS receive special training on how to interview children. Children, particularly young children, can be influenced by improper interview or investigation techniques. Once a child's memory has been influenced by improper interview techniques it can be next to impossible to ever find out what really happened. This is also why it is important that mandated reporters who are not forensically trained interviewers make reports and not conduct investigations on their own. Many an investigation has been compromised because of well-intended but improper questions posed by people who wanted to help a child they suspected was being abused or neglected. Forensic interviewing of children is handled in more detail in Chapter 7.

Often, mandated reporters may be aware that CPS is already involved with a particular family. This does not relieve the mandated reporter from making a report of suspected abuse or neglect. Mandated reporters sometimes think they do not need to make a report because they are aware that CPS is already involved with a family.

CPS workers can have different levels of contact with different families. CPS workers may check in on some families twice a week, while other families may be checked in on as rarely as once a month or every other month. Mandated reporters may have far more contact with a particular child or may see the child in a different setting, which gives them a different, and sometimes better, perspective on whether abuse or neglect might be occurring.

For example, someone who cares for a toddler at a day care center sees a particular child every day. The caregiver changes the child's diapers and often the child's clothes. Therefore the caregiver is in a far better position to observe cuts, bruises, or other possible signs of abuse than a CPS worker who comes by a home once a week to see an older child in the family. In addition, the caregiver sees the child and likely the parents in a very different setting, which may allow them different insights.

Every mandated reporter statute requires reporters to report a new suspicion. None of the statutes have an exception that says no report is required if CPS is already involved with a family. In other words, if CPS is already involved with a family and a mandated reporter fails to report suspected abuse or neglect, the mandated reporter has broken the law.

Consider This

If you work at an agency that has a "designated reporter" who is tasked with making mandated reports, and the person does not make a report in a case you have referred—are you free from your responsibilities to make the call yourself? (Believe it or not, this is not always easy to answer, though many experts say you maintain the duty.)

COMMON REASONS MANDATED REPORTERS DO NOT REPORT

Years ago there was a case that involved two young parents. Both parents had developmental disabilities. The couple had a 3-year-old daughter and twin 8-month-old girls. Both parents loved their children but caring for three young children was more than they could manage on their own. A local agency was involved with the family trying to help them. The caseworker was a nice well-meaning young person who tried to be very supportive of the parents' efforts to care for the infants. The caseworker was concerned that reporting neglect would destroy the family unit as the twins would likely be taken away from their parents. The caseworker did not report that the babies were constantly filthy. The caseworker did not report that the babies were severely underweight. And the caseworker did not report diaper rash so severe that their skin was rotting and falling off. One hot summer's day the caseworker went to visit the home and the mother refused to let her in. The caseworker left and came back a couple hours later. The mother still would not let the caseworker in. The caseworker became very worried. A short time later the babies were found dead in an upstairs bedroom, having died from dehydration and exposure to high temperatures. Even several years later the caseworker was still devastated by the deaths of these two children. The caseworker thought that keeping the family together and keeping the twins with parents who loved wanted them was the right thing to do. Nothing could have been more wrong. Although this is an extreme example of what can happen when mandated reporters fail to report, it is an important reminder of why it is so important to make a report when there is evidence of neglect.

Mandated reporters have lots of reasons why they decide not to report. Next we examine some of the more common reasons. The law requires mandated reporters to make a report when they have a reasonable suspicion of abuse or neglect. There is a reason why there are no exceptions to the requirement that a report must be made. Stories like the one earlier make it clear that when a mandated reporter decides not to report, even when they think they have a good reason, the consequences can be tragic.

- Reporting will only make it worse for the child.
- Fear of retaliation.

- Reporting will destroy a relationship of trust between a child and the mandated reporter.
- The CPS system is broken.
- Reporting will destroy the family.
- What if I am wrong?

First and foremost it is a crime not to report. Later in this chapter we discuss what can happen to mandated reporters who fail to report. Making a report of suspected abuse or neglect is not passing judgment on other people, their ability to parent, or their lifestyle. Making a report of suspected abuse or neglect is fulfilling your legal obligation to report the facts and circumstances as you perceive them. By choosing a career that makes you a mandated reporter you have accepted the responsibility to protect children. Failing to report is not only a crime, it is also a failure to live up to that responsibility.

Reporting Will Only Make It Worse for the Child

The goal behind reporting suspected abuse or neglect is that things will improve both for the family and for the child. Most parents who are abusive or neglectful regret their actions. If you were to ask most of them they would tell you quite honestly they do not want to hurt their children—the problem is they do not know how to stop. Contact with CPS or other social services is often the best opportunity for many parents to learn how to be better parents.

Many people who abuse or neglect their children suffer from drug or alcohol addiction or have significant mental health problems. Other people who abuse or neglect their children simply do not know how to be good parents. Many of the people who need help either do not know that help exists or are too embarrassed to ask. Contact with CPS and the possibility of losing their children is often either the first opportunity or the necessary incentive people need to make positive changes in their lives.

Reporting abuse or neglect is far more likely to help a child than to harm them. Certainly being removed from an abusive parent and placed into a group home is traumatizing for any child but they are far better off than if they remained in a home where neglect or physical abuse could leave them with permanent injuries. The babies in the example at the beginning of this section would have been taken away from parents who truly did love them. The decision not to report the neglect they were suffering was far worse—it cost them their lives.

Fear of Retaliation

It is possible a family will consider retaliation against a reporter. Families who are reported to CPS do often seek to determine who reported them with an eye toward intimidating the reporter. Instances of intimidation of mandated reporters are far less common than those situations where the family believes it is a family member, co-worker, friend, or neighbor who called.

Most families who interact with CPS understand mandated reporters have a duty to report. Many statutory schemes prohibit the disclosure of the identity of the caller, without court order, to maintain the anonymity of the reporter. The entire purpose behind allowing reporters to remain anonymous is to allow mandated reporters to make reports without fear of retaliation.

If you made a report and the family confronts you with whether you reported them, there is no requirement you answer their questions or that you answer them truthfully. Each mandated reporter will have to decide how to handle these situations. You have the right to insist on the confidentiality of your identity and deny the accusation, even if you were the one who called. Alternatively, you can explain you are a mandated reporter and the law requires you to report suspicions of abuse or neglect. You have no choice in the matter.

If the behavior of the family is threatening, harassing, or intimidating, it is critical to report the behavior to CPS and report it to the police. The courts can and will issue a restraining order to protect you if necessary. The local district attorney's office can prosecute family members for harassment or threats. Fortunately actual instances of threats or harassment are very rare.

Reporting Will Destroy a Relationship of Trust Between a Child and the Mandated Reporter

Some mandated reporters worry that reporting suspicions of abuse or neglect that involve a child with whom they have an ongoing relationship will destroy the trust between them. Some children make disclosures of abuse or neglect only after they have made the mandated reporter promise to keep a secret. If you find yourself in this situation you have to remember that we as a society treat children differently than adults for a reason. Society has decided children cannot drink alcohol, become soldiers, serve on juries, vote, or even see certain movies. Society has decided children are vulnerable and require our protection—that is why we have mandated reporters. There is a significant body of scientific research that supports the notion that people are not fully developed until late in adolescence. As the adult in the situation, as well as being the mandated reporter, you are the one society expects to make the right decision. Yes, the child may think you violated their trust. But in reality you are acting both in accordance with the law and in accordance with the trust society has placed in you in your capacity as a mandated reporter. You are doing it to help a child—a person who is not yet mature enough to decide what is best for them.

In many situations the child may never know who made the report. Most mandated reporters are allowed to maintain their anonymity. CPS or other social service workers generally do not disclose the specifics of the report they received. When they first contact a family they are generally vague about the reasons why they are there. If a child asks you if you made the report you are free to respond to that question however you like. Just as there is no requirement for you to tell a family, there is no requirement for you to disclose you were the reporter to a child.

Depending on the age of the child and your relationship with them, you can decide to explain to the child that you are legally required to report your suspicions. You can tell them this prior to or after making the report. Some children are likely to understand you are legally required to make the report. Other children may never understand. Regardless of how children or their family perceives your conduct, your legal obligation is the same.

Consider This

Imagine that you believe your good friend has lost her temper and seriously (but not fatally) abused her child, a child in your school. Think about the duties you would have, the requirements you face, but also the ramifications you may need to endure. Mandated reporters need to consider such personal costs before they enter a field with mandated reporting requirements.

WHEN AM I SUPPOSED TO MAKE A REPORT?

Almost every, if not all, mandated reporter statutes require the report to be made *immediately*. The only exception to this requirement is if doing so would put the mandated reporter in danger.

Although there are a litany of "reasons" mandated reporters might want to wait to make their report, none of those "reasons" are exceptions to the requirement that the report be made immediately; for example, if a mandated reporter is uncertain and wants to go over the situation with a supervisor who has not been available all day, or the mandated reporter is not familiar with the rules and protocols to know when a report is supposed to be made. Sometimes a mandated reporter thinks someone else involved was going to make the call. Other times, there are protocols in place that require taking this information to a supervisor or designated agent and that person is unavailable. The purpose of making the call is to allow CPS to investigate the suspicion. In order for an investigation to be effective it needs to begin as soon as the suspicion of abuse or molestation exists. Again, almost every, if not all, mandated reporter statute requires the report to be made *immediately*.

WHAT INFORMATION DO I PROVIDE TO THE HOTLINE CALL TAKER?

Most agencies have forms delineating what information should be provided in a hotline call. The form outlines the information the call taker will try to learn from the person making the call. Most mandatory reporter statutes provide lists of information the call taker will want. You must call in suspicion of abuse or neglect even if you cannot answer all the questions on the list. The more specific information you can provide, the better start the children's division or child protective services has on the investigation of your suspicion.

Below is a list of what information a call taker will commonly ask for:

- The names and addresses of the child and his parents or other persons responsible for his care, if known.
- The child's age, sex, and race.
- The nature and extent of the child's injuries, abuse, or neglect, including any evidence of previous injuries, abuse, or neglect to the child or his siblings.
- The name, age, and address of the person responsible for the injuries, abuse or neglect, if known.
- Family composition.
- The source of the report.
- The name and address of the person making the report, the reporter's occupation, and where the reporter can be reached.
- Any actions taken by the reporting source (such as photographs or X-rays).

There are specific reasons why a call taker seeks certain information during the call. First, most child welfare statutes require the CPS worker who goes out to check on a family to check on *all* the children in the family. Certainly it is possible a situation exists in a family or household that only affects one child, but often there are issues and circumstances affecting all the children. The first call is an opportunity to investigate the well-being of all of the children in a home.

Second, the call taker wants the child's age, sex, and race, if known. Age is extremely important for a call taker to know. In most cases it is probably perfectly acceptable for a 15-year-old to be left home alone for a few hours. However, it is never acceptable to leave a 15-month-old baby home alone for any length of time. One situation would not require a CPS investigation whereas the other situation would certainly require an investigation. The other reason to provide basic identifying information is to make it easier for a call taker to find the child, or family, in the computer system, assuming the family has had prior involvement with the children's division or child protective services. Lastly, if this is a family that is not known to the authorities, the identifying information may help locate the child and the family to make contact.

The third factor to provide to the call taker is the "nature and extent of the child's injuries, abuse or neglect, including any evidence of previous injuries, abuse or neglect to the child or his siblings." This information is important for several reasons. First, it aids CPS and law enforcement in determining the appropriate response. If you called in and said you saw a child being severely beaten by a parent, CPS and law enforcement would want to respond immediately. On the other hand, if an 8-year-old child told you that a few months ago her parents left her and her teenage brother home alone for 3 days, CPS may not act on this report instantly because the child is not currently in grave danger.

It may be the case that you are mandated to make multiple reports regarding the same child or the same family. If that is the case it is very helpful if you can inform the call taker that you have made reports about the family or the child previously.

The fourth piece of information on the list is "the name, age, and address of the person responsible for the injuries, abuse or neglect, if known." If you know or have reason to suspect you know the identity of the person who abused or neglected a child, you need to provide that information. If the identity of the perpetrator is known this can provide a lot of useful information to CPS and law enforcement. If the perpetrator has a criminal history of abuse this may indicate to CPS and law enforcement that they need to move more quickly in their investigation. Or say that the hotline received a call that children were being neglected. When the call taker looked up the criminal history of the parents they discovered that one of the parents had multiple drug- and alcohol-related arrests. A neglect call regarding the children of a person who is addicted to drugs or alcohol might suggest that the parent's drug addiction was interfering with their ability to parent.

Do not guess and do not investigate. Only provide this information if you have a basis for the information. If children told you they were hit by their parent you have a basis for the information. On the other hand, if you see a severe burn on the hand of a 4-year-old and the child does not want to talk about the burn, do not try to ask more questions. Report the injury, report how you discovered it, and report that the child is reluctant to discuss the details. Hotline call takers and child protective service workers are all trained in the proper next steps. Remember, you have to report suspected abuse and neglect even if you have absolutely no idea who caused the abuse or neglect.

Fifth, a common area hotline takers are likely to ask about is "family composition." In other words, who lives in the household with the child. This is important for several reasons. Remember, most abuse or neglect affects all of the children in a home, not just one. If there are five children living in a home and you are reporting neglect, the call taker needs to know that potentially five children are at risk. This information also informs a follow up CPS worker on the best approach to take with the family. For example, a mandated reporter suspects a child is not getting enough food at home and makes a report of suspected neglect. The mandated reporter is also able to tell the call taker that the family has recently immigrated to the United States, the entire extended family is living together in a small apartment, and they are very poor. This is a very different situation than a neglect call where a child is not being supervised because one parent is a known drug dealer and is out on the streets all night selling drugs. In both instances the mandated reporter has to make the report but knowing the family composition is going to provide a lot of information to CPS about the best way to help and protect the child.

Sixth on the list is the source of the report. Imagine the following set of facts taken from a real case (the names and identifying details have been changed). A 14-year-old girl, Jamie, was talking to her friend, Sarah, who was the same age. Jamie told Sarah that their mutual friend Kennedy's dad had molested Jamie. Sarah said Kennedy's dad molested her also. Jamie and Sarah know that Kennedy often hung out with a girl named Shirley. Jamie and Sarah called Shirley and asked if Kennedy's dad had molested her. Shirley said no. Jamie and Sarah told Shirley that Kennedy's dad had molested them. Shirley worried about her friends. Shirley told her mom. Shirley's mom was a teacher and a mandated reporter. The mom did the right thing and did not ask Jamie and Sarah any questions, she just called the hotline and reported. This situation is very different from a situation in which a child discloses abuse directly to an adult who was a mandated reporter. The situation where multiple people have been talking about a situation generally raises red flags for child protective services workers. At a minimum, it tells them they are going to have to conduct their investigation much more carefully to make sure they are getting each individuals' recollection of events. In other words, when a CPS worker contacts Jamie and investigates the claim, the CPS worker is going to ask Jamie about what happened to her and what Jamie knows separate and apart from what Jamie may have learned from her conversations with Sarah. If there were ultimately a criminal prosecution, the success of that prosecution could hinge on how well CPS managed to disentangle each witness' independent recollections.

When a child makes a disclosure of abuse or neglect directly to a mandated reporter CPS the caseworkers do not have to focus their investigation on parsing out the potential influence of other witnesses.

Seventh on the list: the contact information for the person making the report. Not every state requires a mandated reporter to provide this information. It is up to you to know the laws of your state. Regardless of whether you are legally required to give this information, the call taker at the hotline may ask you for this information because you are an important resource for follow-up on the report. If CPS or law enforcement has questions in the course of their investigation it is very helpful for them to be able to go back and contact the person who made the report.

The eighth on the list: any actions taken by the reporting source (such as photographs or X-rays). Almost all mandated reporter statutes include people who work in the medical field as mandated reporters. They may have X-rays of a child that show a broken arm for which the child was brought into the emergency room. But the X-rays may also show previous traumas that the parent and/or the child deny but that appear suspicious. Other states require people who process film to report suspected abuse or neglect. These people may come across images of child pornography or pictures of a child who appears underfed and ill-cared for.

WHAT HAPPENS AFTER A REPORT IS MADE?

Regardless of the nature of the report, some kind of an investigation is conducted into the report. Exactly what kind of investigation and how quickly that investigation occurs depends on the nature of the report.

Earlier in this chapter was an example of a child not getting enough food at home and a mandated reporter made a report of suspected neglect. The child and his family have recently immigrated to the United States, the entire extended family is living together in a small apartment, and they are very poor. This is not the kind of case where law enforcement needs to respond immediately with lights and sirens blaring. This is the kind of situation where within a few days of the report someone from child protective services will go to the apartment, ensure that other children living in the residence are okay, and start working with the family to address the fact that perhaps all of the children are hungry.

Another example earlier in this chapter was about a mom of twin babies who refused to open a door to a social services worker. When that social services worker returned to the home and was refused admission she became gravely concerned and immediately called her supervisor as well as law enforcement. Within a few short minutes local law enforcement was at the front door of the apartment and paramedics and fire fighters were en route.

Child protective service workers are generally well versed on the appropriate reaction to a report of suspected abuse or neglect. CPS workers have the discretion to decide how to handle a report based on the nature of the report and the seriousness of the situation. This is why it is so important to provide as much detailed information as possible when making a report.

In one form or another, the court system often becomes involved in reports of suspected abuse or neglect. In most places courts are split into lots of different divisions. The courts most likely to address issues of abuse and/or neglect are juvenile dependency or criminal courts. The different kinds of courts and their functions are discussed in detail in Chapter 11. Basically juvenile dependency courts exist to help children. Criminal courts punish people who have either criminally neglected a child or abused a child.

What Happens If I Do Not Report Suspected Abuse or Neglect?

Most states make failing to report abuse or neglect a crime, generally a misdemeanor. Misdemeanors are generally punishable by no more than one year in county jail and a fine. In addition to potentially going to jail, a criminal conviction for failing to report suspected abuse or neglect will almost certainly cause mandated reporters to lose their job. This makes sense. Mandated reporters are required to report because by nature of their occupation they have assumed a special position of trust. They fulfill an important social role to protect children. Failing to fulfill this important social role means that mandated reporters did not do their job and, more importantly, are not worthy of the trust society has placed in the reporters.

If mandated reporters are also professional license holders, such as a doctor, dentist, or, in most states, a teacher they may lose the license that they spent years going to school to obtain. For professional license holders the conviction of a crime, particularly one related to their license, generally means they will be reviewed by their state licensing board. Think about a teacher who was convicted of failing to report abuse and was convicted of a misdemeanor. In most states that teacher's license would be reviewed by state teacher's licensing board. It is unlikely that teachers, people who spend every day with children, who were convicted of failing to report suspected abuse would be allowed to keep their license and potentially endanger additional children in the future.

Failure to report can also result in the imposition of civil fines. The amount of the fines vary greatly from state to state. They can be as small as a few thousand dollars to many thousands of dollars.

Perhaps the worst thing that can happen to you if you do not report is the consequences of your decision not to report. Think about the case of the twins. The caseworker who did not report the neglect thought that not reporting was the right thing to keep a family together. That caseworker now has to spend a lifetime knowing that one phone call, even one day earlier, might have saved the two children. Living with that knowledge is far worse than having to spend time in jail or losing your job.

CONCLUSION

Most people reading this book are likely pursuing a career path that will make them a mandated reporter. A lot of these career paths allow you to have a lot of contact with children—in fact that may be the main reason you are interested in this kind of career.

Working with children brings great joy but it also brings with it great responsibility. Children cannot protect themselves, and most children cannot advocate for themselves. It is your responsibility to know the mandated reporter laws in the state in which you live and work. It is your responsibility to follow the law, not just because your career and potentially your liberty depend on it, but society is depending on you and children are depending on you.

STUDY QUESTIONS

1. What is the difference between statutory law and case law?
2. What is the "reasonable cause" standard of evidence and how does it apply to reporting of child abuse?
3. What is a legal communication "privilege" and what types of people generally have such a privilege?
4. What is mandated reporting and what types of people may be determined to be mandated reporters?
5. Describe the kinds of events that might "trigger" a need for mandatory reporting.
6. Describe what types of things might be required in a mandated report of child abuse.
7. Discuss the occasional difficulty in distinguishing legally acceptable corporal punishment from physical abuse, including the "four-part test."
8. Describe a common way mandated reporters might make a report to authorities.
9. What are some reasons that a mandated reporter might decide to not make a report?
10. What information must be provided to a hotline during a mandated report?
11. What might be expected to happen after a report is made?

GLOSSARY

CAPTA (Child Abuse Prevention and Treatment Act) Passed in 1974, CAPTA has no federal mandatory reporting provision but requires states to pass their own mandatory reporting provisions in order to receive federal grants to obtain funds to investigate and prosecute child abuse.

case law Law based on how previous court decisions have established the interpretation of law, or precedent.

corporal punishment Physical punishment that includes aversive actions against the body of a child (e.g., spanking). Many states distinguish between allowable corporal punishment and abuse.

Fifth Amendment privilege People cannot be compelled to provide evidence that would tend to incriminate them.

legal privilege A concept that eliminates reporting needs of specific professional parties. It is designed to allow people to freely communicate with their lawyer, clergy, doctor, or therapist. Members of these professions may be prohibited from disclosing communication unless danger to self or others is clear and imminent.

mandated reporter People who are legally required to report possibilities of child abuse, including doctors, nurses, dentists, psychologists, psychiatrists, social workers, day care workers, members of the clergy, teachers and school employees, members of law enforcement, or any other person with the responsibility to care for a child. Alaska and Illinois both include people who process or produce visual or printed materials.

reasonable cause to believe An intentionally low standard of evidence that triggers a mandatory reporting of possible child abuse by specific people. For example, "when a reasonably prudent person would believe a certain event may have occurred."

statutory law Law voted on and passed by the legislative branch of the government (i.e., federal, state, or local).

REFERENCES

Child Welfare Information Gateway. (2011). *About CAPTA: A legislative history*. Washington, DC: U.S. Department of Health and Human Services, Children's Bureau.

Child Welfare Information Gateway. (2012). *Mandatory reporters of child abuse and neglect*. Washington, DC: U.S. Department of Health and Human Services, Children's Bureau.

Christian Scientists found liable in death. (1993, August 19). *New York Times*.

Delaronde, S., King, G., Bendel, R., & Reece, R. (2000). Opinions among mandated reporters toward child maltreatment reporting policies. *Child Abuse & Neglect, 24*(7), 901–910.

In re Jerry M., 59 Cal. App. 4th 289 (1997).

Planned Parenthood Affiliates v. Van de Kamp, 181 Cal. App. 3rd 245, 260–261 (1986).

Sege, R., Flaherty, E., Jones, R., Price, L. L., Harris, D., Slora, E., … Child Abuse Recognition and Experience Study (CARES) Study Team. (2011). To report or not to report: Examination of the initial primary care management of suspicious childhood injuries. *Academy of Pediatrics, 11*(6), 460–466.

13

Juveniles and the Justice System

GOALS OF THIS CHAPTER:

1. To provide a basic understanding of juvenile delinquency and dependency courts.
2. To understand the different terminology often used in juvenile court systems.
3. To understand the important difference in consequences between the adult and juvenile court systems.

OVERVIEW

The juvenile justice system is divided into two separate branches: delinquency and dependency. **Juvenile delinquency courts** deal with minors who have committed crimes and in many regards is the same as a criminal adult court. The aim of the juvenile delinquency court is very different from that of the adult criminal court. Most adult criminal courts have two goals in sentencing offenders: just punishment and rehabilitation. On the other hand, **juvenile dependency courts** generally have only one goal: rehabilitation. Juvenile delinquency courts exist for the sole purpose of trying to ensure that juvenile offenders do not become adult offenders.

Juvenile dependency courts assist minors when their parents, for one reason or another, cannot adequately care for their children. There are many, many ways in which minors might find themselves involved in dependency proceedings.

When juvenile courts first came into being in the late 1880s there was only one juvenile court. It was not until the reform movements of the 1960s that the juvenile court system split into the two branches that exist in some form in all states today.

The purpose of this chapter is to give you a basic understanding of both systems, explain how they work, and allow you to familiarize yourself with some of the common terminology. Lawyers are frequently surprised how confusing and overwhelming many people find the legal system. As confusing as the legal system is to adults, it is even more confusing and often scary to children. Perhaps the most important reason you need to understand the basic workings of the delinquency and dependency systems is so you can explain to the children you work with that the legal system is there to protect them and help them.

In most if not every state, it is illegal for nonlawyers to give out legal advice. That means that when you are talking with the children and potentially the families involved in this system you have to be careful to make sure you are explaining the system to people—not giving them advice on what they should do. If people ask you for legal advice you can and should tell them that it is against the law for you to give out legal advice. Most court systems have self-help centers—places for nonlawyers to get help with legal questions. It is perfectly acceptable for you as a nonlawyer to refer people to self-help centers. Self-help centers frequently offer assistance in multiple languages both via interpreters and documents published in different languages.

JUVENILE DELINQUENCY

As with all other areas of the law, the laws pertaining to juveniles are constantly evolving and changing as society changes. Not all crimes committed by juveniles are prosecuted in juvenile delinquency courts. Almost every state has a system in place that allows prosecutors to decide whether a child should be prosecuted as an adult or as a juvenile. Many states have a list of crimes, which, if committed by a person under the age of 18, can be prosecuted in adult court. Generally these lists consist of very serious crimes such as murder, rape, mayhem, or crimes involving the use of dangerous weapons such as guns. Prosecutors have wide discretion in deciding if they think a case should be prosecuted in adult court in or juvenile court.

When children are prosecuted in the adult system they face the same punishment adults face with some narrow exceptions. In *Romer v. Simmons* (2005), the U.S. Supreme Court held juveniles cannot be sentenced to the death penalty regardless of the crime for which they were convicted. This ruling settled what had been an ongoing debate in the law.

Since the mid-1980s laws prevented the imposition of the death penalty on anyone under the age of 16. In the *Romer* case, the U.S. Supreme Court spent a lot of time discussing why young people are frequently not as morally culpable for crimes they commit. The Supreme Court relied on evidence that young people's brains are not fully developed and in particular things like decision making and impulse control are among the last phases of development between being a child and being an adult. The U.S. Supreme Court's decision in 2005 is important not only because it settled an issue that had been the subject of debate for many years, but also because it provided clear guidance for lower courts about how they are supposed to treat juvenile offenders, and why children are to be treated differently by the legal system.

Premise Behind the Juvenile Justice System

Traditionally the juvenile delinquency system was based on a rehabilitative model—the goal was to reform youthful offenders. In the 1950s and 1960s people began to wonder if the traditional rehabilitative model was really able to prevent youths from committing crimes. The 1970s and 1980s saw a response to these concerns when a number of states passed laws that allowed for juveniles to be treated more like adults in criminal courts, allowed for longer sentences, and carried far more severe consequences. Juvenile offenders were not deemed to be as responsible as adults for their crimes but they were no longer viewed as innocent children (Scott & Grisso, 1997). Although many states favored this "tough on crime" stance it became increasingly clear that juvenile laws focused on punishment and not rehabilitation, treated minors too much like adults, and brought about a number of problems as well as failing to account for basic science.

Many laws passed during the 1970s and 1980s that increased penalties for juvenile offenders have come under increasing attack. People worry that sentences are too severe and children are being punished too harshly. Many states are trying to seek a balance between the original rehabilitative model of juvenile justice with a model that also provides punishment for criminal behavior.

Somewhere in states' statutory schemes they have language describing the purpose of their juvenile delinquency courts. Approximately 20 state statutes contain language that indicates that among the purposes of the juvenile delinquency system is rehabilitation. At least six states, Connecticut, Hawaii, North Carolina, Texas, Utah, and Wyoming, have juvenile delinquency systems that are more similar to adult criminal justice systems in that they stress community protection, offender accountability, crime reduction through deterrence, or outright punishment, either predominantly or exclusively. The majority of the remaining states have blended the goals of rehabilitation and punishment.

It is important for you to understand the purpose of the juvenile delinquency system in the state in which you live and work for a few reasons. First, if you are working in the court system as a probation officer or social worker you need to understand what the juvenile delinquency system is trying to teach the children you work with in order to effectively reinforce the justice system's message. Second, you need to be able to explain the purpose to the children and families with whom you are working. When they ask why a child is being ordered to do volunteer work you need to be able to answer that question. The only way you can correctly and effectively answer that question is if you understand the model on which your state operates.

Regardless of the state in which you work and which model that state operates on, the children and the families you work with need to understand that crimes committed by juveniles can have very severe consequences. Children were, and still are, being sentenced to lengthy prison terms, even in states that largely subscribe to a restorative or rehabilitative model of juvenile justice.

Consider the following scenario taken from the facts of a real case that occurred in one of the 20 states that focuses on a rehabilitative model of juvenile justice. Michelle, a 15-year-old girl, had been talking and flirting with an older boy named Jason who was 19. Michelle was from a good home, she did well in school, and had never been in trouble with the law. Michelle learned that Jason had marijuana in his car. She told her 17-year-old friend, Ashley. Michelle asked Ashley to ask Ashley's cousin, Oliver, to rob Jason and take his marijuana. Oliver was 20 years old, had a lengthy criminal record, and generally carried a gun. Michelle generally knew that Oliver had been in trouble with the law before but did not know the specifics of how much trouble he had been in, nor did she know that he usually carried a gun.

Oliver agreed to do the robbery. Michelle persuaded Jason to go a park and said she and Ashley would meet him there. Instead Oliver and another boy met Jason at the park. As Oliver approached the car Jason arrived in Oliver thought Jason reached down to pull a gun. Oliver reached for his gun and shot and killed Jason.

During this crime Michelle never left her house. It took law enforcement several weeks to put the entire chain of events together. They figured out Michelle and Ashley's involvement in the crime by looking at telephone records, when Michelle called Jason, when Ashley called Oliver, and when Michelle called Oliver. Michelle and Ashley were charged with conspiracy to commit murder. Oliver was charged with conspiracy to commit murder and murder. When Michelle went to trial she was nearly 17 years old. Because of the nature of the crime with which she was charged the prosecutor was forced to charge her as an adult. Michelle was convicted at trial and received a sentence of 15 years to life. The court had no discretion to sentence her to any lesser sentence. Fifteen years to life means the first time she will be eligible for parole will be 15 years from when she was sentenced.

Whether Michelle's sentence is fair or appropriate is open to debate. Certainly Michelle should be held accountable for her actions regardless of the fact that she was a child. A sentence that will likely require her to spend the rest of her life in prison for something she did when she was 15 years old ignores the fact that she probably lacked the foresight to consider how dangerous her plan was or the potential, horrible consequences of her actions.

Michelle's case demonstrates what the children and families you work with need to understand—the law treats crimes committed by children very, very seriously. If you are working in the juvenile justice system part of your job will be to impress on people the potential seriousness of the situation or the fact that if children graduate to more serious crimes the consequences can be far greater than most children or their families can imagine.

The Effect of Modern Psychology

As modern psychology has continued to advance so has our understanding of juvenile development. Modern psychology provides indirect proof that adolescents are cognitively and socially less mature. That immaturity affects their decisions to engage in criminal conduct as well as their decisions as defendants in criminal proceedings.

Youth crime has a high social cost. Those costs can be lessened with policies that ensure that the impact of punishment on youthful offenders will not affect their future lives. Incarcerating youths who are likely to soon outgrow their criminality is a waste of young lives. This is not to say juvenile offenders should not be bear any consequences from their actions; however, intervention and rehabilitation benefit both the youth and society far more than incarceration. Society should recognize that there is some class of youths that may be better served by treatment and counseling.

During the past decade juvenile laws have begun to return to a more rehabilitative model of juvenile justice. This shift has been advocated by many in the social sciences as well as advances in the understanding of human development. This paradigm shift is also due at least in part to the U.S. Supreme Court decision in *Romer v. Simmons* and the express recognition that children, their personality traits, and their decision-making abilities are not as well formed as those of adults:

> [T]he personality traits of juveniles are more transitory, less fixed. [Citation omitted.] These differences render suspect any conclusion that a juvenile falls among the worst offenders. The susceptibility of juveniles to immature and irresponsible behavior means "their irresponsible conduct is not as morally reprehensible as that of an adult." [Citation omitted.] Their own vulnerability and comparative lack of control over their immediate surroundings mean juveniles have a greater claim than adults to be forgiven for failing to escape negative influences in their whole environment. [Citation omitted.] The reality that juveniles still struggle to define their identity means it is less supportable to conclude that even a heinous crime committed by a juvenile is evidence of irretrievably depraved character. From a moral standpoint it would be misguided to equate the failings of a minor with those of an adult, for a greater possibility exists that a minor's character deficiencies will be reformed. (*Romer v. Simmons*, 2005)

It is important to understand that in *Romer v. Simmons* the U.S. Supreme Court was interpreting the U.S. Constitution's Eighth Amendment, the constitutional amendment that prohibits cruel and unusual punishment. When the U.S. Supreme Court is interpreting the federal Constitution all states and all courts are bound by the Supreme Court's ruling. In other words, since the U.S. Supreme Court has decided that minors, because of the fact they are still children, must be treated differently in the juvenile justice system, all states must act consistently with this decision.

How the Juvenile Delinquency Court Works

The juvenile court has original jurisdiction over any crime involving a minor. The term *original jurisdiction* means the juvenile court is the only court with the legal authority to hear the case. Juvenile courts can only hear cases that involve minors. Each state is free to define how old a person can be and still be a "minor." New York and North Carolina define a juvenile as anyone under the age of 15. Georgia, Illinois, Louisiana, Massachusetts, Michigan, Missouri, New Hampshire, South Carolina, Texas, and Wisconsin define a minor as anyone under the age of 16. All other states as well as the District of Columbia define a minor as anyone under the age of 18 (Office of Juvenile Justice and Delinquency Prevention, n.d.).

As mentioned earlier, most, if not all states, have lists of certain crimes that, if committed by a minor, can be prosecuted in adult court. Other states allow for prosecution of minors in adult court based on the prior record of the minor. In these instances the juvenile courts do not have "original jurisdiction," they have **concurrent jurisdiction** with the adult courts. The system that allows for certain crimes to be prosecuted in adult court is also referred to as *prosecutor discretion* or *direct file jurisdiction*.

Many states have structured their juvenile delinquency courts to allow the court to hear a case until a defendant has reached their mid-20s. In other words, if people are prosecuted in juvenile court when they are a minor but they are still on probation when they are 19 or 20 years old, they are still under the supervision of the juvenile court system as opposed to the adult system.

Some states have statutes that set the lowest age of juvenile court delinquency jurisdiction. Other states rely on common law or previous legal decisions. These laws frequently refer to *infants*. The laws defining the minimum age at which a child can be prosecuted have their roots in the British legal system from the 1700s and 1800s. Then the term *infant* was used to describe children as old as 5 or 6 years old. The basic concept is that below a certain age children are incompetent to form the necessary intent to commit crimes and are therefore exempt from prosecution. Most crimes require some form of intent, usually referred to broadly as *criminal intent*. The vast majority of crimes are either general intent or specific intent crimes. The other two, less common kinds of intent, are criminal negligence and strict liability crimes.

General intent means people have to intend the act but they do not have to intend the result of the act. Specific intent means the person had to intend the result. Murder is a specific intent crime—when the person pulls the trigger of a gun the intent is to kill another person. The intent is not merely to pull the trigger. Battery is a general intent crime—someone hits another person. The crime is committed as soon as people throw a punch. It does not matter whether they actually hit the person or if the recipient of the punch is actually injured. Children below a certain age are not capable of truly understanding what they are doing or engaging in truly intentional conduct in the same manner as an adult. Think about a preschool-age child. They are often incapable of predicting the consequences of their actions. They act extremely impulsively. Regardless of their conduct, prosecuting a young child would serve no social or penological purpose.

The definition of criminal negligence varies from state to state. Generally it can be defined as more than ordinary carelessness or mistake in judgment. People act with criminal negligence when they act in a way that creates a high risk of death or bodily harm and reasonable people would have known that acting in that way would create such a risk. Strict liability crimes are very rare and usually only occur in connection with regulatory offenses.

How the Juvenile Delinquency Process Starts

How juvenile delinquency cases are initiated varies greatly from state to state and even from community to community. When a minor allegedly commits a crime, law enforcement has two options: *initiate juvenile delinquency proceedings* or *divert the matter into some form of diversion program.*

There are numerous kinds of **diversion programs.** Many schools have their own student-run judicial process where students prosecute minor crimes committed by other students, conduct trials, and impose sentencing. For minor crimes this is a common way to keep children out of the juvenile justice system. Other diversion programs can include drug treatment programs or community service. There are limitless possibilities for diversion programs. The decision to divert is generally based on a number of considerations: the type of alleged criminal conduct, the opinion of the victim of the crime, whether the minor has a prior criminal record, and input from the minor and that minor's parent or legal guardian. The entire purpose of diversion is to keep children out of the justice system while ensuring that they will not commit future crimes. In order for law enforcement to feel confident that these objectives will be met, both the minor and their parents have to be willing to commit to the diversion process.

Law enforcement is not the only entity that can refer a matter to the juvenile delinquency court. In many states, schools, parents, victims, and probation officers have the capacity to refer a matter to juvenile delinquency court, although once the referral is made law enforcement generally is involved in the investigation of the allegations.

Another common informal treatment of juvenile delinquency cases is something called a *consent decree*. A **consent decree** is generally a written contract between a minor and either the prosecutor's office or the juvenile delinquency court. In the contract the minor agrees to certain conditions such as doing or not doing certain things for a period of time. For example, a minor might agree to pay to repair a car they vandalized, attend drug counseling, attend school on a regular basis, or agree to a curfew. Consent decrees are a type of informal probation. Once the minor completes the terms of the consent decree the entire matter is dismissed. If the minor fails to successfully complete the terms of the consent decree or fails their informal probation for some other reason, the matter is referred back to the juvenile delinquency court for formal proceedings.

Once a case is referred to the juvenile delinquency court it goes to *intake*. In most states intake is run either by the prosecutor's office or the probation department. Intake decides if the case should be handled formally or informally. Informal treatment of a case can include referring the matter to diversion. If intake decides to proceed with formal proceedings either because minors failed their informal probation or because the matter was too serious to qualify for informal proceedings, the formal court process begins. Generally it is at this time that intake decides whether a case should be transferred to adult court or if a delinquency petition should be filed in juvenile delinquency court. The filing of a delinquency petition is the filing of a formal legal document that sets forth the crimes the minor allegedly committed.

Although courts, lawyers, and law enforcement often seem rigid and formal, the truth is that many of the adults involved in this process truly seek to help the children involved in the juvenile delinquency system. Unfortunately, although many of these adults want to help they are generally not trained in psychology or child development. This is where the role of people with such training can become very important.

If you are concerned that a judge or a lawyer is missing something important about a child you work with, you should not be afraid to speak up. Most judges are prevented from speaking to you directly about a particular case because of the all rules. However, you can always talk to the lawyers involved—their ethical rules not only allow them to talk to you, if you have something important to tell them about a child or about the facts of a case, they are ethically required to listen to what you have to say. If you feel like you really need to communicate with a judge, ask the judge's clerk the best way to go about it. The clerks usually have close working relationships with the judges they work with and they can give you good insight into the best way to deal with the situation.

Many of the children who end up involved in the juvenile delinquency system are poor, come from single-parent homes, often have untreated mental or emotional problems, have experienced some form of abuse at home, or have faced other challenges that have in some way contributed to their being in delinquency court. Many of the people who work in the juvenile delinquency system lack formal training in recognizing how these factors may have contributed to a child becoming involved in the system. The job of educating lawyers and judges often falls to the social service workers or probation officers.

Some years ago there was a case where a young man, let us call him Michael, kept getting into trouble. Michael lived in a rough neighborhood and his mother worked long hours, which limited her ability to properly supervise her son. Over the course of a few years Michael was in and out of the delinquency court system on countless occasions. Each occasion he was caught engaging in more and more serious criminal conduct. The lawyers who dealt with Michael found him hostile and noncommunicative. Finally, Michael was ordered detained in juvenile hall. It was only then that a trained social worker began to realize what part of the problem was—Michael had an extremely low IQ, so low he was legally incompetent. He was hostile and noncommunicative with the people around him because he did not understand what was going on around him and he was scared. Once the legal system had him evaluated and understood Michael's needs, the system was able to fashion an appropriate solution—a solution that ultimately kept him out of the juvenile delinquency system altogether.

THE PETITION

A **delinquency petition** differs from the charging documents filed in adult court. At the conclusion of an adult criminal case a defendant is either acquitted or convicted. If convicted they are sentenced. Because the goals of the juvenile justice system are historically different, and in many states still are very different than the adult criminal justice system, the purpose of the delinquency petition is very different. At the end of a delinquency petition there is a request that the court sustain the petition and judge that the minor is delinquent and now a ward of the delinquency court.

The term *ward of the court* has a very specific meaning to lawyers and judges. In juvenile delinquency proceedings that term means the court now has the authority to decide what should happen to a minor. In some ways the court has stepped into role of being the minor's parent.

After the delinquency petition is filed the court holds a detention hearing. A **detention hearing** is a judicial determination as to whether a minor will remain in law enforcement custody prior to the adjudicatory hearing. The courts have the authority to order minors remain in a secure detention facility, often juvenile hall, because the minors may be deemed a danger to themselves or to society. The juvenile court also has the authority to fashion specific release conditions before agreeing to allow a minor out of custody. Those release conditions can include ordering counseling; placing the minor on house arrest, which often means they have to wear a GPS tracking device or ankle bracelet;

setting curfews; or any other set of conditions that are calculated to ensure the minor appears in court when ordered and to protect the public.

In most states minors do not have a right to post bail. That means if a court determines that a minor should remain in custody pending their adjudicatory hearing the minor's parents cannot post money to secure the minor's release.

In most states prior to a detention hearing, intake conducts an interview of both the juvenile and their family to determine whether release is appropriate. Different states have different rules about what can and should be asked during this interview. Frequently the court wants to know about the child's home and family life. Many courts specifically instruct the person doing the interview not to ask about the facts of the alleged criminal case as doing so could interfere with the child's Fifth Amendment rights to remain silent. You should be careful to understand your agency's particular policy in this regard.

Once a delinquency petition is filed, an adjudicatory hearing is set. An *adjudicatory hearing* is similar to a trial in adult proceedings but with some significant differences. In *In re Gault* (1967), the U.S. Supreme Court established that under the 14th Amendment, children accused of crimes in a delinquency proceeding must be given many of the same due process rights as adults, such as the right to timely notification of charges, the right to confront witnesses, the right against self-incrimination, and the right to counsel.

(The 14th Amendment was passed after the U.S. Civil War. Prior to the passage of that amendment it was unclear whether the rights protected by the constitution applied in the states or if they only applied with respect to the federal government. For example, the First Amendment states that people who live in the United States have the right to free speech. They can say what they want. However, even though the way the Bill of Rights was first written made it clear that the federal government could not interfere if a person in Ohio wanted to criticize a member of the Ohio state legislature, it was unclear whether the state of Ohio could interfere. The 14th Amendment made it clear that the state could not interfere, that the rights guaranteed by the Bill of Rights bound state governments as well as the federal government. Today it seems obvious that a state cannot abridge a person's rights as secured by the Bill of Rights, but 150 years ago this was the subject of much debate.)

In most states juvenile delinquency proceedings are not public—only the minor's parents have the right to attend. In the vast majority of juvenile delinquency proceedings the determination of whether the petition should be sustained is made by a judge, not a jury. If the prosecutor has decided to charge the child as though the child were an adult, then the proceedings are open to the public and the child has the same rights to a jury trial as an adult.

Prior to an adjudicatory hearing a final determination as to whether the matter should be heard in adult court is made. Once an adjudicatory hearing is held and the court decides whether to sustain the petition the case can no longer be transferred to adult court.

If the judge, or in a limited number of states, the jury, decides not to sustain the petition, that is the end of the case. It is the same as an acquittal in adult court. If the petition is sustained a disposition hearing is set. At the time the petition is sustained the minor becomes a ward of the court. This is the stage at which the court steps into the shoes of being the minor's parent. You might hear the term *in loco parentis*. This is a Latin term that literally means in place of the parent. In place of the parent is exactly how the juvenile court views their role from this point forward. The court now has the authority, or the discretion, to decide where the children live, where they go to school, what time they come home at night, whether the children are allowed to play sports. The court has the ability to make every decision a parent would normally make. All of those decisions will be made at a deposition hearing.

A **disposition hearing** is the same thing as a sentencing hearing in adult court. Probation writes a report and recommends a disposition. Probation has broad discretion regarding what it can recommend for a disposition. Because many juvenile delinquency systems are based on a rehabilitative model, probation's recommendations often include recommendations for drug treatment and counseling. Dispositional recommendations can also include time spent doing community service work, being sentenced to house arrest, serving time in juvenile hall, or serving time in other, more long-term juvenile detention facilities.

Less than a decade ago many states had far more options for probation to recommend for juvenile disposition hearings. For example, probation could recommend placement in halfway houses or group homes as part of a delinquency disposition. Because so many state budgets have been so drastically affected after the Great Recession many of these options no longer exist.

At the dispositional hearing the minors, through their attorney, are allowed to suggest what they think would be an appropriate disposition if they believe something different from what was recommended by probation would be better. The prosecution also has the right to recommend something different from the recommendations made by probation. The court has the authority to accept probation's recommendations, follow the recommendations of the minor and minor's counsel, follow the recommendations of the prosecutor, or come up with a plan of its own.

Often a child's parents have a very limited role at this state. Usually whoever prepares the recommendations interviews the parents about what the parents want to happen to their child. Although the opinion of the parents is considered, the court does not have to follow the parent's desires. Similarly, although many judges will allow parents to speak during the disposition hearing most states do not give the parents a right to speak—meaning the court does not have to let them.

Perhaps more than anyone else, parents are often confused and frustrated by how the court works during a disposition hearing. In some cases it can be important to explain to the parents the reasons why a court has made a certain ruling. Parents may not understand why their children are being ordered to do community service, they may not believe their child has a drug problem, or they may not understand why the child is being detained in juvenile hall for a period of time. It is important for you to understand why the court has made the orders it has so you can explain that to the parents. The child involved has the best chance of successfully exiting the juvenile delinquency system when the parents support the court's actions and encourage the child to do the same.

Collateral Consequences

The juvenile delinquency system uses terminology that is very different from the terminology used in adult criminal court. Petitions are sustained instead of minors being found guilty. There is a juvenile disposition instead of a criminal sentence. Despite these differences the collateral consequences of having a juvenile petition sustained can be very serious and can follow a minor for life.

In criminal law, *collateral consequences* is the term used to refer to the indirect consequences of being convicted of a crime. Lawyers and courts are supposed to inform defendants, both minors and adults, of the most serious potential collateral consequences of being found guilty or having a petition sustained. A common collateral consequence for both minors and adults who are convicted of some kind of a crime is that if they are not a citizen of the United States their conviction may result in them being deported or denied admission into the United States. For a minor this can have devastating effects.

Many minors are brought into the United States illegally as children. They have little or no contact with their native country. They get into trouble in the United States, sometimes serious trouble. Instead of being released back into society, they are sent to a deportation facility and ultimately deported back to their home country. The fact that they are young, cannot speak the language, and have no family contacts left in their native country is irrelevant. They are returned to their native country and left to fend for themselves. Illegal reentry into the United States is a serious federal crime that can carry lengthy terms in federal prison.

Every state now has some form of sex offender registration for those convicted of specific sex crimes. Most states require minors to register as sex offenders if they are the subject of a sustained juvenile petition for a specific sex crime. Depending on a number of factors, including what state the minors are in, their age at the time they committed the offense, and the type of offense, they may be required to register as a convicted sex offender for the remainder of their life.

Many states also have three strikes laws—laws that require a life term in prison if a person has been convicted three times of certain classes of crimes. Again, depending on a number of factors, juvenile strikes can follow a minor for the rest of their life. Many states have wash-out provisions; they do not count felony strikes if a person remains out of trouble for a specific number of years. Other states do not have such provisions and strikes last forever.

It would be inappropriate for you to advise anyone about the potential collateral consequences of sustained petition in a specific case. However, you need to know that these things exist so you can try to warn children whom you think are likely to get into trouble or so you can warn their parents. Sometimes just being able to make children understand how much trouble they could be in is enough to make them think twice.

Minors' Rights

In general minors have the same rights when they are facing criminal accusations as adults. For example, when adults are arrested they have the right to make a phone call, which is generally used to secure legal representation. In many states minors are allowed to call not only a lawyer but also specifically their parents. Although minors generally have the same rights as adults, courts can apply different standards in determining whether a minor's rights were violated. Courts are more likely to find that a minor's rights have been violated when law enforcement uses aggressive tactics to obtain information from a minor—tactics that, depending on the circumstances, might be perfectly acceptable if used on an adult.

Consider the case of Jonathan Doody. Doody was a 17-year-old high school student who was a suspect in a murder investigation. He was originally contacted by law enforcement while participating in a flag ceremony at a high school football game. He voluntarily went with law enforcement to the police station for questioning.

When he arrived at the station police officers purported to read Doody his *Miranda* warnings. *Miranda* warnings are the rights read to suspects in custody, which informs them that they have the right to remain silent, they have the right to be represented by counsel, and that anything they say can be used against them in court. Over the years law enforcement has developed a modified version of these rights to be read to minors, which makes them more understandable to young people.

The officers who interrogated Mr. Doody misrepresented the *Miranda* warnings. A group of law enforcement officers proceeded to question Mr. Doody for more than 12 hours between the hours of 9 P.M. and 10 A.M. the following morning. Mr. Doody was not allowed to sleep or take a break during the questioning. The officers arranged the questioning in a tag team format—as some officers got tired they left the room while other officers took over. Mr. Doody ended up admitting to having committed nine murders.

An appellate court ultimately overturned Mr. Doody's conviction and threw out his confession because law enforcement interrogated a 17-year-old who had never been in trouble with the law for more than 12 hours, completely misconstrued *Miranda* warnings, and essentially overcame the will of an unsophisticated 17-year-old kid (*Doody v. Ryan*, 2011). Many other courts, including the U.S. Supreme Court, have frequently cautioned that confessions by minors are to be viewed with suspicion because they are so easily influenced by adults. The kind of questioning Mr. Doody experienced might be legal if the questioning had been directed at an adult.

In a vacuum it is impossible to set forth a series of bright line rules for what kind of investigatory tactics by law enforcement are acceptable when minors are involved. Because of their youth and lack of sophistication courts will treat minors differently, just how differently depends on a number of circumstances.

Minors Tried as Adults

All states allow minors to be tried as adults for certain crimes. As mentioned earlier in this chapter, minors cannot be sentenced to the death penalty because of their youth. The U.S. Supreme Court has also held that minors cannot be sentenced to life in prison without the possibility of parole. This does not mean, however, that people who committed a crime as juveniles cannot spend the rest of their life in prison—it just means that it cannot be their initial sentence.

Consider the example of Michelle given earlier in this chapter. Her sentence was 15 years to life. Her sentence is referred to as an indeterminate term, meaning that how long she will spend in prison is undetermined but in no circumstance can it be less than 15 years. That means her first hearing before the parole board will be 15 years from when she was sentenced. Most parole boards in most states are reluctant to release people sentenced to indeterminate terms, particularly when they were convicted of crimes such as murder.

The U.S. Supreme Court decision banning a sentence of life in prison without the possibility of parole for a minor occurred within the past couple of years. Given that fact, coupled with an increasing body of scientific literature suggesting that children's brains are less fully developed and that they are therefore less culpable for their crimes, it seems likely that children who have received indeterminate prison sentences may have a greater chance of being released from prison in the future.

JUVENILE DEPENDENCY

Modern juvenile dependency courts exist in large part due to a movement to end child abuse and neglect that began to gain momentum in the late 1960s and 1970s. In 1974 the passage of CAPTA, the federal Child Abuse Prevention and Treatment Act, which marked the beginning of a national move toward Mandated Reporter Laws, also marked the beginning of the dependency court system.

Once this country began to develop child protection laws it needed a way to implement the protections those laws offered. Criminal courts could prosecute parents who abused or neglected their children, but what happened to the children next? Did they return to their parents? Who would oversee the future treatment of the children? By the 1960s and 1970s juvenile delinquency courts were full to capacity dealing with children who had allegedly broken laws. Dependency courts began as an effort to address the needs of children who had not broken laws but were the victims of abuse or neglect.

Dependency Court

A case can get started in juvenile dependency court whenever there are allegations of parental abuse or neglect. Frequently the department of social services or law enforcement will make a referral to dependency court because of concern about potential abuse or neglect of children in a particular home. Criminal charges do not have to be initiated against a parent or parents for the juvenile dependency court to have jurisdiction. Another common way parties arrive before the dependency court is when one or both parents are facing or have been convicted of criminal allegations.

Sometimes the criminal allegations may be related to abuse or neglect of a child. However, there are countless other circumstances that may give rise to dependency proceedings. For example, if a parent is convicted of possessing drugs the matter may be referred to dependency court for a determination of whether it is safe for the children to remain in the home. In other cases the parents may have been sentenced to lengthy prison terms for wholly unrelated conduct. The courts may intervene to make sure there is a safe place for the children to live, and, in some cases, may terminate an individual's parental rights depending on their underlying criminal conduct.

Dependency Court Process

When the dependency process begins, an initial determination is made by law enforcement or social services as to whether the children should be allowed to remain in the home. If the children are not in immediate danger of neglect or abuse, and are living with a parent, relative, or friend, they may be allowed to remain there pending the court proceedings.

When children are left in the home it is frequently on condition that the family will agree to supervision of social services as well as other terms such as counseling or treatment for drug or alcohol abuse.

If a child is removed from the home there are time limits on how long the juvenile dependency court has to act. Most states have laws requiring juvenile dependency courts to have an initial hearing within 72 hours after a child has been removed from a home. Children who are removed from the family home are taken into protective custody and are usually taken to some kind of children's receiving home. Law enforcement officials who place children into protective custody are acting in the best interest of the children and making sure they are not in danger. However, this can be a terrifying experience for children. Even if their home life is less than ideal it is at least familiar. Being taken from their homes and thrust into a new and unfamiliar environment can be a very difficult experience for many children.

When children are taken into protective custody, law enforcement officers or social workers will immediately attempt to notify the parents or guardians.

The juvenile dependency system is premised on the belief that it is best for children to remain with their families if at all possible. An investigation is triggered when children are taken from the home and placed in protective custody. The purpose of the investigation is to decide whether the children can be safely returned to the home from which they were taken. This initial investigation is made by social workers. In many states these social workers work for the intake unit of the department of social services.

The social worker must decide whether the children were at significant risk for abuse or neglect. If the social worker decides it is safe for the children, the children can be released to the parent. No formal court action is taken. However, as mentioned earlier, the parent may have to sign an agreement agreeing to certain conditions to keep the children in the home. In some cases this agreement can mark the end of the dependency proceedings.

In cases in which the abuse or neglect was minor or where the social worker believes the parents can rectify the situation with the help of social service workers, social service workers have the discretion to fashion an agreement that states if the parents meet certain conditions, including no further reports of abuse or neglect over a specified period of months, no further action will be taken.

In other instances the social worker may decide that the children should remain in the home if the parents are willing to agree to certain conditions during the pendency of the court proceedings.

If the social worker decides the children are at risk and the children are removed from the home, the social worker must file a petition with the juvenile dependency court. The petition must include both necessary legal information as well as a statement telling why a dependency proceeding is necessary for the safety of the children. In response to the petition, a detention hearing is held before a judge or referee. (A referee is a lawyer who is appointed to act in a similar capacity as judge. Referees have very limited jurisdiction. A referee in juvenile dependency court can only hear certain limited matters. Often referees in dependency proceedings are lawyers who have spent many years practicing in a particular field, such as child and family law.)

First Hearing

If children were removed from the home, the first hearing in dependency court will be a kind of a detention hearing. Different states use different terms to describe this hearing. In some states it is simply called the *first hearing*. In other states it is called an *initial detention hearing*.

If the children were not removed there is still some kind of a first hearing. When this is the same the formal name of the first hearing makes clear that the hearing is not to determine where the children will reside while the abuse or neglect allegations are handled.

Regardless of whether the children have been removed from the home, one of the main objectives of this first hearing is to advise parties of the allegations, appoint counsel (if necessary), and set a future hearing. It is very important the parents understand why they are in dependency court and what they did or did not do to cause the government to be concerned about the safety of their children. Depending on the age of the children involved, sometimes the children are allowed to be present during these hearings. If they are present the court will often try to explain to the children what is happening.

If the children had been taken out of the home and are not returned to the parents, the children remain in protective custody. All dependency courts have investigators, although different jurisdictions call the investigators by different names. The role of the investigator is to meet with the parents, investigate the allegations of abuse or neglect, and write a report for the court hearing. In most states the investigators work for the court and report directly to the court—they typically are not members of law enforcement.

It is common for parents to be reluctant, even hostile, to work with the court investigator. Think about it from the parents' perspective: Someone has just come and taken their children away. The parents may not understand the legal system, they may be frightened, and they are likely concerned about their children's health and safety.

Think about the following from a real case: A young woman and her husband illegally grew marijuana. Their home was raided by FBI and DEA agents early one morning. Law enforcement agents took the couple's three young daughters away from them. The young woman had recently emigrated from China and did not speak English. She was from rural China and had very little education. She later told someone she was terrified because all she could think about was China's one child policy and the fact that she had three daughters. She did not know if the United States had a policy regarding how many children people could have. She did not know where her children were or even if they were being cared for. She did not understand the role of the social workers or why they kept asking her questions.

If you are in the role of the court investigator or social services worker you have to keep in mind that the people you are trying to help may not understand the system and may not realize you are trying to help them. People from other countries may bring with them fears from other political systems, fears that were well founded in their homelands but which make it much harder for you to work with them in this country.

The report is an evaluation of the case. Whenever possible the report contains a reunification plan along with recommendations to the court regarding where the children should be placed. When reunification is not possible the report still will make recommendations about where the children should live.

If the court approves, the investigator arranges visits between the parents and their children. The court investigator can also arrange for services such as counseling, job training, parenting classes, drug and alcohol treatment, anger management classes, or any other services that will help reunite the family.

Courts frequently follow the recommendations in the report. Writing the report is a big responsibility.

Jurisdiction Hearing

After the first hearing the court sets a jurisdiction hearing. The purpose of this hearing is to determine whether the allegations of abuse or neglect are true. The evidentiary standard used at this hearing is a preponderance of the evidence. This is the lowest evidentiary standard in the U.S. legal system. This standard has been described as 50% plus a feather or 50% plus a peppercorn.

It is often very difficult for people to understand that in order to send a person to prison the prosecutor has to prove guilt beyond a reasonable doubt. But in order to remove children from their parent there just has to be a preponderance of the evidence. (Removing a child from a home is different than terminating parental rights. A termination of parental rights requires clear and convincing evidence.)

In dependency court there is no right to a jury trial. All decisions are made by the judge. The judge's decisions are subject to review by appellate courts. If the court decides that abuse or neglect has been proven by a preponderance of the evidence the court sustains the petition and makes a finding that it has jurisdiction. Jurisdiction in this instance simply means that the court finds it has authority to intervene to protect the child.

Right to Counsel

When and under what circumstances a parent has the right to be represented by legal counsel in juvenile dependency proceedings can be a difficult question to answer. In all states, if parents can afford to retain their own legal counsel they cannot be denied the right to be represented by a lawyer in court. On the other hand, if parents cannot afford to retain their own counsel, determining when they are entitled to appointed legal counsel can be difficult.

Some states, either by statute or prior case law, have determined that before people's parental rights can be terminated they have the right to be represented by appointed counsel. Other states follow a complex system that makes a case-by-case determination of whether a parent is entitled to an appointed lawyer.

In the early 1980s, in *Lassiter v. Department of Social Services of Durham County* (1981), the U.S. Supreme Court decided that there is no right to appointed counsel in every case. The Supreme Court stated that whether a parent should be entitled to an appointed lawyer is a decision that should be made by the judge in each dependency case based on all of the surrounding circumstances. Although it is easier to have a clear and simple rule about when the court has to appoint a lawyer, justice is better served by allowing judges to tailor their decisions to the facts of each case.

Appointing a lawyer in the case of every dependency proceeding would cost a lot of money and a lot of resources. In *Lassiter* the mother had been convicted of murder and sentenced to a lengthy prison term. If she got out of prison, it would be long after her son was an adult. In that instance no one was well served by the mother having appointed counsel; not the mother, not the child, and not society.

It would be next to impossible in the context of this book to explain all the times parents are and are not entitled to have appointed lawyers to represent them in dependency court. The rules vary greatly from state to state.

Children and the Right to Be Heard

Courts have consistently held for many years that children do not enjoy the same rights and privileges as adults. For example, children do not have the same rights as adults when it comes to free speech under the First Amendment. As discussed earlier in this chapter, children have the same rights as adults in criminal proceedings. In addition, children have specific rights in dependency court, which can be greater than the rights of the adults.

The children who are involved in dependency proceedings are the ones who are the most significantly impacted by the court's decision. It is the children who have the greatest interest in the outcome. Children's rights to remain with their family is probably more important than adults' rights to keep their child. Among the most important things to children is a sense of stability, which allows their minds and their character to grow. Uncertainty about where they are going to live, who they are going to live with, and what is going to happen to them is counterproductive to their growth and development.

Courts are in the difficult position of having to balance a child's needs and wants with the court's responsibility to make sure that a child is not the victim of abuse or neglect. In order to meet these sometimes competing goals most states have a system that allows for children to have their own advocates.

Court Appointed Special Advocates or CASA is a group of highly trained volunteers. CASA started in the late 1970s when a judge in Washington state found himself having to make a decision on behalf of abused and neglected children. He was concerned that the only information he had was from child protective services. Although child protective services had the best interests of the child at heart, the judge was concerned that the children had no voice in the process. The judge decided that volunteers could be assigned to a case, meet with the children, and speak on their behalf. About 50 people responded to the judge's first request. Today CASA exists in every state in the nation.

Among the goals of CASA is to ensure that all abused or neglected children in the dependency court system have their own advocate. Once a child is assigned a CASA advocate that person stays with the child through the entire court process and often beyond. The CASA advocate is often the only constant adult presence in some of these children's lives.

CASA advocates are trained to do more than just advocate for what the children want because that may not always be in the child's best interests. The advocates also explain the court process to the children and help them in other ways outside of the court process. A lot of research has been done on the effectiveness of the CASA program. That research has consistently shown that children involved in the CASA program do better in school and adjust to their new surroundings far better than their peers who were not assisted by CASA.

CONCLUSION

Navigating delinquency and dependency courts can be an overwhelming challenge both for children and their families. Judges and lawyers often use words and phrases that are totally foreign to people who have never been involved in the system. In modern times delinquency and dependency courts handle enormous case loads. It will likely fall to you to explain to the children and families you work with how the system works and the goals of these two very different branches of the court.

If you are working with children involved in the juvenile delinquency court it is important that you familiarize yourself with the theory behind your state's delinquency court, whether it is based on a rehabilitative model or a punitive or punishment model. If you are working in the dependency system, you will be faced with the tough task of helping children who may be separated from their parents against their will and as a result of something the parents, not the child, did.

There are numerous programs throughout the country to help children who are dealing with both the delinquency and dependency systems; only a couple of examples have been discussed in this chapter. If you are working in an agency setting, hopefully that agency will a list of local programs that will aid you in your effort to assist the children with whom you are working.

Whatever the case, you need to keep in mind that the children you are working with likely view you as the adult authority figure and the person they can rely on to guide them through this process. The more you know and understand, the more you will be able to successfully assist both children and their families.

STUDY QUESTIONS

1. What are the differences between juvenile delinquency and dependency courts?
2. What is the basic purpose behind the creation of a different court system for juveniles?
3. Who, in addition to law enforcement, can refer cases to a juvenile justice system court?
4. Describe the process of the juvenile justice system after referral.
5. In what types of cases is the juvenile dependency system used?
6. Some terminology is different between the juvenile and adult courts, though they share similar functions. Name some examples.

GLOSSARY

concurrent jurisdiction When two different courts have the legal ability to rule on the same case. For example, when a juvenile court and an adult court both can rule on a criminal case involving a minor.

consent decree A written contract between a minor and either the prosecutor's office or the juvenile delinquency court.

delinquency petition At the end of a *delinquency petition* there is a request that the court sustain the petition and judge that the minor is delinquent and now a ward of the delinquency court. This differs from adult court, which will yield either conviction or acquittal.

detention hearing A judicial determination as to whether a minor will remain in law enforcement custody prior to the adjudicatory hearing.

disposition hearing Similar to a sentencing hearing in adult court.

diversion programs Programs designed for juveniles to keep them from adult systems of punishment and corrections. These programs must ensure as much as possible that future crimes will not happen.

juvenile delinquency courts   Deal with minors who have committed crimes and are essentially the same as a criminal adult court, with more palpable goal of rehabilitation.

juvenile dependency courts   Assist minors when their parents, for one reason or another, cannot adequately care for their children.

REFERENCES

Doody v. Ryan, 649 F.3d 986 (9th Cir. 2011).

In re Gault, 387 U.S. 1 (1967).

Lassiter v. Department of Social Services of Durham County, 452 U.S. 18 (1981).

Office of Juvenile Justice and Delinquency Prevention. (n.d.). *OJJDP Statistical Briefing Book.* Available at www.ojjdp.gov

Romer v. Simmons, 543 U.S. 551 (2005).

Scott, E. S., & Grisso, T. (1997). The evolution of adolescence: A developmental perspective on juvenile justice reform. *Journal of Criminal Law and Criminology, 88,* 137.

Author Index

Subject Index

Page numbers followed by *g* indicate glossary term; Page numbers followed by *t* indicate table.